Incorporating the Internet of Things in Healthcare Applications and Wearable Devices

P. B. Pankajavalli
Bharathiar University, India

G. S. Karthick
Bharathiar University, India

A volume in the Advances in Medical
Technologies and Clinical Practice (AMTCP) Book
Series

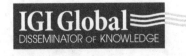

Published in the United States of America by
IGI Global
Medical Information Science Reference (an imprint of IGI Global)
701 E. Chocolate Avenue
Hershey PA, USA 17033
Tel: 717-533-8845
Fax: 717-533-8661
E-mail: cust@igi-global.com
Web site: http://www.igi-global.com

Library of Congress Cataloging-in-Publication Data

Names: Pankajavalli, P. B., 1979- editor. | Karthick, G. S., 1990- editor.
Title: Incorporating the internet of things in healthcare applications and
    wearable devices / PB Pankajavalli and GS Karthick, editors.
Description: Hershey, PA : Medical Information Science Reference, [2020] |
    Includes bibliographical references and index. | Summary: "This book
    examines the implementation of the internet of things in healthcare
    applications and systems"--Provided by publisher.
Identifiers: LCCN 2019024248 (print) | LCCN 2019024249 (ebook) | ISBN
    9781799810902 (h/c) | ISBN 9781799810919 (eISBN)
Subjects: MESH: Telemedicine | Internet | Wearable Electronic Devices |
    Mobile Applications | Remote Sensing Technology | Electronics,
    Medical--trends
Classification: LCC R855.3 (print) | LCC R855.3 (ebook) | NLM W 83.1 |
    DDC 610.285--dc23
LC record available at https://lccn.loc.gov/2019024248
LC ebook record available at https://lccn.loc.gov/2019024249

This book is published in the IGI Global book series Advances in Medical Technologies and Clinical Practice (AMTCP) (ISSN: 2327-9354; eISSN: 2327-9370)

British Cataloguing in Publication Data
A Cataloguing in Publication record for this book is available from the British Library.

For electronic access to this publication, please contact: eresources@igi-global.com.

Advances in Medical Technologies and Clinical Practice (AMTCP) Book Series

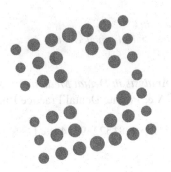

Srikanta Patnaik
SOA University, India
Priti Das
S.C.B. Medical College, India

ISSN:2327-9354
EISSN:2327-9370

MISSION

Medical technological innovation continues to provide avenues of research for faster and safer diagnosis and treatments for patients. Practitioners must stay up to date with these latest advancements to provide the best care for nursing and clinical practices.

The **Advances in Medical Technologies and Clinical Practice (AMTCP) Book Series** brings together the most recent research on the latest technology used in areas of nursing informatics, clinical technology, biomedicine, diagnostic technologies, and more. Researchers, students, and practitioners in this field will benefit from this fundamental coverage on the use of technology in clinical practices.

COVERAGE

- Medical Informatics
- Clinical Nutrition
- Medical Imaging
- Patient-Centered Care
- E-Health
- Biomechanics
- Clinical Studies
- Clinical Data Mining
- Clinical High-Performance Computing
- Nutrition

IGI Global is currently accepting manuscripts for publication within this series. To submit a proposal for a volume in this series, please contact our Acquisition Editors at Acquisitions@igi-global.com or visit: http://www.igi-global.com/publish/.

The Advances in Medical Technologies and Clinical Practice (AMTCP) Book Series (ISSN 2327-9354) is published by IGI Global, 701 E. Chocolate Avenue, Hershey, PA 17033-1240, USA, www.igi-global.com. This series is composed of titles available for purchase individually; each title is edited to be contextually exclusive from any other title within the series. For pricing and ordering information please visit http://www.igi-global.com/book-series/advances-medical-technologies-clinical-practice/73682. Postmaster: Send all address changes to above address. Copyright © 2020 IGI Global. All rights, including translation in other languages reserved by the publisher. No part of this series may be reproduced or used in any form or by any means – graphics, electronic, or mechanical, including photocopying, recording, taping, or information and retrieval systems – without written permission from the publisher, except for non commercial, educational use, including classroom teaching purposes. The views expressed in this series are those of the authors, but not necessarily of IGI Global.

Titles in this Series

For a list of additional titles in this series, please visit:
https://www.igi-global.com/book-series/advances-medical-technologies-clinical-practice/73682

Handbook of Research on Clinical Applications of Computerized Occlusal Analysis in Dental Medicine
Robert B. Kerstein, DMD (Tufts University School of Dental Medicine, USA & Private Dental Practice Limited to Prosthodontics and Computerized Occlusal Analysis, USA)
Medical Information Science Reference • copyright 2020 • 1356pp • H/C (ISBN: 9781522592549) • US $765.00 (our price)

Early Detection of Neurological Disorders Using Machine Learning Systems
Sudip Paul (North-Eastern Hill University Shillong, India) Pallab Bhattacharya (National Institute of Pharmaceutical Education and Research (NIPER) Ahmedabad, India) and Arindam Bit (National Institute of Technology Raipur, India)
Medical Information Science Reference • copyright 2019 • 376pp • H/C (ISBN: 9781522585671) • US $265.00 (our price)

Incivility Among Nursing Professionals in Clinical and Academic Environments Emerging Research and Opportunities
Cheryl Green (Southern Connecticut State University, USA)
Medical Information Science Reference • copyright 2019 • 181pp • H/C (ISBN: 9781522573418) • US $195.00 (our price)

Computational Methods and Algorithms for Medicine and Optimized Clinical Practice
Kwok Tai Chui (The Open University of Hong Kong, Hong Kong) and Miltiadis D. Lytras (Effat University, Saudi Arabia)
Medical Information Science Reference • copyright 2019 • 290pp • H/C (ISBN: 9781522582441) • US $245.00 (our price)

Advanced Classification Techniques for Healthcare Analysis
Chinmay Chakraborty (Birla Institute of Technology Mesra, India)
Medical Information Science Reference • copyright 2019 • 424pp • H/C (ISBN: 9781522577966) • US $285.00 (our price)

Tele-Audiology and the Optimization of Hearing Healthcare Delivery
Elaine Saunders (Blamey Saunders Hears, Australia)
Medical Information Science Reference • copyright 2019 • 274pp • H/C (ISBN: 9781522581918) • US $225.00 (our price)

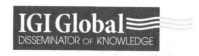

701 East Chocolate Avenue, Hershey, PA 17033, USA
Tel: 717-533-8845 x100 • Fax: 717-533-8661
E-Mail: cust@igi-global.com • www.igi-global.com

Editorial Advisory Board

Table of Contents

Detailed Table of Contents

Chapter 1
IoT in Healthcare: Ecosystem, Pillars, Design Challenges, Applications, Vulnerabilities, Privacy,
and Security Concerns 1

V. Jeevika Tharini, Bharathiar University, India
S. Vijayarani, Bharathiar University, India

One of the best-known features of IoT is automation. Because of this, IoT is a much-needed field for many applications, namely emergency and healthcare domains. IoT has made many revolutionary changes in the healthcare industry. IoT paves the way to numerous advancements for healthcare. The possibilities of IoT have reached their peak in the commercial industry and health sector. In recent years, serious concerns have been raised over the control and access of one's individual information. Privacy and security of the IoT devices can be compromised by intruders. Apart from the numerous benefits of IoTs, there are several security and privacy concerns to consider. A brief overview of different kinds of security attacks, solution for the attacks, privacy and security issues are discussed in this chapter.

Chapter 2
Internet of Things in Healthcare: An Extensive Review on Recent Advances, Challenges, and
Opportunities 23

Rajasekaran Thangaraj, KPR Institute of Engineering and Technology, India
Sivaramakrishnan Rajendar, KPR Institute of Engineering and Technology, India
Vidhya Kandasamy, KPR Institute of Engineering and Technology, India

Healthcare motoring has become a popular research in recent years. The evolution of electronic devices brings out numerous wearable devices that can be used for a variety of healthcare motoring systems. These devices measure the patient's health parameters and send them for further processing, where the acquired data is analyzed. The analysis provides the patients or their relatives with the medical support required or predictions based on the acquired data. Cloud computing, deep learning, and machine learning technologies play a prominent role in processing and analyzing the data respectively. This chapter aims to provide a detailed study of IoT-based healthcare systems, a variety of sensors used to measure parameters of health, and various deep learning and machine learning approaches introduced for the diagnosis of different diseases. The chapter also highlights the challenges, open issues, and performance considerations for future IoT-based healthcare research.

Chapter 3

G. S. Karthick, Bharathiar University, India
P. B. Pankajavalli, Bharathiar University, India

The rapid innovations in technologies endorsed the emergence of sensory equipment's connection to the Internet for acquiring data from the environment. The increased number of devices generates the enormous amount of sensor data from diversified applications of Internet of things (IoT). The generation of data may be a fast or real-time data stream which depends on the nature of applications. Applying analytics and intelligent processing over the data streams discovers the useful information and predicts the insights. Decision-making is a prominent process which makes the IoT paradigm qualified. This chapter provides an overview of architecting IoT-based healthcare systems with different machine learning algorithms. This chapter elaborates the smart data characteristics and design considerations for efficient adoption of machine learning algorithms into IoT applications. In addition, various existing and hybrid classification algorithms are applied to sensory data for identifying falls from other daily activities.

Chapter 4

M. Sridhar, Bharathiar University, India
N. Priya, Bharathiar University, India
A. Muniyappan, Bharathiar University, India

Wireless body area networks (WBANs) are valuable solutions for healthcare lifestyle monitoring applications which allow the continuous screening of health data and constant access to patients despite their current locality or activity, with a fraction of the cost of regular face-to-face examination. In such environments, entities are equipped with intelligence-embedded devices to collect data for providing pervasive information. WBANs can serve as passing reference for huge audience instance systems for architects, practitioners, developers, medical engineers, etc. In particular for the medical field, devices fixed inside the human body measure and transfer real-time data to the caregiver through the communication network. Many technologies have showed their efficiency in secondary WBANs application such as biofeedback, remote sensing, and QoS requirement. This chapter highlights the major applications, design, and security of WBAN.

Chapter 5

Sumathi V., Sri Ramakrishna College of Arts and Science, India

Wireless network led to the development of Wireless Sensor Networks (WSNs). A Wireless sensor network is a set of connected devices, sensors, and electronic components that can transmit the information collected from an observed field to the relevant node through wireless links. WSN has advanced many application fields. It can change any kind of technology that can modify the future lifestyle. WSNs are composed of tiny wireless computers that can sense the situation of atmosphere, process the sensor data, make a decision, and spread data to the environmental stimuli. Sensor-based technology has created several opportunities in the healthcare system, revolutionizing it in many aspects. This chapter explains in detail wireless sensor networks, their protocol, and performance metrics. The impact and role of the Biosensor in a wireless sensor network and healthcare systems are depicted. The integration of the computer engineering program into the WSNs is addressed.

Chapter 6

R. Vadivel, Bharathiar University, India
J. Ramkumar, VLB Janakiammal College of Arts and Science, India

Internet of Things (IoT) is a technology which accommodates the hardware, software, and physical objects that collaborate with each other. IoT-based healthcare applications are increasing day by day and are never going to be decreased. Healthcare applications work in an ad-hoc manner to collect patient data and send it to corresponding persons so they can take just-in-time action. The routing protocols designed for general ad-hoc networks and applications are not supported by IoT-based, ad-hoc networks. Hence, there exists a need to develop a routing protocol to support IoT-based, ad-hoc networks. This chapter focuses to develop a routing protocol for an IoT-based, cognitive radio ad-hoc network by utilizing bio-inspired concept with the objective of reducing the delay and energy consumption. NS2 simulation results reflect the proposed routing protocol's performance in terms of benchmark performance metrics.

Chapter 7

Kameswara Rao M., Annamalai University, India
S. G. Santhi, Annamalai University, India

The sturdy advancements of internet of things are being changed into a methodology of associating smart things. E-health applications in this vision are a standout amongst IoT's most energizing applications. Indeed, security concerns were the fundamental boundary to the establishment. The encryption of various interlinked substances and the classification of the swapped information are the real concerns which should be settled for clients. This chapter proposes an e-health application using lightweight verification mechanism. The proposed model utilizes nonces as well as keyed-hash message authentication (KHAC) for checking the validity of verification trades.

Chapter 8

N. Geetha, PSG College of Technology, India
A. Sankar, PSG College of Technology, India

Healthcare monitoring has grown drastically in the world. People are provided with modern treatments and continuous monitoring of physiological changes in their body. Many technologies are merged into the medial field to bring in this revolution. Many solutions are provided and are commonly used in hospitals and by patients. An IoT-based intelligent healthcare monitoring system provides a continuous health monitoring for tribal people. The system collects data from a patient and loads it into the cloud storage. The doctors have the privilege to view the patients' data and suggest the prescriptions or send an alert message in case of any emergency. A prototype model is developed and tested. This system helps to provide a healthcare solution for tribal community.

Chapter 9

Most of the elderly citizens are either living by themselves or locked up at home when the rest of the family members go to work. Health of the elderly deteriorates gradually with age, but people fail to notice these changes in everyday life. The elderly are at risk of not receiving attention immediately in the case of emergencies. Internet of things can be used to alert family members and health personnel immediately when an abnormality in the elderly person's health is sensed to prevent discovery of illness at an irrecoverable stage. Internet of things can monitor parameters like heart pulse rate, body temperature, body movement, position, and location, and raise an alert to take immediate preventive actions. Making this system portable is one of the most necessary requirements because it will be worn by the user. That introduces various conditions in itself. For instance, the system should not disturb the patient or be heavy.

The objective of IoT in healthcare is to empower people to live healthy lives by wearing connected equipment. The healthcare industry has perpetually been in the forefront in the adoption and utilization of information and communication technologies (ICT) for the efficient healthcare administration). Detection of atrial fibrillation is done by checking the variations in the period of the heart rate. If a patient has atrial fibrillation, the period between each heartbeat will vary. A gas sensor is used to check the quality of air and a MEMS sensor to detect the fall of the body. The MEMS sensor is a compact device that collects comprehensive physical information and uses the gateway and cloud to analyze and store information.

The objective is to build an IoT-based patient monitoring smart device. The device would monitor real-time data of patients and send it to the Cloud. It has become imperative to attend to minute internal changes in the body that affect overall health. The system would remotely take care of an individual's changes in health and notify the relatives or doctors of any abnormal changes. Cloud storages provide easy availability and monitoring of real-time data. The system uses microcontroller Arduino Nano and sensors – GY80, Heartbeat sensor, Flex sensor, and Galvanic Skin (GSR) sensor with a Wi-Fi Module.

Chapter 12

Ibrahim Taiwo Adeleke, Federal Medical Centre, Bida, Nigeria
Qudrotullaah Bolanle Suleiman Abdul, University of Ilorin Teaching Hospital, Nigeria

IoMT has helped to improve health safety and care of billions of people and at least, health-related parameters can now be monitored from home in real time. This chapter deployed a cross-sectional design to determine perceptions of Nigerian healthcare providers toward medical confidentiality and cyber security in the wake of electronic health records and IoMT. Participants' opinions on the workings of EHRs in Nigeria include: security of health records (79.4%); aiding effective healthcare data backup (88.2%); enhancement of medical confidentiality (89.2%); speeding up documentation process (93.1%); and that EHRs will generally bring about positive changes in the country healthcare system. Nearly a third (31.4%) of participants have heard about audit trail, which they admitted (43.1%) have the capabilities to facilitate effective medical confidentiality. Healthcare providers in Nigeria have some concerns over security of patient health information on the Cloud, but are hopeful of the workability of IoMT for its promises to improve healthcare quality.

Chapter 13

Amine Boulemtafes, Research Center on Scientific and Technical Information, Algeria
Nadjib Badache, Research Center on Scientific and Technical Information, Algeria

Continuous monitoring generally imposes a set of constraints including form factor, energy consumption, and mobility support in order to enable anywhere and anytime monitoring. Sensors, within this context, play an important role as the first building block of such systems and the main entry point for the monitoring process. Therefore, to experiment continuous health-monitoring systems in real-like conditions, sensing platforms need to meet a number of related requirements and constraints, especially for mobility factor. This chapter aims to present an overview of popular sensing platforms meeting appropriate constraints, allowing experimenters and researchers to start prototyping and experimentation projects for continuous health monitoring. For that, a number of requirements and constraints for continuous monitoring prototyping are firstly identified, then sensing platforms are classified into three proposed and compared categories, namely, ready-to-use, ready-to-compose kits, and do-it-yourself platforms. On that basis, a set of interesting platforms are reviewed and compared under each category.

Chapter 14

Isakki Alias Devi P, Ayya Nadar Janaki Ammal College, India

IoT seriously impacts every industry. The healthcare industry has experienced progression in digitizing medical records. Healthcare services are costlier than ever. Data mining is one of the largest challenges to face IoT. Big Data is an accumulation of data. IoT devices receive lots of data. Big data systems can do a lot of data analytics. The tools can also be used to perform these operations. The big health application system can be built by integrating medical health resources using intelligent terminals, internet of things (IoT), big data, and cloud computing. People suffer from many diseases. A big health system can be applied to scientific health management by detecting risk factors for the occurrence of diseases. Patients can have special attention to their health requirements and their devices can be tuned to remind them of their appointments, calorie count, exercise check, blood pressure variations, symptoms of any diseases, and so much more.

The chapter covers the challenges faced in real-world healthcare services such as operating room bottlenecks, upcoming newborn medicines, managing datasets, and sources. It includes future directions that address practitioner difficulties. When IoT is merged with predictive techniques, it improves the medical service performance rate tremendously. Finally, the chapter covers the case studies and the tools that are in use to motivate the researchers to contribute to this domain.

Foreword

Internet of things (IoT) is an emerging concept and enabler that has the potential to completely reshape the future of the industry. Since the inception of the IoT, It has been making a serious impact on every industry. It has extensive applicability in numerous areas, including healthcare. It has been widely identified as a potential solution to alleviate the pressures on healthcare systems and has thus been the focus of much recent research. But, IoT remains a relatively new field of research, and its potential use for healthcare is an area still in its infancy.

The editors of this book have taken a timely initiative to go for extensive research in the field of IoT-based health care systems, as the steadily aging population and the related rise in chronic illness are placing a significant strain on modern healthcare systems. We could see the editors' deep passion for the technology—IoT—and their desire to understand how it can help improve everyone's quality of life. We are glad to see their passion for IoT bear fruit through this book.

It is evident from the articles and the chapters of the book that the researchers are striving to reach the goal of developing an end-to-end healthcare systems for general or specific purposes through the development of a wearable, IoT-based system for the provision of emergency healthcare that incorporates health sign monitoring, machine learning for diagnostics, and long-range communications to notify emergency service providers when a patient needs urgent help.

There is no doubt that this book will be a pioneer in guiding and providing research exposure to the researchers, academicians, students, faculty, scientists and industry professionals in the field of IoT in healthcare. We wish the research articles of this book transformed into real products which will make healthcare easier and lessen the strain on healthcare systems.

V. Krishnaveni
Kongu Arts and Science College, India

K. G. Santhiya
Kongu Arts and Science College, India

V. Krishnaveni *received both B.Sc. and M.Sc degrees in Computer Science from Madurai Kamaraj University, Madurai, Tamilnadu, India, in 1991 and 1993 respectively, M.Phil degree in Computer Science from Mother Teresa University, Kodaikanal, Tamilnadu, India in 2002 and Ph.D. degree in Computer Science from Madurai Kamaraj University, Madurai, Tamilnadu, India, in 2014. She has 25 years of experience in collegiate education and currently working as an associate professor in the Department of Computer Science, Kongu Arts and Science College (Autonomous), Erode, Tamilnadu, India. Her current research interests include Soft computing, machine learning, data mining, and big data analytics. Dr.V.Krishnaveni has published her research*

Papers in Scopus indexed and peer-reviewed journals including IEEE Explore, Springer and Computer Systems Science & Engineering. Currently, she is accomplishing a Research Project funded by University Grants Commission, New Delhi, India.

K. G. Santhiya *received B.Sc., M.Sc and M.Phil degrees in Computer Science from Bharathiar University, Coimbatore, Tamilnadu, India, in 1998, 2000 and 2004 respectively, and a Ph.D. degree in Computer Science from Mother Teresa Women's University, Kodaikanal, Tamilnadu, India, in 2014. She has a total experience of 19 years in collegiate education. Her areas of research include routing in mobile ad-hoc networks and wireless networks. Dr.K.G.Santhiya has published her research papers in Scopus Indexed and peer-reviewed journals including Elsevier.*

Preface

BACKGROUND

Innovation and development in sensing technology, smart devices, wireless sensor networks, device miniaturization, data analytics, and actuations are rationalizing the awareness on the Internet of Things (IoT). IoT is applied on a wide variety of applications including the environment, buildings, industries, agriculture, healthcare and so on (Li et al., 2015). Especially, IoT devices and services have created a new pathway towards the generation of efficient services for saving human lives and time with a high degree of accuracy (Reis et al., 2016). Constant growth in remote healthcare area has led to the invention of handy healthcare devices. IoT technology facilitates the development of numerous prototypes for a comprehensive view of a patient's vital signs, which transforms the healthcare domain with efficient and better patient monitoring systems (Ahmed et al., 2017). Such applications of IoT technology in healthcare domain is highly accepted by both patients and medical practitioners. The ability of healthcare systems to communicate with the connected devices has been considered as a game-changing feature because it empowers the patients to concentrate on their health status. Also, it has the capability to enhance the medical practitioner's healthcare delivery ratio.

The connected healthcare device generates a terrific amount of data which is difficult to make sense of by the medical practitioners. Parallelly another research challenge comes to the picture- the need for the tremendous data to be secured, particularly during the data exchange between IoT devices (Kvedar, 2015). This created a new trend of offering personalized healthcare services by building new protocols for developing the proficient ubiquitous pool of healthcare services. On the other hand, the application of IoT in the healthcare domain is still suffering from various drawbacks that include cost, accuracy, architecture standards, and interoperability issues. Therefore, the success rate of IoT healthcare system entirely depends on the device interoperability ratio and the coupling ratio of devices with machine learning concepts, which standardizes the decision-making functionality of IoT devices.

ABOUT THIS BOOK

The above-addressed challenges and requirements endow a wide range of opportunities to discover and examine new conceptual theories, algorithms, intelligent medical systems and applications in IoT-based healthcare domain. The goal of this book is to bind the researchers and practitioners into a single medium, to capture the state-of-the-art IoT in healthcare applications, to address how IoT improves the proficiency of the healthcare domain with respect to wireless sensor networks, addressing the challenges and issues, examining the machine learning algorithms which assists in prediction of high-level information from real-time healthcare data and also giving a vision for research and development. It explores possible automated IoT solutions in daily life, including structures for healthcare systems that manage large amounts of data (big data) to improve clinical decisions. This book will prove to be invaluable for professionals who want to improve their understanding of the recent challenges in the IoT healthcare domain. The individual chapter addresses diversified aspects of IoT systems which include design challenges of IoT, theory, various protocols, implementation issues, and a few case studies. Moreover, the book will be very useful for postgraduate students and researchers to understand and implement IoT in the healthcare domain.

TARGET AUDIENCE

IoT-based healthcare systems gained attention worldwide since the last decade. Researchers, academicians, students, faculty, scientists and IT sector professionals will find this book beneficial for research exposure and new ideas in the field of IoT with respect to healthcare applications.

ORGANIZATION OF THE BOOK

This book is organized into 15 chapters. Introduction section reveals how the connected IoT-enabled healthcare devices are stepped up even under the presence of stumbling blocks. All the contributors to this book are the upcoming researchers in the field of IoT. The summary of the chapter contents is as follows:

Chapter 1 presents an overview of IoT in healthcare in various aspects which includes the IoT ecosystem, supporting technologies, design challenges, applications, security issues, and concerns.

Chapter 2 does a detailed study on IoT-based healthcare systems, a variety of sensors used to measure vitals of human, the challenges, open issues, and opportunities in healthcare research.

Chapter 3 depicts how an IoT based system must be architected with the support of machine learning algorithms and also this chapter discusses the smart data characteristics, design considerations for efficient adoption of machine learning algorithms into IoT applications. In addition, various existing and hybrid classification algorithms are applied to sensory data for detecting accidental falls.

Chapter 4 highlights the importance of Wireless Body Area Networks (WBAN) in terms of requirements, characteristics, design considerations, and challenges.

Chapter 5 explains about the wireless sensor networks, its protocol and performance metrics. The impact and role of the biosensor in a wireless sensor network and healthcare systems are also discussed.

Chapter 6 delves about the research work that went into developing a routing protocol for IoT-based cognitive radio ad-hoc network by utilizing a bio-inspired concept with the objective of reducing the delay and energy consumption.

Chapter 7 explains the most recent lightweight E-health authentication in which a protected channel is built up between sensor hubs. In this, the base station validates each item with a keyed-hash message confirmation, and then the framework utilizes nonce's and ensures the honesty of both the different exchanges.

Chapter 8 elaborates an IoT based intelligent healthcare monitoring prototype system which provides continuous health monitoring for tribal people.

Chapter 9 depicts the prototype system designed for detecting abnormalities in the health condition by monitoring the parameters like heart and pulse rate, body temperature, body movement and position, location and raising an alert to take immediate preventive actions.

Chapter 10 elaborates about the prototype system which detects atrial fibrillation, accidental falls and air quality using IoT technologies.

Chapter 11 presents a framework for endless remote-monitoring of patient's health parameters to avoid deep deterioration.

Chapter 12 explores the major concerns over the security of a patient's health information on the cloud in Nigeria.

Chapter 13 presents an overview of popular sensing platforms meeting appropriate constraints allowing experimenters and researchers to start prototyping and experimentation projects for continuous health monitoring.

Chapter 14 clearly illustrates how big data analytics gained its importance in the development of IoT-based healthcare applications.

Chapter 15 provides a summary of how predictive modeling enhances IoT healthcare applications.

The contributions compiled in this book presents the review reports, discussions, issues, implementation strategies, most recent research, as well as case studies focusing on the design and development of IoT-based healthcare systems.

P. B. Pankajavalli
Bharathiar University, India

G. S. Karthick
Bharathiar University, India

REFERENCES

Ahmed, Begum, & Raad. (Eds.). (2017). Internet of Things Technologies for HealthCare. Västerås, Sweden: Springer Publisher.

Kvedar, J. C. (Ed.). (2015). *The Internet of Healthy Things*. Internet of Healthy Things Publisher.

Li, S., Da Xu, L., & Zhao, S. (2015). The internet of things: A survey. *Information Systems Frontiers, 17*(2), 243–259. doi:10.100710796-014-9492-7

Reis & da Silva. (Ed.). (2016). Internet of Things and Advanced Application in Healthcare. IGI Global.

Acknowledgment

Writing this part is probably the most difficult task. Although the list of people to thank heartily is long, making this list is not the hard part. The difficult part is to search the words that convey the sincerity and enormity of our gratitude and love.

First of all, we would like to thank the almighty.

Acknowledgment when sincerely given is a reward without price. We are thankful to the publishing team at IGI Global for accepting to publish this edited book. We would like to thank the entire development editor team, for helping us in bringing this project to a successful end.

We would like to express our deepest appreciation to Editorial Advisory Board members for extending their valuable suggestions and support to accomplish this task in a successful manner.

The editors would like to express appreciation and thank the reviewers for their careful reading of our manuscript and their many perceptive comments and suggestions. We want to acknowledge the authors for their valuable contributions and hereby we convey sincere thankfulness.

Editor Dr. P. B. Pankajavalli would like to thank her family members, friends, and scholars for extending their constant support.

Editor Mr. G. S. Karthick owes his sincere thanks to his grandparents who are always blessing him from heaven. He express the deepest gratitude to his parents Mr.G.Selvaraj and Mrs.S.Saraswathi for their moral support, blessings, and encouragement throughout his life. He would like to thank his research supervisor and co-editor of this book, Dr.P.B.Pankajavalli, for her patient guidance, encouragement, and advice she has provided throughout the completion of this task. He has been extremely lucky to have a supervisor who cared so much about his work, and responded to his questions and queries so promptly. He is greatly indebted to his co-scholar Mr.M.Sridhar and other family members for their constant support in every aspect of life and also responsible for encouraging him to finish this book.

P. B. Pankajavalli
Bharathiar University, India

G. S. Karthick
Bharathiar University, India

Introduction

Modern technology has interrupted every domain including healthcare, agriculture, industries and so on. Healthcare is a withstanding domain which adopts the evolving technological transformations to upgrade the diagnosis and treatment procedures. While considering the recent Internet of Things (IoT), it provides a whole host of advantages like improving the efficacy and service quality by deploying it in healthcare systems. The following statistical discloses the usage of IoT in healthcare and its impact on the healthcare industry (Parker, 2018).

- ❖ 60% of the healthcare organizations have implemented IoT devices into their services
- ❖ Almost 73% of healthcare organizations adopted IoT for patients health monitoring and management
- ❖ Nearly 87% of healthcare organizations have planned to implement IoT by 2019 which is 85% higher than the other industries
- ❖ Totally 64% of healthcare organizations using IoT for patient monitoring alone
- ❖ 89% of healthcare organization continued to run under IoT oriented security breach

Generally, interconnected devices are used in the process of acquiring data from various diversified sensor terminals which may include blood glucose level, blood pressure level, body temperature level, activity monitors and so on. Though, most of these applications require constant healthcare providers to follow up. Most of the healthcare organizations are focusing on providing smart amenities. In particular, while adopting IoT in healthcare domain major concerns such as privacy and security issues may arise. Therefore, the success rate of IoT strongly depends on how the widely accessible, personalized and on-time healthcare services offered to everyone.

The crucial benefit of adopting IoT in the healthcare domain is cost reduction. Healthcare providers make use of remote health monitoring facility and provide treatment recommendations in the absence of patient at the hospital. In hospitals, the inpatients are meshed up with various medical devices such as heart monitors, intravenous (IV) sets and respiratory monitors. Then the operating and recording of data from such medical devices may prone to errors and it consumes a lot of times. But with the assistance of IoT technology, health data can be automatically conveyed to electronic health records (EHR) systems. This may increase the accuracy of health data and also the healthcare providers can spend more time for caring the patients.

On the other hand, healthcare providers have to interpret the acquired data to take a decision for further treatments. But the increase in medical devices was arriving at an accurate decision becomes a tedious task for healthcare providers. With the power of IoT data analytics, the healthcare providers can easily gain insights on patient's health. Even though the IoT is ground-breaking in the healthcare domain, there are many challenges that must be kept in mind. The identified major challenges of IoT in healthcare are:

- ❖ Security Threats
- ❖ Multiple Device Integration
- ❖ Inferring information from huge data

The traditional healthcare research suffers from the lack of real-time information resources. Whereas, IoT creates a pathway to generate a pool of valuable information through real-time data analysis and testing. As a result, the healthcare domain yields improved solutions to the issues that were experienced previously. Therefore the following chapters in this book empower researchers to use their knowledge and training in a superior way to solve healthcare problems.

P. B. Pankajavalli
Bharathiar University, India

G. S. Karthick
Bharathiar University, India

REFERENCES

Parker, R. (2018, January 13). *Internet of Things in Healthcare: What are the Possibilities and Challenges?* Retrieved June 24, 2019, from https://readwrite.com

Chapter 1
IoT in Healthcare:
Ecosystem, Pillars, Design Challenges, Applications, Vulnerabilities, Privacy, and Security Concerns

V. Jeevika Tharini
Bharathiar University, India

S. Vijayarani
Bharathiar University, India

ABSTRACT

One of the best-known features of IoT is automation. Because of this, IoT is a much-needed field for many applications, namely emergency and healthcare domains. IoT has made many revolutionary changes in the healthcare industry. IoT paves the way to numerous advancements for healthcare. The possibilities of IoT have reached their peak in the commercial industry and health sector. In recent years, serious concerns have been raised over the control and access of one's individual information. Privacy and security of the IoT devices can be compromised by intruders. Apart from the numerous benefits of IoTs, there are several security and privacy concerns to consider. A brief overview of different kinds of security attacks, solution for the attacks, privacy and security issues are discussed in this chapter.

INTRODUCTION

Internet of Things (IoT) is one of the emerging technologies of the present era with a combination of several different computing devices, physical object, Human beings, and animals. Every object in the IoT system is provided with a unique number to represent every individual object is called unique identifiers. IoT can transfer the data from one object to another over the network without any centralized system. Our day to day life is gradually led to an imaginary world with the arrival of computer technology. From anywhere and anytime people can do their daily chores in the virtual world provided by the network. New advancement necessitated the integration of imaginary space and the real-world

DOI: 10.4018/978-1-7998-1090-2.ch001

on the same platform is called as IoT. Based on available low-cost sensors, wireless sensor networks, and wireless communication puts forward a new demand for IoT. Internet technology-based products enrich and simplify human's daily life through connected smart devices and make context-aware. IoT has diminished the manpower in many fields. IoT can improve efficiency in transportation, manufacturing, enacted advanced technologies in hospitals and developed a new education system. Development in IoT accelerates the growth of new industries and start-ups in manufacturing, cloud computing, automation, machine learning, artificial intelligence, and cyber-security. One of the largest obstacles in IoT is adoption. There are numerous definitions and descriptions for IoT by different authors, companies, and researchers (Berte, D. R. 2018).

IoT earns its full potential support by utilizing the key role of smart objects which use numerous actuators and sensors. Objects in the system can perceive the situation of the environment. Through the perceived data, the networking capability is established to the open-source internet services and interact with the human world (Kumar, J.S., and Patel, D. R. 2014). IoT constructs the entire world as connected at the same time safe and comfortable. IoT has influenced many applications among that IoT plays an eminent role in the field of healthcare. Several IoT healthcare products like the wearable health bands, fitness tracking shoes, smart meters, RFID based smart devices, real-time monitoring equipment's, and other smart objects embedded with IoT. Also, the smart-phone based application helps in tracking a medical record with real-time alerts and facilitate to provide emergency services. Smart hospitals consist of a complete system that communicates between network connected systems, apps and devices. Interaction among healthcare professionals, patients, and smart devices is established through the network is improved day by day. These advancements provide easiness to patients as well as to doctors. IoT based healthcare system can help the care-takers of patients and doctors to monitor, track, record patient's essential, sensitive medical information. The power of IoT made the possibility of collecting real-time data from various sources and several types of patients over a long period of time has become very easy and fast. The potential of IoT for medical devices and health care services are established by bio-sensors and other smart sensors (a microcontroller and sensor). Basic and essential biological signal recording sensors such as heart rate, pulse rate, oxygen, the glucose level in blood and blood pressure. These sensors can accurately measure, analyze and monitors a diverse health status of every individual patient.

The healthcare services are getting better and cost-efficient when healthcare is incorporated with ever-growing technology IoT in the real world (Gupta et al., 2016). For example, various smart medical devices have smart sensors embedded into the IoT device that allows collecting the raw data through sensors from physical objects that will be stored, analyzed and conduct tests. Results obtained from the test are used by medical experts to take proper decisions. In healthcare, the consumers, patients, and other health experts need to think of some innovative and more reliable methods to accomplish the technology as the real-time to take the full advantage of IoT and make sure reliable results with reduced time which will be of maximum benefit. The potentials of IoT are unlimited and ever-increasing. IoT will bring enormous changes to future society and can change the way of lifestyle, business strategies as well as the style of business. Internet of Things offers potentials to recognize and hook up the worldwide physical objects into a combined system (Kumar, J.S., and Patel, D. R. 2014).

Figure 1. IoT ecosystem

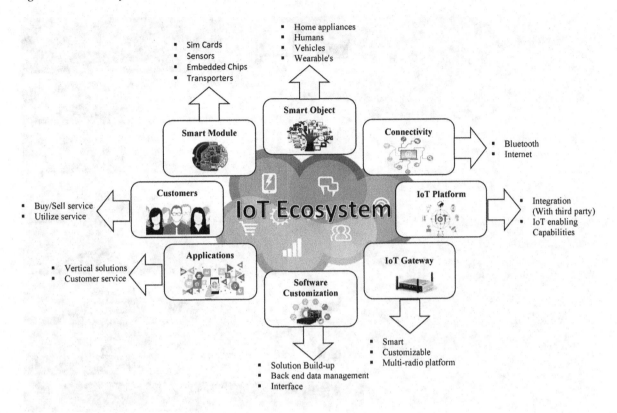

IoT ECOSYSTEM

IoT is a network of interconnected devices and objects such as humans, physical devices, smart objects, and other items. The connected physical devices/objects are embedded with network connectivity and software which enables the device to gather and exchange data or information among the network. The key desire of IoT is to interconnect all things that play a major role in every-day life.

IoT makes the objects intelligent and programmable to make the objects to think, take decisions according to the situation and made act smart. By making the devices intelligent, IoT devices are proficient in exchanging information from one to many persons. IoT allows exchange data or information and communicating among the connected devices. The data collected by the sensors and other devices will provide us various applications to machine goal or common user or. The choice of IoT is not limited just to interconnecting and establishing communication among things to the Internet (J Vojas 2016).

Layers of IoT Ecosystem

The term IoT describes a broad and diverse ecosystem that includes a wide range of different kinds of network connectivity and usage scenarios that dependents on the need or place of deployment. Therefore, discussing the complete Ecosystem is helpful to understand better about IoT and necessary to split the system into layers based on the services (Mattern, F., and Floerkemeier, C. 2010).

Figure 2. IoT world forum reference model (IoTWF 2017)

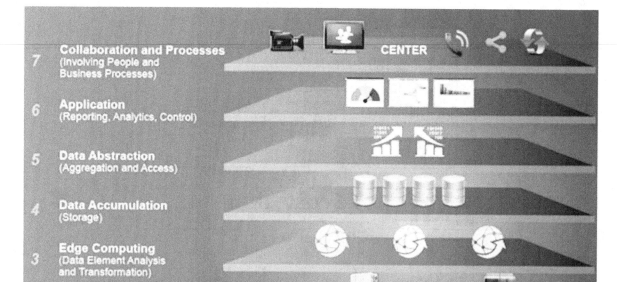

The IoT ecosystem consists of seven horizontal layers. These layers are essential and common to all use cases of IoT. The description of these layers and the components are described as follows,

Physical Devices and Controllers - All the physical objects that belong to the internet of Things are placed in the physical layer. From a systems perspective of design, the "things" are the sensors, related IoT, and devices that are directly managed by the architecture of IoT. Edge Intelligence is one of the important IoT concepts which allows low latency reaction to the field events and higher levels of autonomy. The distributed processing is also implemented in physical layer.

Connectivity - The layer connectivity is spanned from the "middle" of an edge node and device up through and then transmits the data to the cloud. Connectivity maps the field data to the logical and physical technologies which is act as a backhaul to the cloud and further layers.

Edge Computing - The next layer is Edge Computing, interfaces the data and controls the data transfer to the further layers of cloud or other enterprise software. Edge computing performs operations like protocol conversion, routing the information to higher layers of software and speeds the path of logic for low latency decision making.

Data Accumulation - Accumulates the data of IoT systems that provide incoming data for subsequent integration, normalization, processing, and preparation for upstream applications is accomplished by data accumulation layer.

Data Abstraction - Collection of information's from multiple IoT sensors and organize into the appropriate schema. Further the data is allowed for upstream processing. Abstraction layer also performs the dynamic combination of new devices into the IoT ecosystem and expedites the processing.

Application Layer- The application layer is liable for data formatting and representation. Application layer comprises of custom applications, which uses the data generated by smart objects.

Collaboration and Processes - The final process of the application is presented to all the end-users and the data's whichever processed at lower layers are integrated with business applications. Collaboration and processes layer is about human interaction with all the other layers of the IoT system where economic value is delivered. The final layer includes the end-users namely people, businesses, industry and several other users. Collaboration and decision making based information's derived from IoT fraternize the end-users (Juxtology 2018).

FOUR PILLARS OF IoT

Internet of Things (IoT) had spread across a large number of industry sectors and some of the technologies have been used for many years. The expansion of IoT based applications in these sectors is unbalanced to a certain extent. The four pillars of IoT are M2M, RFID, WSNs, and SCADA.

M2M: The Internet of Devices

Machine-to-Machine (M2M) communication is a type of data communication system that integrates one or many entities together.M2M does not require any human interaction or administration for the process of communication and any decision making. M2M is also called Machine Type Communication (MTC) in the 3rd Generation Partnership Project (3GPP).M2M communication could be processed over mobile networks (e.g. GSM-GPRS, CDMA EVDO networks). In the M2M type communication, the part of a mobile network (wireless communication) is largely circumscribed to serve as a transportation network.

RFID: The Internet of Objects

Radio Frequency Identification (RFID) uses electromagnetic waves to transmit data from an electronic tag attached to any type of object and a central system through the RFID's reader. The purpose of RFID is to identifying and tracking any type of object. RFID is a non-contact based technology that's widely used in many places for tasks such as tracking books in libraries, personnel tracking, supply chain management, access control, tollgate systems and so on. RFID uses the radio waves generated by a reader to perceive the presence of an RFID tag. Tags can be embedded in small items like buttons, cards, or tiny capsules.

WSN: The Internet of Transducers

Wireless sensor network (WSN) contains spatially distributed self-governing sensors to monitor environmental situations such as motion, temperature, pressure or pollutants. There are several reports on the overlaps or coverage differences when WSN was compared with M2M and RFID, SCADA or smart system was not mentioned in the report. WSN is a collection of small, low-priced with constrained power

Figure 3. Four pillars of IoT (Zhou, H. 2012)

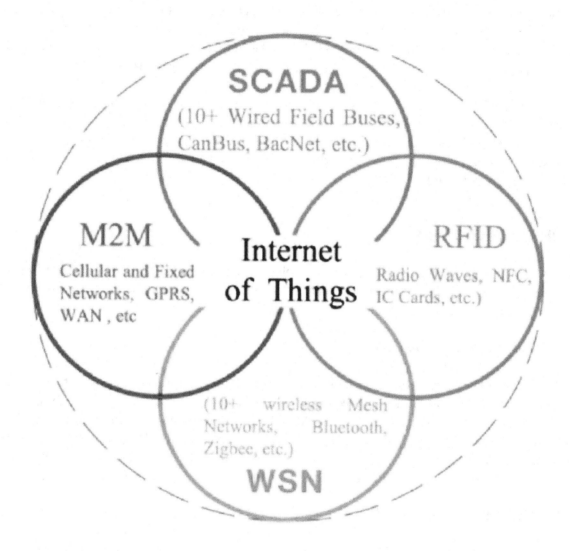

consumption devices. Devices are organized in a cooperative network. Nodes communicate wirelessly in multi-hop routing and dynamically changing network topology.

Body Sensor Network (BSN)

Body Sensor Network is an application of wearable computing devices that permits wireless communication between several tiny body-sensor units. BSN is a single body central unit, which is worn on the human body to transmit needed and important biological signs. Medical practitioners or caregivers make use of those signals for decision making and further analysis. BSN plays a prominent role in the healthcare domain. Application of BSN is used for constant monitoring for patients suffering from chronic diseases such as asthma, diabetes, and heart attacks.

Figure 4. Body sensor network (Reuters 2017)

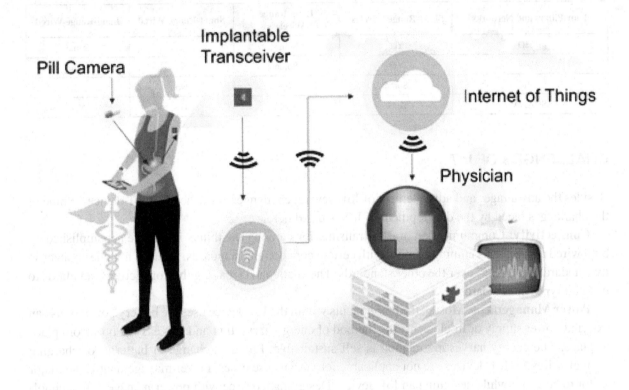

Visual sensor networks are utilized by several fields of research, including image or vision processing, networking, communication, embedded and distributed system processing. Applications include surveillance, environmental monitoring, smart homes, virtual reality, and others. With the development of WSN, recent technological advances have led to the emergence of distributed wireless sensor and actuator networks (WSANs) that are capable of observing the physical world. Observed data is used for decision making and performing appropriate actions.

SCADA: The Internet of Controllers

Supervisory Control and Data Acquisition System (SCADA) is an independent system based on closed-loop control theory. SCADA is also called a smart system or a Cyber-Physical System (CPS) that connects, supervises and manages the equipment through the network. Industrial activities cannot be supervised or controlled manually. Advanced smart and automated technology is needed which can administrate, collect, analyses the data and reports are generated based on the nature or result of the data. A distinctive solution is introduced to face all the requirement of the SCADA system (Hassan Mehmood Khan 2018).

Table 1. Four pillars of IoT and their relevance network

Four Pillars and Networks	Short-Range Wireless	Long-Range Wireless	Short-Range Wired	Long-Range Wired
RFID	Yes	Some	No	Some
WSN	Yes	Some	No	Some
M2M	Some	Yes	No	Some
SCADA	Some	Some	Yes	Yes

CHALLENGES OF IoT

Besides the advantages and advancement of IoT, several challenges were faced by IoT devices. Some of the challenges faced by the development of IoT is listed here,

Connectivity: Communication or data transmissions among the things in IoT are accomplished by both wired and wireless communication with certain connectivity standards. There is not one connectivity standard that "wins" over the other standards. The challenge is making the connectivity standards to meet all types of standards.

Power Management: Most of the components within the IoT device uses the battery power or use an external power supply or implements the method of energy harvesting and it is easy to port from place to place. The energy harvesting method is self-sustainable. Frequent change of batteries or charging through wires for IoT devices are not applicable for various use cases. Power management is the major factor to consider while designing an IoT device. Designing a device with power management technology is one of the biggest challenges in IoT.

Security: Security is one of the important credentials for every product. Data security is important for the amount of data being sent and shared within the IoT system. Built-in hardware security and the use of connectivity security protocols are essential factors for securing the IoT system. Another challenge is simply educating the consumers about security standards that are integrated into the IoT devices.

Complexity: Ease of design and development is essential to get more things connected. Additionally, the end-users and common people have to aware of the IoT technological set-up. IoT devices must be familiar with all kinds of people.

Rapid Evolution: The development of IoT is showing a gradual change in its nature and evolving every day. More devices are being added every day to make human life easy and even though the industry is still in its naissance. The challenges facing the industry is about unknown devices, unknown use cases, and unknown applications. Industries have to be flexible in all facets of the development of IoT based devices and relevant applications. Developers need to show consideration while selecting sensors and power-management technologies and required to provide an energy-friendly user interface for the user while designing an IoT device (Chase, J 2013).

INTERNET OF THINGS IN HEALTH CARE AND ITS APPLICATIONS

Due to the urbanization, declining birth-rate, economic growth, socially unbalanced resource utilization and tremendous increase in population, etc. seems to be an evident concern in the field of healthcare. These are some of the factors that led to the advent of IoT in Healthcare.

- The inability of responding to an emergency is a critical social problem in most of the Hospitals.
- The shortage of medical staff is one prominent factor to concern.
- Inadequate institutional facilities and medical supplies are another concern especially in rural areas and lack of medical facilities with a low level of treatment leads to an ineffective healthcare system.
- To safeguard the health of the peoples becoming a heavy burden for every economy, individuals, families, and states are due to the flawed disease prevention system are the national strategy requirements.
- The shortfall of early disease detection capability and poor disease prevention is also a serious factor in Health care.

Internet of Medical Things

A healthcare application in IoT technologies is termed as the Internet of Medical Things (IoMT) which envisions the network of connected physical devices that sense essential data from the real-time. IoMT enables personalized living environments with higher standards of personalized care, attention and living through the data-driven based treatment as well as optimize devices and customize to handle psychological and physiological needs among individuals. IoT in the medical field has brought forward many changes and challenges in modern healthcare systems. One of the leading technology, Machine learning is applied to process the data involved in IoMT for later medical analysis and diagnosis of disease.

In the past decade, the advent of the IoMT has fascinated many researchers from the healthcare and IT industry (Y Yin et al., 2016). Many IoMT-based platforms, applications, and services for remote health monitoring, chronic diseases, elderly care products, and fitness programs have been introduced recently. The growth of IoMT has upgraded the traditional medical systems in several aspects namely the analysis and diagnosis of various kinds of diseases (M Orsini et al., 2017). IoMT also offers alternative feasible solutions to solve problems met by the traditional medical systems, such as the lack of nurses, doctors, healthcare resources and research data. Big data technology is implemented to IoMT, to analyze and process the health data since the size of data gathered is also growing massively for every second. The popularity of IoT influenced the healthcare system and terminal devices in many aspects.

Applications of IoMT

Remote Monitoring and Management Platform of Healthcare Information (RMMP – HI)

Remote Monitoring and Management Platform of Healthcare Information (RMMP-HI) designed to handle the early detection of lifestyle diseases and prevention (W Zhao et al., 2011) which helps in monitoring as well as managing the patients in the medical field. In spite of all the limitations of the traditional

Figure 5. IoT in healthcare (Data Flair 2018)

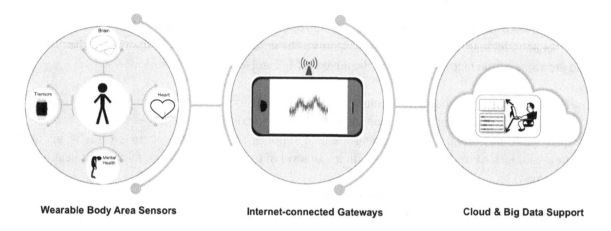

Wearable Body Area Sensors   **Internet-connected Gateways**   **Cloud & Big Data Support**

medical system such as time, location, and maintaining the user's activity state, RMMP-HI can collect medical information on the human body and can maintain the patient's information efficiently. RMMP-HI rectifies the limitations of the medical system. All the needed facilities for the patients are done in time through various medical sensors loaded in and around the human body. The data can be extracted by data encryption and then stored for further process. Comparative analysis and other needed processing are done using the stored information. The initial detection and prevention can be done by notifying the users when an abnormal appearance is found in the human state. Through real-time observing, the possibility of improving medical emergency treatment and response capacity. Prevention and decision-making are the basic key factors for any kind of disease, epidemic and regional disease which can be done through continuous monitoring, comparing the analyses and proper processing healthcare information of the associated groups. By the development of national health management records, capabilities to prevent disease, early detection and treatment are improved extensively.

Medical Body Area Network (MBAN) consists of medical sensors that can register and delete biological signals automatically based on the requirement. Sensors can record the biological signals of the human body that is a piece of human medical information transmitted to the mobile phone or home gateway. Medical information is uploaded to the data storage unit and processing center. Then stored data is subjected to analytical processing by the expert system and the results obtained from the system are further sent to the inspection of professional medical staff. Important health guidance will be sent to the patient, family members of patients or medical institutions in time. RMMP-HI collects medical information from a human's body on time through various medical sensors which are connected to the human and extracts useful information without considering the restrictions of state, time, and location. In emergencies, first-aid notification is delivered to both medical institutions and the caretakers of the patients by health service centers. The notification may contain first aid tips, nearby hospital information, the exact status of the patient, etc., to the caregivers.

Vulnerabilities in the Healthcare IoT

Patient Privacy and Protection of Intellectual Property

IoT is exposed to many vulnerabilities and attacks. Hackers and eavesdroppers able to breach the security codes or lock from the unprotected mobile and may leads to the loss of several personal data. Patient's health data may be stored in different locations such as personal cloud, health cloud, and local storage (health-related IoT mobile app's local storage). Apple's IOS has a closed privacy policy which involves the official store whereas Android has an open policy about application deployment. Due to the openness of the Android applications, it allows third-party stores and also allows the installation of apps via Android application package (APK) files from the un-trusted websites and may cause security threats to mobile.

Open source architecture renders the platform to be structurally vulnerable and makes it easy for the intrusion of malicious behavior in the devices since the Android platform is easy to repackage an application in the device. For example, a malicious agent may intrude on the application and can examine the application's exact functional area. When the user installs the application, users are asked for permission to access certain features of the mobile. Most of the users are unaware of the importance of access permissions in mobile phones and android applications. Many of the mobile users do not know the access permission's importance. Granting of access permission results in various threats and issues. The Android permission system does not adequately protect users from malicious applications and intruders. These types of vulnerabilities in the IoT devices, as well as applications, lead to tampering of the codes, data theft, reverse-engineering and privacy violations of personal data. Patient's sensitive information now being transferred from hand to hand, IoT systems should prepare early and create security policies and procedures regarding the use of wearable gadgets.

Patient Safety

The threat level for data is increasing day by day due to the increase of cybercriminals and hackers. Intruders targeting organizations via IoT devices and their relevant mobile applications such as fitness trackers, VR Headsets, etc. are rated the levels from medium to high. The applications communicate with wearable health gadgets may be intruded by hackers in many ways that may cause physical harm to the users. The biometric data of the patients which is collected from wearable IoT gadgets offers opportunities for hackers to access sensitive information that may lead to the patient's life to risk. Usually, the captured data is transmitted from the wearable gadgets to smartphones using Bluetooth network or other modes of network and these devices are likely to be attacked for security breaches and are may be prone to additional threats. Both the physical and virtual lives of patients are at risk when using such devices. It becomes crucial for health caregivers to implement an effective method to ensure the security of such devices without malfunctions while used by the end users.

Key Tampering and Unauthorized Access

Internal Medical Devices (IMD) may also be exposed to malicious attacks that are created by external adversaries and some unintended software developers or firmware designers. These devices consist of a radio transceiver to communicate with an external device or gadget. Programmers of IMDs executes all the external activities and implements the needed operation based on a user query. An IMD program-

Table 2. Applications of IoT in healthcare

S.No	Title of the Paper - Application	Author Name	Uses
1.	Smart nursing home patient monitoring system	K. Motwani, D. Mirchandani, et al 2016	Sensors on peripheral device gathers the pulse rate, blood glucose level, respiratory level, blood pressure, and other medical related biological data. The gathered data is sent wirelessly to caregivers, doctors, and nurses. Possible problems can be noticed immediately by the professionals and the concerned caregivers are immediately alerted.
2.	Internet of things in sleep monitoring: An application for posture recognition using supervised learning	G. Matar, J. Lina, et al 2016	The author has proposed an Internet of Things (IoT) for remote medical monitoring. The pressure occurred in the body is achieved through a pressure sensing mattress that is placed under the person's body, gathered data is transmitted to a computer workstation for further processing, and results have conversed for diagnosis and monitoring.
3.	RFID technology combined with IoT application in medical nursing system	C. H. Huang and K. W. Cheng 2014	Medical Nursing System which is based on NFC, RFID, and WSN technology. Medical Nursing System promotes the conditions in a nursing home and upgrades the accuracy of drug supply.
4.	IoT-Based smart rehabilitation system	Y. J. Fan and Y. H. Yin 2014	With the incorporation of ontology reconfigures medical resources and rehabilitation strategies according to patient's definite needs automatically and quickly.
5.	An approach of a decision support and home monitoring system for patients with neurological disorders using internet of things concepts	I. Chiuchisan and O. Geman 2014	An integrated intelligent system for Parkinson's disease analysis. The Home monitoring system and decision Support designed to assist physicians in diagnosis, rehabilitation, medical treatment, home monitoring, medical prescriptions, and the progress of patients with Parkinson's disease.
6.	Home Telehealth by internet of things (IoT)	S. S. Al-Majeed, I. S. Al-Mejibli et al 2015	Telehealth is a combination of sensing, communications, imaging, and interaction technologies that targeted at monitoring, diagnosis and giving treatment patients without troubling the lifestyle standard. The device is a low-cost analytics, communication, and medical sensing device.
7.	IoT based health monitoring system for autistic patients	K. B. S. Kumar and K. Bairavi 2016	IoT based health monitoring system gives an automatic monitoring framework, which uses sensors. IoT device collects the biological signals from the persons affected by autism. The analytics are achieved using the sensor data and a constant reminder is sent to their care-takers.
8.	Computer Aided Abnormality Detection for Kidney on FPGA Based IoT Enabled Portable Ultrasound Imaging System	K. D. Krishna, V. Akkala et al 2016	In remote areas the availability of radiologist is not in a sufficient number. Tele-radiology is employed to diagnose and give treatment using the scanned ultrasound data. Availability, scalability, and communication facility are the limitations of tele-radiology. To overcome the limitation Computer Aided Diagnosis (CAD) is used which is favorable in analyzing the patients with minimal intervention.
9.	ECG - Remote patient monitoring using cloud computing	P. Chavan, P. More et al 2016	A mobile-based android application called "ECG Android App" for the healthcare domain, which incorporates the concept of cloud computing and the Internet of Things (IoT). ECG android app visualizes the patients Electro Cardiogram (ECG) record. Medical records were stored in the medical cloud or user's private cloud. Stored records are used for further monitoring and analyzation.

Figure 6. Healthcare monitoring (Data Flair 2018)

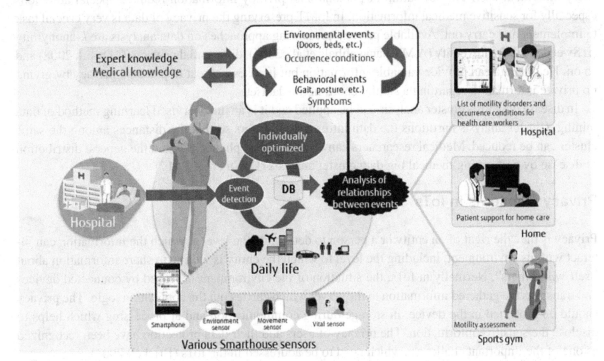

mer sends the concerned commands to configure IMD settings and to retrieve the needed medical data from the user's gadgets. IMDs are remotely monitored and operated via networks or the internet by the patient's health caregivers. IMDs are wireless communication technology and networking capabilities are a major area of security risks. The transmitted packets may be eavesdropped and also expose patient privacy like forging, tampering and replaying the messages. Also, since the patient data is remotely accessed there is also a possibility of cyber-attacks on the patient data or user credentials. Two kinds of adversaries may attack an IMD. Firstly, an active adversary may tamper the messages and send unauthorized commands. Secondly, passive adversary may eavesdrop the messages exchanged. Current IMD access control methods focus on two generic attack models. In the first type of attacks, the medical data residing in the IMD is accessed by an unauthorized programmer that sends malicious commands or modifies the device configurations. In the subsequent attack, an unauthorized programmer illegitimately accesses IMD and thereby initiates the continuous execution of authentication computations to drain the battery. Additionally, it may come with the result of denial-of-service (DoS) which can even prevent authorized emergency treatments (Nausheen, F., & Begum, S. H 2018).

PRIVACY AND SECURITY CONCERNS IN IoTS

Information obtained from IoT devices are analysed and the results are used by doctors and medical researchers for better diagnose of diseases, treatment of patients, study about the causes of diseases and thus medical services are promoted. If the collected data is not properly handled, the collection and analysis of the health data may leak user's privacy information because the health data is linked with every individual user. The revelation of personal and privacy information requires special attentions especially for sensitive medical information. In IoMT preserving the privacy of data is very crucial task to implement and carry out. Available privacy-preserving approaches on data analysis are *k*-anonymity (L Sweeney 2002), *l*diversity (A Machanavajjhala et al., 2006), differential privacy (C Dwork 2008) and so on. Health data can provide valuable information but it poses a threat to personal privacy by giving up private information regarding a single record in the dataset.

In disease diagnosis cluster analysis can be applied and it is an unsupervised learning method of data mining. Cluster analysis partitions the data into several clusters so that the distances among the same cluster can be reduced. Medical researchers can obtain clinical phenotypes and the general distribution of disease by performing medical big data cluster analysis (D Wu et al., 2017)

Privacy Concerns in IoTs

Privacy is the "the right of an entity or a person to determine the level at which the information can interact with its environment, including the level to which the entity is willing to share information about itself with others". Normally in IoTs, the situation of the environment is sensed by connected devices and transmits the gathered information to the server which carries out the application logic. The privacy should be protected in the device, in storage during communication and at processing which helps to disclose the sensitive information. The privacy of users and their data protection have been recognized as one of the important challenges which need to be addressed in the IoTs (Brickell 2004).

- Privacy in device
- Privacy during communication
- Privacy in storage
- Privacy at processing

Privacy in Device

The sensitive information of the user may be disclosed in case of any illegal manipulation or handling of hardware and software components in the IoT devices. For example, an intruder can "re-programme" a surveillance camera to sends data not only to the legitimate server but also to any other third party server. Robustness and tamper-resistance are especially important for devices that accumulate sensitive data. IoTs ensures trusted security computing technologies including device authentication, integrity validations, tamper-resistant modules, and trusted execution environments. To provide privacy in the devices, the designer has to consider the existing problems while designing a device. Problems faced by device users such as

- Location privacy of the device holder
- Non-identifiability means protecting the identification of the exact nature of the device and the sensitive information
- Protecting the personal information in case of the device theft or loss and
- Resilience to side channel attacks

Location Privacy in WSN is attained by using the algorithm multi-routing random walk in the wireless sensors. Privacy algorithm protects the displayed privacy, Personal Identifiable Information (PII), device loss, antitheft can also be achieved by having QR codes (Quick Response Code) technique. Attack on the mobile is in the form of Non-identifiability or side channel, randomness or noise will be added (Hongsong et al., 2011). Several advanced techniques and algorithms were implemented for providing privacy for the devices to meet the needs of the users.

Privacy during Communication

Data confidentiality is assured during the transmission of the data. The most common approach to attain the confidentiality is encryption. Encryption adds certain unique information to data packets in certain times which provides a way for tracing the data e.g. sequence number, IPsec- Security Parameter Index, etc. During the communication, to perform encryption pseudonyms are replaced by real values. This method is not feasible for securing the device's identity or user's to decrease vulnerability. Devices should communicate or transmit data only when there is a need. In 3GPP machine type communications, the devices will detach itself from the network after a certain period of inactivity in order to evade the collection of unnecessary location information with the active device.

Privacy in Storage

For protecting the privacy of information while storing, the following principals should be considered.

- Only the least probable amount of information and the needed information should be stored
- Using authentication to prevent the intruders from accessing the data
- Mandatory or personal information retained in the storage
- Information is brought out based on "need-to-know"

To hide the real identity tied with the stored data, pseudonymization and anonymization could be used for the security purpose. Without disclosing any specific record or user's personal information, a database could allow access only to statistical data (sum, average, count, etc.) to legitimate users. To ensure the output (typically aggregate queries) is independent of the absence or presence of a particular record adds noise called differential privacy could be the appropriate technique.

Privacy at Processing

Privacy at processing is mainly of two folds. Firstly, personal data must be treated in a way that it should be simple with the intended purpose. Secondly, without explicit acceptance and the knowledge of the data owner, their data should not be disclosed or retained to third parties. By considering the points mentioned above, the most suitable Digital Rights Management (DRM) systems (Sweeney et al) controls the utilization of any kind of commercial media and defends against re-distribution illegally to third parties. To secure the information, one can define privacy policies for personal data in a rights object or license instead of excising principles for commercial media which must be obeyed during the data processing. DRM requires trusted devices, secured devices to work efficiently and effectively. User's permission and their awareness are requirements for the distribution of personal data to others. User notification aids to avoid any kinds of abuse.

Security Concerns in IoTS

A virtual network in IoT allows real-time interaction between humans in day to day life is the most prominent feature of the IoT system in today's real world. IoT has unique characteristics, subscription and deployment contexts in the initial stage of the development. Machine to Machine is a broad field that can be used to define any type of technology that enables devices among the network to interchange information and perform actions without any manual assistance and administration of humans. Even though it helps to improve social efficiency to a certain extent, it may lead to information security and privacy concerned issues. The biggest security challenges of IoT are data transmission that is the data transmission happens in the absence of direct human-machine interaction and remote management of devices. Hence, there is a high chance for information loss. There are three ways to analyze the existing information security of the IoT:

- Front- End Sensors and Equipment
- Network
- Back End IT Systems

Front-End Sensors and Equipment

To achieve networking services of multiple connected sensors they obtain data through the built-in sensors and transmit data through the modules. This will involve the security of machines with node connectivity and business implementation.

- Internet of Things in the Local Security Threat and Analysis: In the Internet of Things nodes are deployed in the absence of any monitoring scenarios. So the intruder can easily access these devices, thus it causes damage or information loss. The analysis of possible threats is faced by the wireless interface between the equipment's terminal and in services (Camenisch 2004).
- Unauthorized access to data: An intruder can access or loot the personal information of the user by hacking their device and can also accomplish by obtaining confidential information key. Intruders control data through signaling data, eavesdropping user data and control data on the wireless link or steal the signal or exposes in public places. Therefore, a two-way authentication mechanism for network and implementing the designed encryption algorithm. This prevents eavesdropping or unauthorized accessing to the data on wireless links for good health equipment.
- Threat and analysis to the internet: The integrity protection mechanism should be strengthened and the equipment in the device should be of encrypted when transmitting the personal user data. Since the attacker can cause harm to the transaction information by deleting, modifying, inserting, or replaying the legitimate user data in a wireless link.
- The attack of denial of service: Attacker interferes with the user's data during the transmission through the physical layer or protocol layer to achieve denial of service (DoS) attacks of the wireless link. Stubborn and good health algorithm should be designed to resist or mitigate the DOS

attacks or tracking mechanism to quickly identify the location of an attacker can also reduce the damage on the network.

- Internet of Things in the Local Security and Analysis: IoT devices having the capability to operate without any supervision by humans for extended periods and to communicate over the wireless area network (WAN) or WLAN. As the IoT equipment may be connected to the network before deployed network infrastructure and that leaves the IoT nodes unattended. So the configuration of the remotely signing information and health-related information is a problem. The communication terminals are directly involved in the management of people rarely, so there are many chances of attacks towards devices.

Network

A network's role is to offer a more comprehensive interconnection capacity, effectiveness, and economy of connection, as well as the reliable quality of service. The denial of service attacks happens mostly when data spread across the network because a large number of nodes in IoT and to exist in groups and also since a large number of machines sending data leads to network congestion.

- Threat and Analysis of Unauthorized Access to Data: When entering into the service network, an intruder may listen to the user data and access the stored data within the system network elements. Certification technology with the encryption algorithm can be used against unauthorized data access, so an attacker cannot perform malpractices to services data on the network.
- Threat and Analysis of Unauthorized Access to Service: To prevent unauthorized access to services, the relying party directly assesses the validity of the device based on the evidence for the verification received in Remote Validation. Local verification is only passive, just measuring the integrity values of the loaded and started components (Leicher et al., 2009). A Stored Measurement Log (SML) must be conveyed to the lying party who makes all policy decisions. In remote evidence, a Trusted Computing Group (TCG) platform shows an SML and platform configuration register (PCR), in a signed message to the relying party. The signing keys are ephemeral, certified by a privacy certification authority (PCA), which acts as an identity provider for validation. Pseudonymity of remote attestation may not be adequate in all security cases. TCG has additionally described direct anonymous attestation (DAA).DAA is based on zero-knowledge proofs (Brickellet al., 2004).
- Viruses or Mal-ware Attacks: An attacker may access the application software and signing information by malware, Trojans or other means of virus and then replicated in other connected devices to restore the fraudulent use. Through virus attacks or malicious software, information's can be changed, inserted and removed by the user's communications data. Anti-virus software can reduce viruses and malware on IoT equipment.
- Analysis of Networking Security: The heterogeneous, multi-hop, distributed network consisted of four categories of a network for transmission namely length/short distance of cable and length/ short distance of wireless. They are interconnected networks that lead to difficulty in achieving the bridging and transition of data in a unified security system. Data transmission is prevented from reaching the end of service, so the attacker can obtain user data. Physical theft or online listening aims at unauthorized access to data. Secure communications between heterogeneous network systems established by using the existing technology called Trust chip, an embedded chip, which pro-

vides a security architecture that operates as a security service to any type of application. During manufacturing, uniquely serialized to achieve ease of implementation. There are no certificate servers to deploy, configure or maintain the Trust chip.

Back-End of IT Systems

Back-end IT system forms on the IoT gateway, application or middleware, which is enriched with high-security requirements. It collects, analyses the sensor data in real-time or pseudo-real-time to increase usage of smart device and its relevant applications.

- Safety Management of Code Resources: The security of the Internet of Things system has eight major standards. They are access control, privacy protection, user authentication, no arrived patience, data confidentiality, communication layer security, data integrity, and availability at any time. Most particularly concerned issues in the Internet of Things are "privacy" and "credibility" (data integrity and confidentiality). To safeguard the privacy and confidential information's of the users, many researchers begin to focus on designing privacy-preserving techniques such as, for example, k-anonymity, data transformation/randomization, and so on.
- Security Threat Occurs When the Replacement of Operator: Since several operators are there to carry out the IoT based operations. While changing the operator, certification information and the key may be faced with the threat. Due to the improper behavior when they exchange them between operators, causing user's personal or health-related information to leakage and lead to privacy loss. For such threats, the Government should introduce suitable legislation to standardize and regulate the behavior of operators and the use of contracts may reduce the risk when switching carriers. Besides, operators should also provide a specialized process to transfer the key and other useful information while changing the operators, to ensure the security for user information.

SECURITY AND PRIVACY REQUIREMENTS

The efficient security mechanism is not equipped with the devices connected to the internet and is susceptible to various privacy and security issues e.g., integrity, authenticity, and confidentiality, etc. Malicious attacks can be prevented only when certain credentials and some security requirements must be fulfilled in the IoT. Here, some of the most prominent and required capabilities of a secure network are briefly discussed.

- Resilience to attacks: During data transmission among the network, it may meet with any of the crashes, the network has to be capable enough to recover by itself from the occurred crash. For an example, a server is equipped for a multiuser environment. Working capability must be intelligent and sufficiently strong to defend itself from an eavesdropper or an intruder. Without any intimation to the users about the down status, the server can recover itself from the issue is an aid to be resilience.
- Data Authentication: Authentication is the verification of the reputed user. To ensure security and privacy for the users, the data and the associated information must be authenticated. An authenti-

cation mechanism is used to allow data transmission from only authentic devices and the relevant users of the information.

- Access control: Only authorized persons (legitimate users) are allowed and provided with access control to their account of information. The system administrator only allowed to control the ac-

Table 3. Summary of different types of attacks and their threat levels, their nature and suggested solutions

Type of Attack	Level of the threat	Behavior of the attack	Suggested Solution for the attack
Active	High	Active attack effects on the confidentiality and integrity of data. Hostile in the network can modify or change the integrity of messages, block messages, or may re-route the messages to any other location. An active attacker should be an internal attacker. Example: Worms, Viruses, malware, Denial of Service attacks (DOS), and password crackers	By ensuring both the integrity and confidentiality of data. Maintenance of data confidentiality is achieved by symmetric encryption and authentication mechanism. Authentication only lets the authorized user access the information.
Passive	Low	Confidentiality of the data is breached in the passive attack. Intruder in the network silently listens to the exchange of information for their benefit. The attacker won't commit any interchange or intercept any information. Example: Passive eavesdropping and Traffic analysis	By using symmetric encryption techniques and ensuring the confidentiality of the data and can be taken to the safe hands.
Man in the Middle (MIM)	Low to medium	In MIM type of attack, intruder relays in secret and change the data that is communicated between the parties. They can sense silently to know the type of transmission medium and can change the data if encryption or any other security measures is not applied. They can steal and manipulate the information that is being exchanged. Example: Insertion of data into a flow which creates the traffic and intercepts or injects the fake information.	Apply data confidentiality techniques and proper integration methodology on data to ensure integrity. Encryption can also be applied so that no one can loot or modify the transmitted information or encode the false information before transmission.
Eavesdropping	Low to medium	Stealthily listening to private communication, such as a message, phone call, fax transmission or video conference without the consent of the relevant person. For example: in the medical environment, the privacy of a patient may be leaked.	Apply encryption techniques on all the devices that perform communication especially on Android phones.
Privacy	High	Sensitive information of an individual or group may be disclosed by the attacker. Such attacks may lead to the exposure of privacy. Example: Intruding the private information of the users	Ring signature and blind signature applied to rectify privacy risk.
Interruption	High	In interruption, network service is ruined and affects the availability of data. Interruption makes the network unavailable for the genuine user. Example: Eavesdropping on communication and Wiretapping telecommunications networks.	A strong authorization mechanism has to be implemented and only authorized users are allowed to access specific information to accomplish a certain operation.
Routing diversion	High	Routing diversion is implemented by poisoning of the routing table. The route is diverted showing the huge traffic and the response time is increased. Example: ISP diversion and creating internet traffic.	To avoid the network diversion, connectivity based approach is ensured.
Blocking	Extremely High	Blocking is a type of DoS, jamming, or malware attacks. During data transmission large streams of data which may lead to jamming or flooding of the network. Example: Different types of viruses like Trojan horses, worms and other programs can disturb the network.	To avoid blocking turn on the firewall, apply packet filtering, anti-jamming, active jamming and install the updated antivirus programs.
Fabrication	Extremely High	Fabrication affects the authenticity of user information. An intruder can inject false data and can destroy the authenticity of genuine user's information. Example: Breaching the user's authentication information	Data authenticity can be applied to safeguard that no information is changed during the transmission of data.
DoS	Extremely High	Intruders may change the packets or resend a packet again and again or send a bulk message on the same network. Example: Making the system to malfunction	Apply cryptographic techniques to ensure the security of the network. Authenticity is implemented to detect the malicious user and block them permanently.

cess of various users by managing, organizing their usernames and passwords based on authentication. By defining their access rights, different users can access an only relevant portion of their database or programs from the huge data.

- Client privacy: The data and information about the users should be in safe a hand that it must be stored in a confidential place. Personal data should only be accessed by an authorized person to maintain the privacy of the client. Irrelevant or any unauthorized user from the system have no access permission to the private information of the client (Razzaq et al 2017).

CONCLUSION

Emergent technological solutions are being explored in the healthcare industry complements the existing services with the effective utilization of many IoT potential. The advent of IoT in Health care has brought many advantages to the medical sector. Affordable, wearable, and implantable health care gadgets were developed in IoT with the incorporation of healthcare. In this chapter the advancements, research activities, impact, the importance of IoT in healthcare with its security and privacy challenges were described. Also, the vulnerabilities that result when the sensitive data of patients are being stolen by the hackers through the mobile application are discussed and different access control mechanisms are presented to understand how the implantable medical devices can be safeguarded against unauthorized access by appropriate protection of keys.

REFERENCES

Al-Majeed, S. S., Al-Mejibli, I. S., & Karam, J. (2015). Home Telehealth by internet of things (IoT). *Proc. Canadian Conference on Electrical and Computer Engineering.* 10.1109/CCECE.2015.7129344

Berte, D. R. (2018, May). Defining the IoT. In *Proceedings of the International Conference on Business Excellence* (*Vol. 12*, No. 1, pp. 118-128). Sciendo. 10.2478/picbe-2018-0013

Brickell, E., Camenisch, J., & Chen, L. (2004, October). Direct anonymous attestation. In *Proceedings of the 11th ACM conference on Computer and communications security* (pp. 132-145). ACM.

Camenisch, J. (2004, September). Better privacy for trusted computing platforms. In *European Symposium on Research in Computer Security* (pp. 73-88). Springer.

Chase, J. (2013). *The evolution of the internet of things.* Texas Instruments.

Chavan, More, Thorat, Yewale, & Dhade. (2016). ECG - Remote patient monitoring using cloud computing. Imperial Journal of Interdisciplinary Research, 2(2).

Chiuchisan, I., & Geman, O. (2014). *An approach of a decision support and home monitoring system for patients with neurological disorders using internet of things concepts* (Vol. 13). Wseas Transactions on Systems.

Dataflair. (n.d.). Received from https://data-flair.training/blogs/iot-applications-in-healthcare

Dwork, C., & Smith, A. (2009). Differential privacy for statistics: What we know and what we want to learn. *Journal of Privacy and Confidentiality*, *1*(2), 135–154.

Fan, Y. J., & Yin, Y. H. (2014, May). IoT-Based smart rehabilitation system. *IEEE Transactions on Industrial Informatics*, *10*(2).

Gupta, P., Agrawal, D., Chhabra, J., & Dhir, P. K. (2016, March). IoT based smart healthcare kit. In *2016 International Conference on Computational Techniques in Information and Communication Technologies (ICCTICT)* (pp. 237-242). IEEE. 10.1109/ICCTICT.2016.7514585

Hassan Mehmood Khan. (2018). Received from https://iotlearners.com/windows-10-for-the-internet-of-things/

Hongsong, C., Zhongchuan, F., & Dongyan, Z. (2011, July). Security and trust research in M2M system. In *Proceedings of 2011 IEEE International Conference on Vehicular Electronics and Safety* (pp. 286-290). IEEE. 10.1109/ICVES.2011.5983830

Huang, C. H., & Cheng, K. W. (2014, January). RFID technology combined with IoT application in medical nursing system. *Bulletin of Networking, Computing, Systems, and Software*, *3*(1), 20–24.

IoTWF. (2017). Received From https://www.iotwf.com/

Juxtology. (2018). Received From https://juxtology.com/iot-transformation/

Krishna, K. D., Akkala, V., Bharath, R., Rajalakshmi, P., & Mohammed, A. M. (2016). *Computer Aided Abnormality Detection for Kidney on FPGA Based IoT Enabled Portable Ultrasound Imaging System.* AGBM, Published by Elsevier Masson SAS. doi:10.1016/j.irbm.2016.05.001

Kumar, J. S., & Patel, D. R. (2014). A survey on internet of things: Security and privacy issues. *International Journal of Computers and Applications*, *90*(11).

Kumar, K. B. S., & Bairavi, K. (2016). IoT based health monitoring system for autistic patients. *Proc. Symposium on Big Data and Cloud Computing Challenges, Smart Innovation, Systems and Technologies*. 10.1007/978-3-319-30348-2_32

Leicher, A., Kuntze, N., & Schmidt, A. U. (2009, May). Implementation of a trusted ticket system. In *IFIP International Information Security Conference* (pp. 152-163). Springer.

Machanavajjhala, A., Gehrke, J., Kifer, D., & Venkitasubramaniam, M. (2006, April). l-diversity: Privacy beyond k-anonymity. In *22nd International Conference on Data Engineering (ICDE'06)* (pp. 24-24). IEEE. 10.1109/ICDE.2006.1

Matar, G., Lina, J., Kaddoum, G., & Riley, A. (2016). Internet of things in sleep monitoring: An application for posture recognition using supervised learning. *Proc. International Conference on IEEE Healthcom*. 10.1109/HealthCom.2016.7749469

Mattern, F., & Floerkemeier, C. (2010). From the Internet of Computers to the Internet of Things. In *From active data management to event-based systems and more* (pp. 242–259). Berlin: Springer. doi:10.1007/978-3-642-17226-7_15

Motwani, Mirchandani, Rohra, Tarachandani, & Yeole. (2016). Smart nursing home patient monitoring system. Imperial Journal of Interdisciplinary Research, 2(6).

Nausheen, F., & Begum, S. H. (2018, January). Healthcare IoT: Benefits, vulnerabilities and solutions. In *2018 2nd International Conference on Inventive Systems and Control (ICISC)* (pp. 517-522). IEEE.

Orsini, M., Pacchioni, M., Malagoli, A., & Guaraldi, G. (2017, September). My smart age with HIV: an innovative mobile and IoMT framework for patient's empowerment. In *2017 IEEE 3rd International Forum on Research and Technologies for Society and Industry (RTSI)* (pp. 1-6). IEEE. 10.1109/RTSI.2017.8065914

Razzaq, M. A., Gill, S. H., Qureshi, M. A., & Ullah, S. (2017). Security issues in the Internet of Things (IoT): A comprehensive study. *International Journal of Advanced Computer Science and Applications*, 8(6), 383–388.

Reuters. (2017). Received from https://www.reuters.com/brandfeatures/venture-capital/article?id=16545

Sweeney, L. (2002). k-anonymity: A model for protecting privacy. *International Journal of Uncertainty, Fuzziness and Knowledge-based Systems*, 10(05), 557–570. doi:10.1142/S0218488502001648

Vojas, J. (2016). Demystifying the internet of things. *Computer*, 49(6), 80–83. doi:10.1109/MC.2016.162

Wu, D., Bleier, B. S., Li, L., Zhan, X., Zhang, L., Lv, Q., ... Wei, Y. (2018). Clinical phenotypes of nasal polyps and comorbid asthma based on cluster analysis of disease history. *The Journal of Allergy and Clinical Immunology. In Practice*, 6(4), 1297–1305. doi:10.1016/j.jaip.2017.09.020 PMID:29100865

Yuehong, Y. I. N., Zeng, Y., Chen, X., & Fan, Y. (2016). The internet of things in healthcare: An overview. *Journal of Industrial Information Integration*, 1, 3–13. doi:10.1016/j.jii.2016.03.004

Zhao, W., Wang, C., & Nakahira, Y. (2011). *Medical application on internet of things*. Academic Press.

Zhou, H. (2012). *The internet of things in the cloud: a middleware perspective*. CRC Press. doi:10.1201/b13090

Chapter 2
Internet of Things
in Healthcare:
An Extensive Review on Recent Advances, Challenges, and Opportunities

Rajasekaran Thangaraj

KPR Institute of Engineering and Technology, India

Sivaramakrishnan Rajendar

KPR Institute of Engineering and Technology, India

Vidhya Kandasamy

KPR Institute of Engineering and Technology, India

ABSTRACT

Healthcare motoring has become a popular research in recent years. The evolution of electronic devices brings out numerous wearable devices that can be used for a variety of healthcare motoring systems. These devices measure the patient's health parameters and send them for further processing, where the acquired data is analyzed. The analysis provides the patients or their relatives with the medical support required or predictions based on the acquired data. Cloud computing, deep learning, and machine learning technologies play a prominent role in processing and analyzing the data respectively. This chapter aims to provide a detailed study of IoT-based healthcare systems, a variety of sensors used to measure parameters of health, and various deep learning and machine learning approaches introduced for the diagnosis of different diseases. The chapter also highlights the challenges, open issues, and performance considerations for future IoT-based healthcare research.

INTRODUCTION

The technological evolution results in the increase of electronic devices in many fields which can be connected over the Internet termed as Internet of Things (IoT). IoT nowadays becomes a huge network

DOI: 10.4018/978-1-7998-1090-2.ch002

of physical devices such as smartphones, sensors, actuators, with global network connectivity in order to store and exchange data. It plays a vital role in many applications including smart homes, smart cities, automotive, smart grid, healthcare etc. Among the wide applications of IoT, it plays a significant role in the healthcare industry. Today, the healthcare industry faces many challenges in the early diagnosis of diseases which is essential for initial treatment to save the lives of patients. In recent days, health monitoring is gaining importance and wearable health monitoring systems have become popular among industries and researchers. The wearable devices collect the patient's health information including heart rate, blood pressure, and blood glucose level. These devices enable patients to monitor their health condition and make a precise analysis related to treatment. Due to the increased population and advancement in technology, the volume of the data generated from healthcare industries is huge. Henceforth, a mechanism is required to store and analyze big medical data over the cloud environment. With huge measures of information spilling out of EMRs, wearable's, and various other new sources, the significance of machine learning and artificial intelligence is intense than other industry. Machine learning accelerates disease diagnosis and classification of health data and empowers physicians to make quick decisions. In addition, machine learning and deep learning methods work in conjunction with IoT to diagnose diseases early. With a detailed history of patient records, an IoT system blended with a deep learning method enables early diagnosis and prediction of numerous diseases.

WEARABLE DEVICES IN HEALTH MONITORING

Information and communication technology (ICT) plays an important role in society nowadays. The impact of recent technology on improving the health and prosperity of people is remarkable, that converse about the digital revolution in the healthcare industry (Birkler and Dahl, 2014). The digital revolution provides an opportunity for individuals in taking care of their own health with the assistance of monitoring devices (Kostkova, 2015; Klonoff, 2013). These devices generate more and more data about individuals, transmit and analyze to monitor the individual health conditions through the technology, Internet of Things (IoT). IoT is defined as the network of physical objects connected through internet. It provides the possibility of continuous and close monitoring of individual healthcare using wearable devices (LeHong and Velosa, 2014). In recent years, wearable devices become popular among the academic and research community (Gao et al., 2016). Wearable devices are autonomous devices that can be mated with the human body for continuous monitoring of individual's activities (Gao et al., 2016). Now-a-days, wearable devices including eyeglasses, splints, bandages, and contact lenses are employed to provide medical functions like medical monitoring, rehabilitation assistance, and medical aid for long term (Barfield, 2015). The objective of this paper is to address the important most important wearable devices.

In today's fastest world, people spend their time in doing various tasks and fail to take care of their health and fitness. And also, a lot of time is needed for making an appointment with the doctor in a clinic. Therefore, people are finding alternative through devices that can be mated on the human body and provides continuous health monitoring of user (Xu et al., 2014). Wearable monitoring devices provide assistance for the treatment of diseases like heart diseases, diabetes, treatment and vital sign monitoring of heart rate, the oxygen level of blood, respiration, and body fat. Such device gathers and broadcast the information related to the person health condition through the wireless connection and provide an instant alert to the health care provider (Bowman and Schuck, 1995). Figure 1 represents the working

Figure 1. Wearable technology in healthcare
Source: Patel, 2012

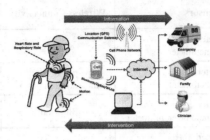

principle of wearable sensor technology in healthcare and some of popular wearable devices with their characteristics are presented in table 1.

Motion Tracker

The human movement tracker has several applications in sports, healthcare vehicles, and aircraft. The sensors such as 3-axis accelerometers, magnetometers, and gyroscopes embedded in the tracker system are employed to recognize the human activity in the ubiquitous computing domain (Haghi et al., 2017). In particular, motion tracking in healthcare is an important application. However, to obtain high accuracy in the medical field, the sensor with the uniaxial accelerometer in motion tracking was introduced by Veltink and Boom (Veltink and Boom, 1995). To improvise the accuracy of the tracker integrated semiconductor-based gyroscopes was introduced in 1997 to bio-mechanical assessments and gait analysis. Later in 1997, Miyazaki, proposed the initial framework for tracking in the 2D sagittal plane with a fusion of accelerometers and gyroscopes. This tracker primarily focuses on gait analysis for clinical applications by employing gravity sensitive accelerometers to estimate the tilt angles between the gravity vector and the sensor's axes (Takeda et al., 2009). In 2006, Roetenberg introduced integrated sensors

Table 1. Features of popular wearable devices

Device	Market price ($)	Weight (g)	Battery life	Characteristic	Mode of communication
Fitbit Flex	100	16.4	4–6 (months)	Small in size Wrist worn Counting of steps	Wi-Fi
Withings Pulse	120	8	6 months	Measuring the heart rate Recording of sleep time Counting of steps	Wi-Fi
Misfit Shine	100	9.4	3 months	Daily calories burnt measurement Sleep tracker monitoring	Bluetooth
Jawbone	100	19	4-6 months	Step counting Daily calories burnt measurement Tracking daily activity Tracking user sleep data	Bluetooth

Table 2. Comparison of motion tracking devices applied in healthcare

Wireless Motion Tracker devices	Sensors	Wireless Connectivity	Sensor network	Weight
Motionnode Bus	3-axis accelerometer, 3-axis gyroscope, 3-magnetometer	802.11g	Yes, up to 20 sensors	10 g Battery:180 g
Opal	3-axis accelerometer, 3-axis gyroscope, 3-magnetometer	Low-power wireless communication protocol	Yes, up to 24 sensors	22 g (with battery)
Shimmer3	3-axis accelerometer, 3-axis gyroscope, 3-magnetometer, altimeter	Bluetooth	Yes	Not specified
Physilog	3-axis accelerometer, 3-axis gyroscope, 3-magnetometer, pressure sensor	Bluetooth	Yes	19 g
MTw development kit	3-axis accelerometer, 3-axis gyroscope, 3-magnetometer, static pressure sensor	Awinda radio protocol	Yes	27 g
Memsense W2 IMU	3-axis accelerometer, 3-axis gyroscope, 3-magnetometer, static pressure sensor, Temperature sensor.	Bluetooth	No	Not specified
STT-IBS	3-axis accelerometer,3-axis gyroscope,3-magnetometer	Wi-Fi, Bluetooth	No	30 g
12M Motion SXT	3-axis accelerometer, 3-axis gyroscope, 3-magnetometer, Temperature sensor	Low power wireless communications protocol	Yes	22 g

(accelerometer, gyroscope, and magnetometer) which provide accurate data with 9DoF using a set of tri-axial accelerometers, tri-axial gyroscopes, and a magnetometer to monitor the human motion. Wearable devices are restricted by various factors such as size, weight, and on-board sensors. Table 2 provides a comparison of all mentioned elements of motion tracking devices used in healthcare.

Vital Signs Measurement

Wearable devices in healthcare monitoring have been used to measure the crucial elements which include electrocardiogram (ECG) measurement, electroencephalogram (EEG) measurement, skin temperature, etc. Recently, a lot of efforts has been made in wearable devices to provide multi-task vital signs measurement. Remote ECG monitoring through wearable devices plays a significant role in health monitoring. In general, these devices are tough to implement and inefficient in performance.

Smart Clothing

Traditional health monitoring has failed to monitor the health conditions of the individuals for the long term, which collect an inadequate number of physiological signals, are not useful in full range health monitoring system for chronic diseases. The primary focus of smart clothing is to monitor individual health through obtaining a numerous number of physiological signals from various sensors, which are integrated into textile clothing. In smart clothing, sensors are deployed on the body which collects the vital signs that are integrated into clothing. To provide efficiency, location of sensor placement, flexible electricity cable layout, sensor quality, weak signal acquisition equipment, low power wireless commu-

Table 3. Sensor placement and its job in smart clothing

Sensor to measure	Sensor placement	Sensor job
Pulse	Wrist	Measurement of pulse wave signals
Body temperature	Under arm	Measurement of body temperature
ECG	Chest, ribs	Measurement of vital sign
Myocardial	Left chest	Measurement of the myocardial signal of the body
Blood oxygen	The muscle of the left or right arm	Measurement of blood oxygen level
EEG	Left or Right forehead, Backside of the left or right head	Detection of abnormalities related to brain activity

nications, and comforts of the worn user are key factors (Spinelle et al., 2015). However, smart clothing has some major drawbacks: Customization is necessary for the physical wearable body; Problem of communicating data collected with smart clothing to the outside world. Table 3 summarizes the position and task of each sensor placed in smart clothing and figure 2 shows the sample picture of smart clothing.

Wired Wearable Devices

In 2015, Sanfilippo and Pettersen introduced a novel wire-based approach to measure many vital signs. This wire based integrated wearable health monitoring system is built with Arduino and Raspberry Pi. The system mainly focuses on monitoring the health condition of individuals with help of various sensors through observing vital signs and motion tracking. The sensors employed in the system collect the data related to EEG, ECG and body temperature of the user for real time monitoring. Figure 3 shows the e-Health sensors enabled Arduino Uno board.

Bottlenecks for Wearable Medical Devices

Wearable medical devices based on IoT address many challenges from other medical devices in healthcare. Validity and reliability of the devices is the main concern (Evenson et al., 2015). The accuracy of the wearable devices in individual activity monitoring is insufficient as of traditional monitoring devices (Price et al., 2017). The accuracy provided by the various wearable devices confirms huge difference with error margin up to 25% (Piwek et al., 2016). User privacy and security are considered as another

Figure 2. Sample smart clothing

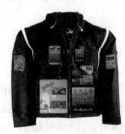 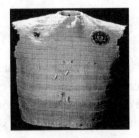

Figure 3. Arduino Uno (enabled with e-health sensor shield)
Source: Escobar, 2016

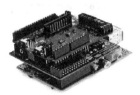

main concern that wearable devices pose (Redmond et al., 2014). Similarly, wearable devices face several other challenges like power consumption which is correlated to numerous parameters such as efficient coding, data packing, encryption and compression and device used in different environmental conditions and handling of the device.

Opportunities for Wearable Devices

Wearable devices present a number of significant forecasts in the future of the healthcare industry. Some of the key features include:

- The growth of wearable medical devices increases the lifetime of individuals through continuous monitoring and support.
- IoT based health monitoring system reduces human intervention in healthcare.
- The automatic remote data collection increases the efficiency of healthcare services.

CLOUD COMPUTING IN HEALTHCARE

Evolution of Cloud Technology

Technology has infiltrated in lives of human so much and it is the vital part of moving our regular life smoothly. Social media plays its strong role on decision making for personal and professional assessments. The blend of growing anticipations and a quick rate of revolution poses a challenge to outmoded tactics for current technology of information. Cloud is a new computing standard which is an on-demand service which is available at anywhere and anytime. In cloud, resources like software, infrastructure, and computing platform are provided as a service by the service providers like Kamatera, phoenixNAP, Amazon Web Services, Microsoft Azure, Google Cloud Platform, Adobe, VMware, IBM Cloud. Cloud services are available for on-demand and at scale in a multi-tenant environment (Gupta et al., 2011).

Characteristic of Cloud Computing

- Delivers services over network based on demand.
- Irrespective of the place and time the service can be availed consistently.
- The scale up and scale down of operating resources is much easier than the traditional system.
- Ability to adopt and handle big data with the support of technology update.

Figure 4. Current adoption of cloud computing
Source: The economist intelligence unit, 2015

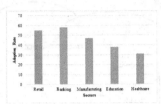

- Possibility of providing multitenant collaborative services.
- Possibility of accessing data through wide range of devices like laptops, smartphones and other devices as per the convenient

There are wide variations in service models of cloud computing such as IaaS (Infrastructure as a Service), PaaS (Platform as a Service) and SaaS (Software as a Service) and in deployment models like private cloud, public cloud, community cloud.IT services for effective handling of health care data will be precisely provided by emerging trend of cloud computing. This technology can play a vital role in enhancing the level and quality of services in the health care sector at the right time as per the demand from patients, physicians, and various healthcare providers, who intend to brand business and widespread adoption at customer place. Implementing cloud computing solutions can make healthcare operations even more expedient and cost effective. Current adoption of cloud in various industries is as shown in Figure 4 below. Microsoft HealthVault and Google Health platform are examples of applications in medical services (Ali et al., 2018).

Here the adoption of cloud computing in healthcare industry is 31%. Currently the level of cloud utilization raised remarkably due to its powerful services towards the enrichment of Electronic Health Record handing techniques (Chatman, 2010).

Healthcare and Cloud

Health care industry basically adopted the technology very slowly due to the difficulties in adoption like dissimilar structure of medical data and its security. Due to increased population and variety of diseases there is a need for moving towards the technology support. Health care providers basically expects the provision for automation of back office systems, payment and reimbursement, digitization of medical records, and business intelligence for regulatory compliance and accreditation.

The cost of investment for the digitization is comparatively low and it can be an additional investment for further equipment as needed on demand for expansion of industry. Cloud-based applications can offer solutions to current problems within healthcare industries like abundant growth of data, secured data maintenance, provision of data and solutions on demand, requirement of cost-effective storage and management infrastructure (Christoph et al., 2015).

Figure 5 shows the simple view of cloud-based health care system where the data from various data sources like hospitals, clinical reports and personal information formulated and entered patients who are aware of technology updates and their periodic health parameters through various handheld devices and gadgets. These data are effectively received by the interface tools like gsutil. Cloud Storage is a

Figure 5. Cloud based health care system

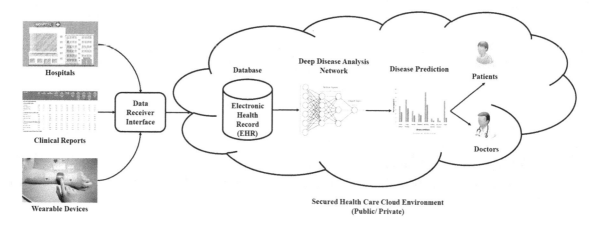

highly-available and robust object store service. It does not have any limit on number of files in bucket storage and each file size should be of maximum 5 TB size. There are variety of cloud storage services are available such as Amazon S3, Oracle Cloud Storage and Microsoft Azure Storage, object storage software like Openstack Swift, object storage systems like EMC Atmos, EMC ECS and Hitachi Content Platform, and distributed storage research projects like OceanStore (Rhea et al., 2001) and VISION Cloud (Rao et al., 2010). When we migrate data from traditional storage to Google Cloud Platform (GCP) a large amounts of data need to be shifted to Cloud Storage. Such information might include:

- Various clinical applications (EHRs, physician enquiries, pharmacy orders, etc.)
- Healthcare management applications to handle income series management
- Patient medical data management

The other GCP services like BigQuery and Cloud Dataflow also helpful for optimized cloud storage and exploration. Which will lead to fruitful insights for current business trends. The figure 6 shows the oracle industry solution for healthcare (Oracle, 2017). The healthcare supporters and innovators can ef-

Figure 6. Oracle industry solution for healthcare
Source: Oracle, 2017

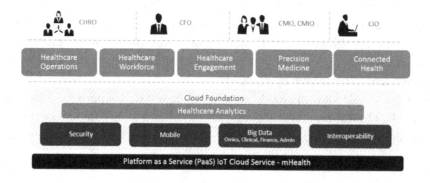

fectively utilize software as a service (SaaS) application of Oracle and other providers for management and exploitation of medical data.

Thus the unbounded support of cloud computing towards infrastructure and software will take the healthcare industries to the next level of expansion. Which will help the growth of industries horizontally as well as vertically with anywhere any time support to customers (Ali et al., 2018). The medical data from various kind of sources like sensors linked with medical devices are compiled together by cloud-based system which can facilitate secured and optimal storage of data, availability and sharing (Rolim et al., 2010). The Dhatri a pervasive cloud initiative supports doctors and other health care takers to admittance patient medical data at any time and at any place (Rao et al., 2010). The cloud based collaborative health care management system can deliver the support to the society in terms of applications which is highly helpful for prediction and prevention of diseases, developing medical software tools and applications, prescriptions and even the support for healthcare education. Best cloud storage of 2019 are IDrive, pCloud, Zoolz Cloud backup, Degoo, Mega (Kolodner et al., 2011).

Benefit of Cloud Computing for Healthcare Providers

Cloud based health care support leverages anywhere any time support to the society through various portable devices as per convenient. It is also very much supportable for the collaborative work of various medical centers through internet (Nate Drake, 2019). The basic cloud service models such as:

Software as a Service (SaaS)

Through this the cloud service providers can provide services which facilitate the instant access of their commercial applications and satisfying Customer Relationship Management (CRM) at right time at right place.

Infrastructure as a Service (IaaS)

This model of cloud services can provide solutions to offer on-demand computing and huge storage for medical services.

Platform as a Service (PaaS)

It can offer a security-enhanced environment for web-based services and the deployment of medical applications for developing and testing.

Risks of Cloud Computing in Healthcare

Though cloud computing provides enormous advantages there are few issues such as security and privacy issues, Technological issues and various other legal issues. The security breaches can be avoided initially by proper selection of cloud service providers who is complete response for the provision of security services as per Health Insurance Portability and Accountability Act (HIPAA) of 1996 (OCR, 2013). With considerable data holes progressively stated in recent years, there is an increasing discomfort between patients who distress that hospitals and doctors that use a cloud service supplier will muddle privacy of their data. There are also concerns of allowing multiple users to share EHRs and to work collaboratively which also causes further more threatening impact on data security and indirectly affects the cost of investment and management (Ahuja et al., 2012). The regulatory body should periodically audit the Cloud Service provider and their metrics to meet customer needs. The technological issue mainly addresses the lack of service delivery. Initially customers are attracted by specific aspects of storage capacity and application support but they are not provided as per the agreement. This should be handled carefully before starting of service utilization. And also data migration between one Cloud Service Provider to another during the closing of previous service provider also highly challenge one.

MACHINE LEARNING AND DEEP LEARNING APPROACHES IN HEALTH CARE

Machine Learning

Machine Learning (Marco Varone, 2017) is an application of Artificial Intelligence (AI) that gives computers an ability to learn without being explicitly programmed. As it is evident from the name, it enables a computer to automatically learn similar to humans and improve from experience. Machine learning aims at developing computer programs that accesses data and uses for self-learning.

The process of learning is called 'training' and the output produced by this process is called a 'model'. It begins with observations or data such as examples, experience, or even instructions, to effectively identify patterns and make better decisions in future. A model can then be provided with a new data so that it can reason about this new information based on what it has previously learned. It is thus clear that machine learning is actively used worldwide, perhaps in most of the fields.

Deep Learning

Deep learning has become a catchword in recent years, but is often misused, in reality it is just a subfield of machine learning related to the algorithms inspired by the structure and function of the brain called 'artificial neural networks'.

A neural network is an algorithm originated from the functioning of human brain, and involves many nodes called 'neurons' that are connected together in layers to form a network. A neural network must have at least two layers – a layer of inputs and a layer of outputs. There can be many 'hidden' layers between the input layer and output layer, and these are used to extract more information by exploiting structure in the data. A network is considered 'deep' if it has more than one hidden layer (Jason Brownlee, 2016).

Though the concepts of neural networks emerged a few decades ago, the advancements and the popularity has come up in the recent decade. Deep learning is a key technology behind driverless cars and voice control in consumer devices like phones, tablets, TVs, and hands-free speakers.

More precisely, deep learning is a computer model that learns to perform classification text, images or sound. These models achieve a greatest accuracy, sometimes exceeding the human-level performance.

Machine Learning and Deep Learning Techniques employed in Healthcare Applications

In earlier days, medical practitioners use hand wrote lab values, diagnoses, and other chart notes on paper during the phase of their training process. This is the area in which technology could help improve the workflow and patient care. While the healthcare sector is being transformed by the ability to record massive amounts of information about individual patients, the enormous volume of data being collected is impossible for human beings to analyze (Orion Health, 2013). The advancements in electronical medical records have been remarkable, but the information they provide is not much better than the old paper charts they replaced. Hence, the technology must help improving the electronic information provided to physicians. In this scenario, machine learning would empower physicians in diagnosing disease and in sorting and classifying health data will speedup decision making, diagnosing disease in clinic (Ed Corbett, 2017).

Similarly, healthcare and medicine seem to get immense benefit from deep learning because of huge volumes of data being generated and the growth of medical devices and electronic medical record systems. Deep learning models have the potential to handle large datasets, and run on a specialized computing hardware. The model can further be improved with more data so that it can perform better than machine learning models. As discussed earlier, the adoption and application of deep learning in healthcare is remarkable. Especially, deep learning has seen massive applications in computer vision which learns from image and video inputs, and helps in object classification, detection, and segmentation. Convolutional Neural Network (CNN) plays a significant role in computer vision (Ed Corbett, 2017). Deep learning has shown promising results in complex diagnostics spanning dermatology, radiology, pathology and ophthalmology. Further, deep learning enables physicians by offering second opinions and flags concerning areas in images.

The following section discusses various research works carried out in healthcare domain that make use of machine learning and deep learning approaches for disease prediction and identification in association with IOT.

In 2018, Jian Yu et al., proposed EdgeCNN model to effectively diagnose atrial fibrillation using electrocardiogram (ECG) recording. EdgeCNN integrates edge computing and cloud computing in order to solve the problems of storing and processing IoT data in the cloud platform. In their work, deep learning method is tied up with smart devices (edge devices) to enable real-time diagnostic capabilities. They implemented a CNN with a dataset published in cardiology challenge announced by PhysioNet in 2017. Their model outperforms the existing models in terms of delay, network I/O, privacy and cost. Developing an open platform for all types of edge devises is still an open challenge of their work.

A deep learning model for on-node Human Activity Recognition (HAR) was developed by Daniele Rav`i et al., during 2016. It combines features learned from inertial sensor data along with complementary information from a set of shallow features. The model is built with an objective of resolving the limitations of low-power wearable devices, real-time on-node computation, and activity classification. In order to achieve this purpose, spectral domain pre-processing is applied to data, before it is passed to deep learning framework. Furthermore, the model is used to classify time-series data and is evaluated with 5 different datasets namely ActiveMiles, WISDM v1.1, WISDM v2.0, Daphnet FoG, and Skoda.

Nowadays, nutrition monitoring systems become more popular. In the year of 2018, Prabha Sundaravadivel et al., proposed a fully automated nutrition monitoring system based on IoT. The model is called Smart-Log and uses 5-layer perceptron neural network and Bayesian Network for accurate meal prediction. The USDA dataset of 8791 food items is utilized obtain nutritional values. It consists of WiFi enabled sensors and a smart phone application for food nutrition quantification and collection of nutritional facts of the food ingredients, respectively. It is deployed on an open IoT platform for data analytics and storage. Moreover, it is an autonomous food logging system, with cost effectiveness and high accuracy.

In, Syed Umar Amin et al., (2019), proposed a model for pathology detection which combines IoT and Cloud technologies. Their model uses a variety of sensors to monitor healthcare data, and a cloud platform where all these data are processed. The major objective of the model is to monitor EEG (electroencephalogram) signals, facial expressions, speech, movements, and gestures through various sensors and take a real-time decision to provide emergency help if the patient is in a critical stage. The model uses two pretrained CNN models, namely, VGG 16 and AlexNet for EEG pathology detection. Investigating other deep learning models for EEG pathology detection will improve the current model.

IoT healthcare data are generated in huge volumes. Even though, a numerous research works have been carried out, which involve cloud and deep learning techniques, still they face network and computational congestion. In order to address this issue, Zubair Md. Fadlullah et al., (2018), proposed a IoT-Deep learning based edge analytics model to support smart healthcare for residential users. The major contribution of the work is to overcome delay-sensitive analytics through edge analytics in order to help senior citizens, and isolated patients. The model is analysed with the help of the heart rate time series database gathered from the Harvard-MIT division of health sciences and technology (MIT-BIH). The model provides best results in terms of low loss rate, and high accuracy.

While there have been several research works carried out in the field of IoT-healthcare, the concern for security and privacy of personal data still remains an open challenge. To focus on the aforementioned issue, Ismini Psychoula et al., proposed a deep learning approach for privacy preservation in assisted living in 2018. Ambience Assisted Living (AAL) aims to provide context-aware services to older people to improve the quality of their lives, and overcome aging problems with an affordable cost. Their contribution focuses on ensuring privacy of the personal data being acquired with the help of deep learning LSTM encoder-decoder, and a special encoding technique to restrict the access level for AAL data. The model is simulated with a use case data, and the privacy is ensured between an older person living in AAL and his/her family members. The proposed model is able to learn the privacy concerns and offers different levels of views for each one. Tokenization of attributes might be taken into account to further enhance the privacy. Table 4 provides the summary of our reviewed research works.

FUTURE RESEARCH DIRECTIONS

As IoT continues to emerge as the next wave for healthcare industry revolution, the challenges are bound to increase. Especially, the data collected by wearable health devices, and other sources continues to increase in volumes, and thus storing and processing such mountains of data pose a serious challenge to the healthcare industry and the researchers. Moreover, the data shared amongst other devices is vulnerable to unauthorized access and many other security issues. Hence, adopting a cloud computing framework for storing and processing voluminous healthcare data is of great significance in future research. On the other hand, the adoption of cloud directly depends on the cost of infrastructure, maintenance, authentication, and counter measures for security breach. Thus, alongside the adoption of cloud, developing secure methods to communicate information to the cloud to ensure the safety and security of healthcare data should be taken into account. Having mountains of healthcare data and a cloud computing framework

Table 4. Summary of IoT based healthcare system using machine learning and deep learning

Ref	Approach	Technique	Sensor(s)	Dataset	Problem addressed
Jian Yu, 2018	DL	CNN	Electrocardiographs, Smart wristbands, Smart watches, Blood pressure meters	ECG	Atrial fibrillation
Daniele Rav`i, 2016	DL	CNN	Inertial sensors (accelerometers, gyroscopes)	ActiveMiles and few more datasets	Human Activity Recognition (HAR)
Prabha Sundaravadivel, 2018	DL	Perceptron Neural Network (PNN)	Food weighing sensor	USDA dataset	Nutrition monitoring
Syed Umar Amin, 2019	DL	CNN	EEG Sensor	Abnormal TUH EEG pathology dataset	Pathology detection and monitoring
Zubair, 2018	DL	CNN	Wearable sensors (in general)	MIT-BIH dataset	Heart rate prediction
Ismini, 2018	DL	RNN (LSTM)	Simulates use cases	Simulated AAL dataset	Privacy preservation

doesn't suffice the intended purpose, while the integration of deep learning with the aforementioned two will. Deep learning assists doctors to accurately analyse a disease with the hidden information available in patients' medical history than the ancient manual methods of analysis. This helps to treat patients even better, thus resulting in improved medical decisions. Thus, the integration of wearable devices of IoT with cloud and deep learning technologies will rule the healthcare industry and an interesting research topic to explore.

CONCLUSION

Healthcare monitoring systems are of great importance in today's world. The role of IoT in these systems is more prevalent. This chapter presented a variety of recent wearable devices used in healthcare industry along with their applications, shortcomings and future opportunities. Furthermore, the use of cloud computing in storing and processing the data gathered from the wearable devices is presented. The challenges in adopting the cloud framework for healthcare industry are also highlighted. In addition, various research works carried out in healthcare domain that make use of deep learning approaches are presented. The study reveals various interesting factors, incorporating which enables healthcare monitoring systems more efficient, reliable and secure.

REFERENCES

Ahuja, S. P., Mani, S., & Zambrano, J. (2012). A survey of the state of cloud computing in healthcare. *Network and Communication Technologies*, *1*(2), 12.

Ali, O., Shrestha, A., Soar, J., & Wamba, S. F. (2018). Cloud computing-enabled healthcare opportunities, issues, and applications: A systematic review. *International Journal of Information Management, 43*, 146–158. doi:10.1016/j.ijinfomgt.2018.07.009

Ali, O., Soar, J., & Shrestha, A. (2018). Perceived potential for value creation from cloud computing: A study of the Australian regional government sector. *Behaviour & Information Technology, 37*(12), 1157–1176. doi:10.1080/0144929X.2018.1488991

Amin, S. U., Hossain, M. S., Muhammad, G., Alhussein, M., & Rahman, M. A. (2019). Cognitive Smart Healthcare for Pathology Detection and Monitoring. *IEEE Access: Practical Innovations, Open Solutions, 7*, 10745–10753. doi:10.1109/ACCESS.2019.2891390

Barfield, W. (2015). *Fundamentals of wearable computers and augmented reality*. Boca Raton, FL: CRC Press. doi:10.1201/b18703

Birkler, J. & Dahl, M. R. (2014). Den digitala patienten. Stockholm, Sweden: Liber.

Bowman, B. R., & Schuck, E. (1995). *Medical instruments and devices used in the home*. The Biomedical Engineering Handbook.

Chatman, C. (2010). How cloud computing is changing the face of health care information technology. *Journal of Health Care Compliance, 12*(3), 37–38.

Christoph, J., Griebel, L., Leb, I., Engel, I., Köpcke, F., Toddenroth, D., ... Sedlmayr, M. (2015). Secure secondary use of clinical data with cloud-based NLP services. *Methods of Information in Medicine, 54*(03), 276–282. doi:10.3414/ME13-01-0133 PMID:25377309

Corbett, Ed. (2017, April). *The Real-World Benefits of Machine Learning in Healthcare*. Retrieved from https://www.healthcatalyst.com/clinical-applications-of-machine-learning-in-healthcare

Escobar, L. J. V. & Salinas, S. A. (2016, August). e-Health prototype system for cardiac telemonitoring. In *2016 38th Annual International Conference of the IEEE Engineering in Medicine and Biology Society (EMBC)* (pp. 4399-4402). Piscataway, NJ: IEEE.

Esteva, A., Robicquet, A., Ramsundar, B., Kuleshov, V., DePristo, M., Chou, K., ... Dean, J. (2019). A guide to deep learning in healthcare. *Nature Medicine, 25*(1), 24–29. doi:10.103841591-018-0316-z PMID:30617335

Evenson, K. R., Goto, M. M., & Furberg, R. D. (2015). Systematic review of the validity and reliability of consumer-wearable activity trackers. *The International Journal of Behavioral Nutrition and Physical Activity, 12*(1), 159. doi:10.118612966-015-0314-1 PMID:26684758

Fadlullah, Z. M., Pathan, A. S. K., & Gacanin, H. (2018, June). On Delay-Sensitive Healthcare Data Analytics at the Network Edge Based on Deep Learning. In 2018 14th International Wireless Communications & Mobile Computing Conference (IWCMC) (pp. 388-393). Piscataway, NJ: IEEE. doi:10.1109/IWCMC.2018.8450475

Gao, W., Emaminejad, S., Nyein, H. Y. Y., Challa, S., Chen, K., Peck, A., ... Lien, D. H. (2016). Fully integrated wearable sensor arrays for multiplexed in situ perspiration analysis. *Nature, 529*(7587), 509–514. doi:10.1038/nature16521 PMID:26819044

Gupta, V. (2011). Cloud computing in health care. Express Healthcare, Sept.

Haghi, M., Thurow, K., & Stoll, R. (2017). Wearable devices in medical internet of things: Scientific research and commercially available devices. *Healthcare Informatics Research, 23*(1), 4–15. doi:10.4258/hir.2017.23.1.4 PMID:28261526

Integrated Cloud Applications & Platform Services. (2017). Retrieved from https://www.oracle.com/assets/hc-cloud-technologies-br-3432373.pdf

Jason Brownlee. (2016, August). *What is Deep Learning?* Retrieved from https://machinelearningmastery.com/what-is-deep-learning/

Klonoff, D. C. (2013). Twelve modern digital technologies that are transforming decision making for diabetes and all areas of health care. *Journal of Diabetes Science and Technology, 7*(2), 291–295. doi:10.1177/193229681300700201 PMID:23566983

Kolodner, E. K., Tal, S., Kyriazis, D., Naor, D., Allalouf, M., Bonelli, L., . . . Harnik, D. (2011, November). A cloud environment for data-intensive storage services. In *2011 IEEE third international conference on cloud computing technology and science* (pp. 357-366). Piscataway, NJ: IEEE. 10.1109/CloudCom.2011.55

Kostkova, P. (2015). Grand challenges in digital health. *Frontiers in Public Health, 3*, 134. doi:10.3389/fpubh.2015.00134 PMID:26000272

LeHong, H. & Velosa, A. (2014). Hype cycle for the Internet of Things. Gartner Group, 21.

Marco Varone. (2017, April). *Machine learning, Technology.* Retrieved from https://www.expertsystem.com/machine-learning-definition/

Miyazaki, S. (1997). Long-term unrestrained measurement of stride length and walking velocity utilizing a piezoelectric gyroscope. *IEEE Transactions on Biomedical Engineering, 44*(8), 753–759. doi:10.1109/10.605434 PMID:9254988

Nate Drake. (2019, June). Best cloud storage of 2019 online: free, paid and business options. *Cloud Services.* Retrieved from https://www.techradar.com/

Office for Civil Rights (OCR). (2013, July 26). Summary of the HIPAA Privacy Rule. *Health Information Privacy.* Retrieved from https://www.hhs.gov/

Patel, S., Park, H., Bonato, P., Chan, L., & Rodgers, M. (2012). A review of wearable sensors and systems with application in rehabilitation. *Journal of Neuroengineering and Rehabilitation, 9*(1), 21. doi:10.1186/1743-0003-9-21 PMID:22520559

Piwek, L., Ellis, D. A., Andrews, S., & Joinson, A. (2016). The rise of consumer health wearables: Promises and barriers. *PLoS Medicine, 13*(2). doi:10.1371/journal.pmed.1001953 PMID:26836780

Price, K., Bird, S. R., Lythgo, N., Raj, I. S., Wong, J. Y., & Lynch, C. (2017). Validation of the Fitbit One, Garmin Vivofit and Jawbone UP activity tracker in estimation of energy expenditure during treadmill walking and running. *Journal of Medical Engineering & Technology, 41*(3), 208–215. doi:10.1080/03091902.2016.1253795 PMID:27919170

Psychoula, I., Merdivan, E., Singh, D., Chen, L., Chen, F., Hanke, S., ... Geist, M. (2018, March). A deep learning approach for privacy preservation in assisted living. In *2018 IEEE International Conference on Pervasive Computing and Communications Workshops (PerCom Workshops)* (pp. 710-715). Piscataway, NJ: IEEE. 10.1109/PERCOMW.2018.8480247

Rao, G. S. V., Sundararaman, K., & Parthasarathi, J. (2010, October). Dhatri-A Pervasive Cloud initiative for primary healthcare services. In *2010 14th International Conference on Intelligence in Next Generation Networks* (pp. 1-6). Piscataway, NJ: IEEE. 10.1109/ICIN.2010.5640918

Ravi, D., Wong, C., Lo, B., & Yang, G. Z. (2016). A deep learning approach to on-node sensor data analytics for mobile or wearable devices. *IEEE Journal of Biomedical and Health Informatics*, *21*(1), 56–64. doi:10.1109/JBHI.2016.2633287 PMID:28026792

Redmond, S. J., Lovell, N. H., Yang, G. Z., Horsch, A., Lukowicz, P., Murrugarra, L., & Marschollek, M. (2014). What does big data mean for wearable sensor systems? *Yearbook of Medical Informatics*, *23*(01), 135–142. doi:10.15265/IY-2014-0019 PMID:25123733

Rhea, S., Wells, C., Eaton, P., Geels, D., Zhao, B., Weatherspoon, H., & Kubiatowicz, J. (2001). Maintenance-free global data storage. *IEEE Internet Computing*, *5*(5), 40–49. doi:10.1109/4236.957894

Roetenberg, D. (2006). Inertial and magnetic sensing of human motion. University of Twente, 18.

Rolim, C. O., Koch, F. L., Westphall, C. B., Werner, J., Fracalossi, A., & Salvador, G. S. (2010, February). A cloud computing solution for patient's data collection in health care institutions. In *2010 Second International Conference on eHealth, Telemedicine, and Social Medicine* (pp. 95-99). Piscataway, NJ: IEEE. 10.1109/eTELEMED.2010.19

Sanfilippo, F. & Pettersen, K. Y. (2015, November). A sensor fusion wearable health-monitoring system with haptic feedback. In *2015 11th International Conference on Innovations in Information Technology (IIT)* (pp. 262-266). Piscataway, NJ: IEEE. 10.1109/INNOVATIONS.2015.7381551

Spinelle, L., Gerboles, M., Villani, M. G., Aleixandre, M., & Bonavitacola, F. (2015). Field calibration of a cluster of low-cost available sensors for air quality monitoring. Part A: Ozone and nitrogen dioxide. *Sensors and Actuators B: Chemical*, *215*, 249–257. doi:10.1016/j.snb.2015.03.031

Sundaravadivel, P., Kesavan, K., Kesavan, L., Mohanty, S. P., & Kougianos, E. (2018). Smart-Log: A deep-learning based automated nutrition monitoring system in the IoT. *IEEE Transactions on Consumer Electronics*, *64*(3), 390–398. doi:10.1109/TCE.2018.2867802

Takeda, R., Tadano, S., Todoh, M., Morikawa, M., Nakayasu, M., & Yoshinari, S. (2009). Gait analysis using gravitational acceleration measured by wearable sensors. *Journal of Biomechanics*, *42*(3), 223–233. doi:10.1016/j.jbiomech.2008.10.027 PMID:19121522

Veltink, P. H. & Boom, H. B. K. (1995, November). 3D movement analysis using accelerometry-Theoretical concepts. In Topical workshop of the concerted action RAFT (pp. 45-50).

Xu, S., Zhang, Y., Jia, L., Mathewson, K. E., Jang, K. I., Kim, J., ... Bhole, S. (2014). Soft microfluidic assemblies of sensors, circuits, and radios for the skin. *Science*, *344*(6179), 70–74. doi:10.1126cience.1250169 PMID:24700852

Yu, J., Fu, B., Cao, A., He, Z., & Wu, D. (2018, December). EdgeCNN: A Hybrid Architecture for Agile Learning of Healthcare Data from IoT Devices. In *2018 IEEE 24th International Conference on Parallel and Distributed Systems (ICPADS)* (pp. 852-859). Piscataway, NJ: IEEE. 10.1109/PADSW.2018.8644604

Chapter 3
Architecting IoT based Healthcare Systems Using Machine Learning Algorithms:
Cloud-Oriented Healthcare Model, Streaming Data Analytics Architecture, and Case Study

G. S. Karthick
Bharathiar University, India

P. B. Pankajavalli
Bharathiar University, India

ABSTRACT

The rapid innovations in technologies endorsed the emergence of sensory equipment's connection to the Internet for acquiring data from the environment. The increased number of devices generates the enormous amount of sensor data from diversified applications of Internet of things (IoT). The generation of data may be a fast or real-time data stream which depends on the nature of applications. Applying analytics and intelligent processing over the data streams discovers the useful information and predicts the insights. Decision-making is a prominent process which makes the IoT paradigm qualified. This chapter provides an overview of architecting IoT-based healthcare systems with different machine learning algorithms. This chapter elaborates the smart data characteristics and design considerations for efficient adoption of machine learning algorithms into IoT applications. In addition, various existing and hybrid classification algorithms are applied to sensory data for identifying falls from other daily activities.

DOI: 10.4018/978-1-7998-1090-2.ch003

INTERNET OF THINGS AND HEALTHCARE INTERNET OF THINGS: AN INTRODUCTION

The IoT is an outcome of the technological revolution which interrelates the unified computing devices, mechanical instruments, hi-tech electronic machines and humans that are equipped with the capacity to exchange data over a network. The IoT was first formulated with the back support of Radio Frequency Identification (RFID) that can be applied to track the location of objects. For example, products in the shopping malls are interconnected to their own network, which enables tracking the location of products and increases the billing process flexible at the point of sales depots. Every individual product is exclusively identified and categorized based on its RFID. This uses machine-to-machine networks and these resemble the IoT through network connected systems and data/information. The likelihood of connecting objects to the network allows tagging, tracking and reading of data from objects with greater technical efforts, the technology of this era established called as IoT.

The essentials that emerged the IoT in current and future applications have been elaborated comprehensively and have been characterized by many authors. Gubbi et al., and Li et al., have discussed the major components and architectural elements in IoT (Gubbi, 2013) (Li, 2015). The millions of sensing elements, actuators, and other devices exist at the lowest level of the IoT. Each of which requires a unique identification and addressing schemes because of their deployment are at large scale and also have a high degree of constraints such as energy and computational resources. Communication is another important element which interconnects 'n' number of heterogeneous devices for providing smart services. Some of the short and long-range technologies used for communications in IoT applications which may include Wireless Sensor Networks (WSNs), Radio Frequency Identification (RFID), IETF Low power Wireless Personal Area Networks (6LoWPAN) and protocols like IEEE 802.11 (Wi-Fi), IEEE 802.15 (Bluetooth). As IoT devices generate a vast amount of raw data, thus increases the need for data storage and analytics. The data analytics, processing and machine learning in most of the IoT applications are deployed via cloud services. The IoT services are classified as identity-related, information aggregation, collaboration-aware and ubiquitous services (Montenegro, 2007). Identity-related services provide unique identification for every deployed thing. Information aggregation services are responsible for collecting and storing the data received from sensors. Collaborative aware services make use of the data provided by information aggregation services to take decisions and to provide smartness to the system. Ubiquitous services enable users to access services without geographical restrictions (Montenegro, 2007). Li et al., 2015 categorized the generic service-oriented architecture as sensing layer, network layer, service layer and interface layer (Al-Fuqaha, 2015).

The healthcare domain is in a state of a highly miserable situation, where its services are becoming more costly than ever before due to an increase in global population and a huge rise of chronic diseases. Even the basic healthcare services are out of reach to the people and this would be prone to chronic diseases. The technological revolution could never eradicate the population from aging and chronic diseases completely. But the accessibility to the healthcare services can be made easier with incomparable innovation and applicability of the Internet of things (IoT) in the healthcare domain. The application of IoT technology in healthcare allows doctors to communicate with their patients via smart wearable gadgets and devices without human interventions. On the other hand, major two crucial purposes of Healthcare Internet of things (HIoT) are: (i) Enhanced disease management that satisfies the patients and offers a better experience. (ii) Offers a higher level of interaction which allows patients to gain more information and medical intervention at every situation.

HIoT consists of medical devices, remote patient monitoring tools, wearables and various sensors which transmit the data to other end devices via the Internet. One of the interesting examples of IoT in healthcare is the automated insulin delivery system that entirely differs from continuous glucose monitoring system which can able to measure the amount of glucose in a patient's blood and intimate the end-users via mobile applications. But automated insulin delivery system automatically adjusts the quantity of insulin delivered to the patient's and thus prevents them from hyperglycemia and hypoglycemia. Such kind of applications generates a vast amount of data that has to be stored, incorporated and analyzed for spawning the useful insights for managing the patients with chronic diseases.

The high-level information extraction requires the application of machine learning techniques which processes the data automatically and intelligently. The efficiency of machine learning techniques tends to evaluate the data recorded by devices continuously in order to identify the stability or condition of patients. This streamlined data processing also helps the medical practitioners to predict the secondary illness in accordance with the patient primary illness. IoT improves the lives of patients through seamless connectivity, intelligent data processing, and remote monitoring. IoT technology tends to reshape the healthcare domain in such a way to reduce the hurdles in accessing healthcare services. Few key areas acknowledged where healthcare is reshaped by IoT are: (i) define the regulations for the industries which manufacture the pharmaceutical and medical devices that comply with patient safety, reliability and flexibility,(ii) aging of population simultaneously increase the demand of medical devices, (iii)the relevant data captured from patient's IoT devices to be communicated autonomously and accurately without data tampering.

HEALTHCARE BENEFITS FROM IoT

The number of healthcare service providers opt the IoT solutions is constantly increasing due to the adherence of the following benefits as shown in Figure 1:

Reporting and Monitoring

Remote health monitoring, diagnosing and patient's deterioration condition alerting. Medical gadgets send useful information on patient's conditions to practitioners or healthcare service providers without any human intervention. For example, HIoT device gathers health data like blood pressure, heartbeat, glucose level and oxygen in blood and temperature and stores the data in the cloud. Then stored data can be made available to the authorized person.

End-to-End Connectivity

Innumerable medical equipment is connected together to the centralized hub that eases monitoring and management. Thus avoid human participation, reduces error and time consumption.

Figure 1. Healthcare benefits from IoT

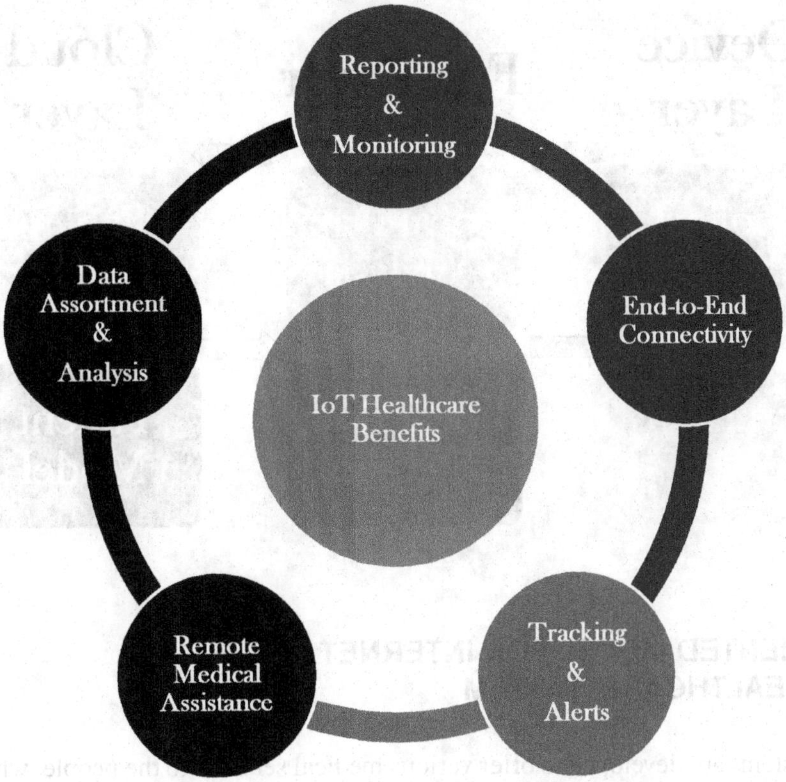

Data Assortment and Analysis

IoT devices generate a huge amount of data in seamlessly and manual analysis of such data is impossible. Therefore, streaming data analytics enables healthcare providers to receive structured data by avoiding data processing distractions.

Remote Medical Assistance

Remote medical device configuration allows the healthcare service providers to change the home-based health monitoring devices which avoid the patient's frequent visits to the hospital.

Tracking and Alerts

IoT-based medical devices drop notifications via mobile applications during life-threatening situations rather than gathering health data. Thus, provides better accuracy, appropriate intervention by healthcare providers and improves the healthcare service delivery.

Figure 2. Cloud-oriented model for Internet of things healthcare system

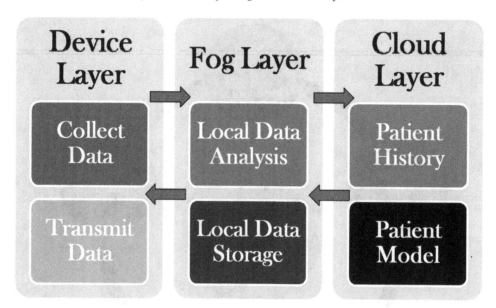

A CLOUD-ORIENTED MODEL FOR INTERNET OF THINGS HEALTHCARE SYSTEM

IoT healthcare systems are developed to offer various medical services to the people, which incorporate reliability, integrity, and security. Furthermore, healthcare applications notify the patient's status by observing the activities of patients and vital signs. A well-formed healthcare system must offer accurate and reliable services in a timely manner for patients, doctors, and caregivers. Existing healthcare model does not guarantee the integrity and confidentiality of data stored in the cloud. Also, there is no reliable communication and latency time is too high. In order to meet all the drawbacks, a new cloud-oriented model is developed for IoT-based healthcare system, which includes fog computing for offering processing and storage services to the users. Figure 2 shows the Cloud-Oriented Model for Internet of things Healthcare System and the functionalities of each layer are explained as follows:

Device Layer

This layer encompassing the 'n' number of physical objects such as medical sensors which are incorporated with the wireless module to gather physiological information of a patient. Every sensory device is enabled with patient identification data tends to capture the physiological patterns from the body. The captured physiological patterns are analyzed and used for predicting patient conditions. These captured patterns are transmitted over wired or wireless communications.

Fog Layer

This layer resembles the fog computing platform which offers storage, computational facility, and network infrastructure between the end devices and cloud. In addition, the main characteristic of fog computing is providing services to the edge of the network. Since IoT generates an enormous amount of data cloud platform is not affordable to maintain these data. To overcome this issue, the edge of the network performs various tasks which include data fusion, data compression, encrypting and local processing and then forwards the data to cloud storage.

Cloud Layer

The cloud layer provides many functions that include data storage, data sharing, and data analysis, where data synchronized periodically to ensure the integrity of the data. In this layer, the patient's information is stored into two groups: public data unit and private data unit. The information stored in the public data unit can be accessible to everyone whereas the private data unit holds the confidential information that cannot be available for public access.

ARCHITECTING IoT SYSTEM WITH MACHINE LEARNING TECHNIQUES

Connected IoT devices generate a huge amount of data which has to be monitored and analyzed continuously without any human intervention. Such kind of analyzes makes the system smarter by the adoption of machine learning techniques. Several machine learning techniques and algorithms are available to analyze the flooding data within a minimum span of time. Techniques like decision trees, classification, clustering, neural network, and fuzzy logic assist the IoT devices to find the patterns in diversified data and make an appropriate decision depends on the analysis. In the case of embedded devices, there is no support for implementing the machine learning algorithms. Without machine learning techniques, it would be a major drawback and the device becomes meaningless.

IoT is still in the state of infancy; it has to flourish in the near future and will play a primary role in walks of our lives. Machine learning can be considered as an important area of computer science domain which has the ability to make any system to act smarter and allows such systems to learn to act autonomously based on the historical inference. In recent times, many factors joined together to make machine learning into reality- heterogeneous data sources, increased processing power required for solving complex computational problems within limited time and the requirement of reliable inference. The primary purpose of embracing machine learning into IoT system is to automate the generation of data analytics models allows the algorithms to learn seamlessly with the help of streaming data. Machine learning can be implemented in any domain other than IoT, which depends on 3W's.

- When expected inference is known in advance - Supervised Learning
- When expected inference is not known in advance - Unsupervised Learning
- When inference depends on the relationship between any specific model and the concerned environment – Reinforcement Learning

IoT without Machine Learning

Even though IoT uses the Internet remarkably, there are some challenges exists in implementing IoT application without machine learning. Traditional procedures cannot handle the huge amount of data generated by multiple devices. Hence some of the challenges that are faced by IoT without machine learning will be discussed in this section.

Diversified Devices and Interoperability

A single domain products and services are developed by diversified manufacturers in the field of IoT. In the case of smart healthcare systems, a wide variety of sensors available from several organizations that measure the body temperature and each of which operates differs in their standards. The integration of such kind of sensors together for accomplishing a particular task becomes a major challenge, which has to be resolved by machine learning techniques.

Device Management

IoT applications are comprised of countless small devices which are connected via the Internet in order to communicate with each other and also deployed over diversified locations. In some cases, the possibility of connecting a few devices together is less due to different communication link issues that require efficient management. For instance, the deterioration condition of patients has to be intimated to the healthcare service providers immediately through the wireless communication links. This requires all possible communication links among the various body sensors and networking devices to be managed for smooth operation.

Multi-Source Data Integration

On deploying the IoT systems, it is anticipated to acquire an abundant variety of data from multiple sources which includes sensors, actuators, mobile devices and so on. To develop an analytics model for data integration and processing of such diversified data might be a major challenge.

Performance and Scalability

IoT systems must be scalable for managing the huge volume of real-time streaming data, as well as the performance of the system, should be equally balanced. Hence, handling and analyzing the real-time streaming data in IoT system is another challenging factor that has to deal with machine learning.

Application Flexibility

Various IoT devices and sensors will tend to evolve with new potentials and enhanced functionalities. This may require more effort to develop new test cases and business models. To develop a flexible IoT system with minimal effort to cope up with the changing requirements, machine learning support is needed for enabling the system to learn varied applications.

How Machine Learning Improves the Efficiency of IoT?

- Traditional data analytics models work on static data and have certain limitations so that they cannot be implemented over dynamic and unstructured data. In the case of IoT, the correlations between enormous sensor data and their external factors must be identified. Traditional data analytics model performs operations on historical data and also requires an expert opinion for identifying the relationship among the variables. But machine learning can able to directly focus on predicting the resultant variable through automatic identification of predictor variables and their relationships. Hence, machine learning really helps in identifying important variables during the decision-making process and thus machine learning becomes a valuable phenomenon.

- Since traditional data analytics models are well suited for static data but various machine learning algorithms are quite simple which accurately predicts the future events. Moreover, machine learning algorithms can be improved constantly due to increased scaling of data. This denotes the algorithms can make better predictions when compared to their historical predictions.
- The predictive abilities of machine learning algorithms are tremendously useful in the healthcare domain. The physiological data gathered from patients from multiple sensors allows the machine learning algorithms to point out the distinctive data and also predicts the abnormality in patients before the condition worsening.

Design Considerations

Some of the IoT system designing factors may affect the decisions made by machine learning algorithms. In order to assure the accuracy of decisions, the following design factors must be considered while developing the system.

Battery Lifetime of IoT Device

The battery power is consumed during the duty cycle (may depend on power modes like active, standby, off) and minimal power is consumed by the sensors, processors and communication interfaces. The power consumption at the communication interface will increase during the raw data transmission from the sensor node to cloud and processors power consumption rate will also increase during local data processing.

On-Time Needs

Most of the IoT systems cannot tolerate the delayed transmission of sensor data to cloud and response from the cloud. So, the systems must afford on-time transmission and response.

Communication Channel Load

The transmission of a huge volume of data to cloud via communication channel may block the entire channel due to traffic. This may sometimes affect the decision-making process.

Sensitivity to the Communication Link Disturbance

Few machine learning algorithms cannot tolerate the communication link disturbance. For example, in a healthcare monitoring system, an emergency alarm must be raised even under the absence of disturbance of the communication link when a patient's condition starts worsening. When the system fails to raise alarm, then the prediction of the patient's condition using machine learning algorithms will be insignificant.

Needy of Algorithms and Multiple Platforms

In many cases, algorithms are needy because the analyst cannot handle the massive amount of IoT data arrival. The algorithm is playing a significant role in processing the IoT data at backend and do a meaningful job (i.e. decision making). Thus, the selection of an appropriate algorithm and attaining accurate results will be a challenging task. Another important challenge is to make algorithms to work on multiple environments without affecting the usual performance of the algorithms.

Agility and Flexibility

Prior to the deployment of IoT devices, the processor capacity and memory size must be fixed. Since they are fixed by default, scaling or replacing the IoT device in terms of computational resources will highly expensive and the degree of complexity will also increase. Meanwhile, using cloud resources and edge resources are more agile in nature. Because it can be scaled up and down depends upon the needs.

Privacy and Security

IoT applications like smart healthcare and smart home are stick on to deal with privacy or sensitive data. For example, transferring entire sensor data to the cloud may expose the IoT device towards the security risks. Instead, incorporating the sensitive wall on the edges will help to filter the sensitive data and transfers the data to the cloud.

SMART DATA CHARACTERISTICS

IoT represents a new paradigm "smart data", which is a challenging domain in the area of computing for researchers. The main challenges are with preparing and processing IoT data. S. Bin et al. proposed four data mining model for IoT data processing (Bin, 2010, April). The first model is a multi-layer model, which concentrates on data collection, data management, event processing, and mining services. The next model is a distributed data mining model which has been proposed for data deposition at various sites. The third model is a grid-oriented model that concentrates on heterogeneous, scalable and high-performance IoT applications. Finally, the fourth model provides the integration functions for the frameworks of the future Internet technologies.

In (Gonzalez, 2006, April), the author has focused on radio frequency identification (RFID) data warehousing with respect to the management and analysis of RFID stream data. F. Chen et al. reviewed many data mining techniques like classification, clustering, association rule mining, time series analysis and outlier detection (Chen, 2015). This work has revealed that the data originated from e-commerce, industries, healthcare, and social media are much similar to that of IoT data. Therefore, it has been identified that traditional data mining algorithms are highly fit for various IoT applications driven data.

C.W.Tsai et al. surveyed many challenges in preparation and processing IoT data using data mining algorithms (Tsai, 2013). They presented their study into three various divisions, which includes the explanation of IoT, data and its challenges existing in building the data mining model for IoT.

In (Zanella, 2014), the authors examined the infrastructure of a smart city in IoT and conversed the advanced communication technologies that support the services provided to the city and citizens. They offered an overview of various enabling technologies, protocols and architectures for smart city and in which the authors studied the data of Padova Smart City.

The IoT devices deployed in the cities generate the data in the streaming manner, signifying that data collected from health, energy management, and traffic applications would provide a huge volume of data. Therefore, the generation of data from various devices, processing of such data with differed generation rates is a major challenge (Qin, 2016) (Costa, 2015) (Jara, 2014, May). As the data generated from heterogeneous devices, the quality of the gathered data is mandatory. The characteristics of IoT data is depicted in Figure 3.

From the study [(Barnaghi, (2015))], it has been identified that the information quality depends on three major factors (i) measurement errors, (ii) device noise and (iii) discrete observation and measurements. The characteristics of smart data collected from smart cities are tabulated in Table 1.

MACHINE LEARNING ALGORITHMS FOR IoT

Machine learning is a major sub-field of computer science, provides the ability to machines, to learn without explicit programming. It has been developed from pattern recognition and computational theory. Frequently used machine learning algorithms for smart data analysis are discussed below. Generally, learning can be of three categories: supervised learning, unsupervised learning and reinforcement learning (Bishop, 2006) (Murphy, 2012)are shown in the Figure 4. A learning algorithm works upon the set of input samples which is termed as a training set.

Supervised learning contains a set of input samples in which each of their samples belongs to a particular target group, known as labels whereas in unsupervised learning labels are not required. Reinforcement learning tends to learn from the appropriate action for a given situation. This review article depicts the supervised and unsupervised learning techniques since it is being commonly applied to IoT smart data analytics. The aim of supervised learning is to learn how to forecast the accurate target group (finite

Figure 3. Characteristics of IoT data

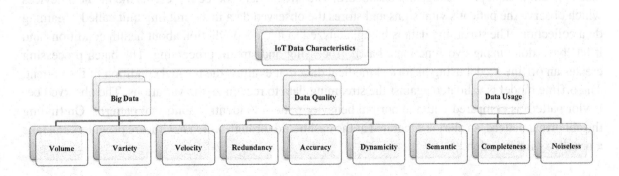

Table 1. Smart city data characteristics

Smart City Use Cases	Type of Data	Data Processing Area	References
Smart Traffic	Stream/Massive	Data Edge	(Kafi, 2013) (Qin, 2016)
Smart Health	Stream/Massive	Data Edge/Cloud	(Toshniwal, 2013, February)
Smart Environment	Stream/Massive	Data Cloud	(Jakkula, 2010, July)
Smart Weather	Prediction Stream	Data Edge	(Ni, 2014, August)
Smart Home	Massive/Historical	Data Cloud	(Souza, 2015)
Smart Air Controlling	Massive/Historical	Data Cloud	(Costa, 2015)

number of distinct categories) for a given input sample and it's called as classification tasks. When the target group is a collection of one or more continuous variables is termed as regression (Goodfellow, 2016). The major aim of unsupervised learning is to predict the clusters of related samples from the set of input data is called clustering. The most frequently used machine learning algorithms for smart data analysis are presented in Table 2 and the various machine learning algorithms that can be applied IoT applications are tabulated in Table 3.

A PROPOSED MACHINE LEARNING ARCHITECTURE FOR STREAMING IoT HEALTHCARE DATA

The increasing ratio of IoT devices analogously generates a huge amount of data; machine learning will provide a wide opportunity to make IoT applications highly effective and intelligent. Applying machine learning on healthcare data helps healthcare providers to improve the quality of patient's life. Additionally, it allows healthcare providers to take more optimal decisions. Machine learning is broadly classified into two types such as supervised and unsupervised machine learning. Supervised learning uses training data for predicting the rules whereas unsupervised learning uses unknown data for predicting the rules. The HIoT systems can be made intelligent combining streaming medical data with machine learning. The application of machine learning into healthcare system allows the doctor to provide smart treatment to the patient's with improved quality at a lower cost. Figure 5 depicts the procedure of applying the streaming data into machine learning, which comprised of four components such as stream data source, data collection, data processing, and dashboard. The stream data source represents the medical devices which observe the patient's vital signs and stores the observed data in assembling unit called streaming data collection. The streaming data is being analyzed to make a prediction about health conditions and it has been done using two functions: batch processing and stream processing. The batch processing creates an offline model using historical medical data that exhibits the normal condition of the patient. The offline model is validated against the streaming data to recognize the variations. The observed behavior pattern is compared with the normal behavior pattern to identify abnormal patterns. On finding the abnormal pattern, an alert is generated at the dashboard through which healthcare providers can take a necessary intervention.

Figure 4. Categories of machine learning algorithms

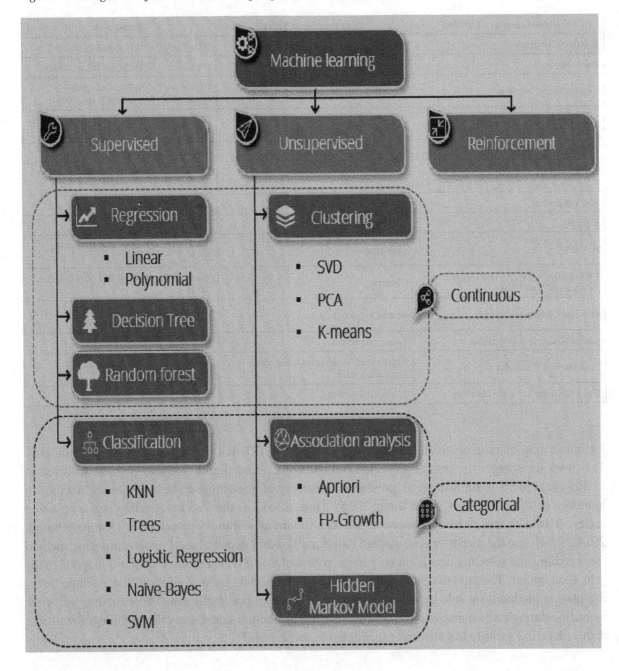

Chiuchisan and Geman proposed the decision support and home monitoring system composed of diagnosis, treatment, prescriptions, rehabilitation for Parkinson's disease (IulianaChiuchisan&Geman, 2014). Thomas Bruschwiler stated that machine learning algorithms can assist doctors and patients to diagnose diseases before worsening. Fizar Ahmed presented an IoT-based architecture for monitoring and it uses the kNN classification algorithm for predicting the number of patients suspected to have a heart attack in the future (Ahmed, 2017) . IBM researchers focused on developing an IoT-based system

Table 2. Machine learning algorithms for smart data analysis – an outline

Machine Learning Algorithm	Data Processing Tasks	References
K-Nearest Neighbors	Classification	(Cover, 1967), (H.V. Jagadish, 2005)
Naive Bayes	Classification	(McCallum, 1998, July), (Zhang, 2004)
Support Vector Machine	Classification	(C. Cortes, 1995), (Guyon, 1993), (Cristianini, 2000), (Scholkopf, 2001)
Linear Regression	Regression	(Neter, 1996), (Seber, 2012), (Montgomery, 2012)
Support Vector Regression	Regression	(Drucker, 1997), (Smola, 2004)
Classification and Regression Trees	Classification/Regression	(Breiman, 2017), (Prasad, 2006), (Loh, 2011)
Random Forests	Classification/Regression	(Breiman, 2001)
Bagging	Classification/Regression	(Breiman, 1996)
K-Means	Clustering	(Likas, 2003), (Coates, 2012), (Jumutc, 2015)
Density-Based Spatial Clustering of Applications with Noise	Clustering	(Ester, 1996), (Kriegel, 2011), (Campello, 2013)
Principal Component Analysis	Feature extraction	(Pearson, 1901), (Hotelling, 1933), (Jolliffe, 2011), (Abdi, 2010), (Bro, 2014)
Canonical Correlation Analysis	Feature extraction	(Hotelling, 1992), (Bach, 2002)
Feed Forward Neural Network	Regression/Classification/Clustering/ Feature extraction	(LeCun Y. B., 1998), (Glorot, 2010), (Eberhart, 2014), (He, 2016),
One-class Support Vector Machines	Anomaly detection	(Schölkopf, 2001), (Rätsch, 2002)

for monitoring chronic obstructive pulmonary disease (COPD) with machine learning technologies. This work encourages the patient-physician communication and slightly reduces the cost involved in healthcare systems. J. Jin Kang et al. presented a new way of predicting the health status by making an inference on the cloud itself (J. Jin Kang, 2015). Thus, it reduces the data overloading issues at sensor nodes. A hybrid density-based clustering for data stream algorithm is proposed in (AmineshAmini, 2014), which use the merits of density-grid based method and density based micro-clustering method for searching and selecting data point only in the potential list. If it is not found, then it is mapped to the grid as an outlier. The growth of IoT is driven by many supporting technologies, in that machine learning plays a predominant role because it makes IoT systems more intelligent. Three fuelling ways are identified through which machine learning shapes the IoT, includes increasing the usability of real-time data, enhancing security features and expanding the scope of IoT.

CASE STUDY: FALL DETECTION USING MACHINE LEARNING ALGORITHMS

Falls are an indisputable medical issue and possibly dangerous for individuals and this case study responds to the challenge of arranging diverse developments as a piece of a framework intended to satisfy the requirement for a wearable device to gather information about fall and nearly fall analysis. Four diverse

Table 3. Machine learning algorithms applied IoT applications

Machine learning Algorithm	IoT Use Cases	Metric to Optimize	References
Classification	Smart Traffic	Traffic Prediction, Increase Data Abbreviation	(M.A. Kafi, 2013)
Clustering	Smart Traffic, Smart Health	Traffic Prediction, Increase Data Abbreviation	(M.A. Kafi, 2013), (D. Toshniwal, 2013)
Anomaly Detection	Smart Traffic, Smart Environment	Traffic Prediction, Increase Data Abbreviation, Finding Anomalies in Power Dataset	(M.A. Kafi, 2013), (V. Jakkula, 2010)
Support Vector Regression	Smart Weather Prediction	Forecasting	(P. Ni, 2014)
Linear Regression	Economics, Market analysis, Energy usage	Real Time Prediction, Reducing Amount of Data	(W. Derguech, 2014)
Classification and Regression Trees	Smart Citizens	Real Time Prediction, Passengers Travel Pattern	(X. Ma, 2013), (W. Derguech, 2014)
Support Vector Machine	All Use Cases	Classify Data, Real Time Prediction	(W. Derguech, 2014)
K-Nearest Neighbors	Smart Citizen	Passengers' Travel Pattern, Efficiency of the Learned Metric	(X. Ma, 2013)
Naive Bayes	Smart Agriculture, Smart Citizen	Food Safety, Passengers Travel Pattern, Estimate the Numbers of Nodes	(X. Ma, 2013), (W. Han, 2014)
K-Means	Smart City, Smart Home, Smart Citizen, Controlling Air and Traffic	Outlier Detection, fraud detection, Analyze Small Data set, Forecasting Energy Consumption, Passengers Travel Pattern, Stream Data Analyze	(X. Ma, 2013)
Density-Based Clustering	Smart Citizen	Labeling Data, Fraud Detection, Passengers Travel Pattern	(X. Ma, 2013)
Feed Forward Neural Network	Smart Health	Reducing Energy Consumption, Forecast the States of Elements, Overcome the Redundant Data and Information	(I. Kotenko, 2015)
Principal Component Analysis	Monitoring Public Places	Fault Detection	(D.N. Monekosso, 2013)
Canonical Correlation Analysis	Monitoring Public Places	Fault Detection	(D.N. Monekosso, 2013)
One-class Support Vector Machines	Smart Human Activity Control	Fraud Detection, Emerging Anomalies in the data	(M. Shukla, 2015), (A. Shilton, 2015)

fall directions (forward, in reverse, left and right); three ordinary activities (standing, walking and lying) and close fall circumstances are distinguished and identified. Fall recognition frameworks are ordered into the accompanying three groups: ambient device, camera-based frameworks, and wearable devices whose pros and cons are depicted in Table 4. Ambiance devices are connected around an area which can recognize falls utilizing the add-on sensors: PIR, pressure, Doppler, amplifier and accelerometer sensors. Computer vision utilizes cameras to follow user developments. A fall might be distinguished when the user is latent for quite a while. Wearable devices which are connected on the user incorporate the following sensors: an accelerometer and a gyrator.

Figure 5. Application of machine learning algorithm on streaming data

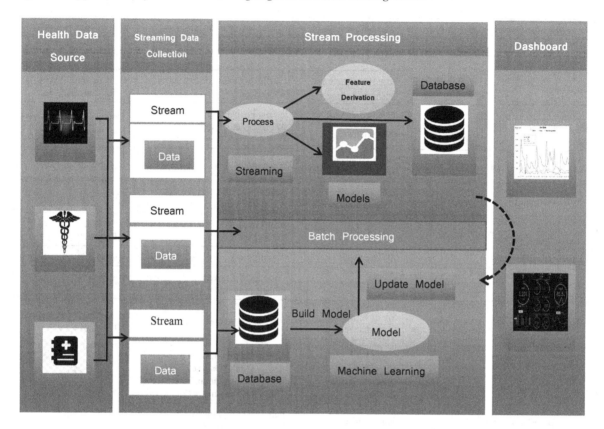

The performance of the framework relies upon the sensors utilized and classification methods. The speed and accuracy of the fall identification classifier are taken into the major considerations of fall detection systems. Components that impact the identification and classification of fall activities and ADLs incorporate difference in movements, environmental conditions and the relocation of the sensor. Classification algorithms can be categorized into two models as supervised and unsupervised models. In a supervised model, the output can be controlled and can be effectively modeled when contrasted with the unsupervised model. Unsupervised models have been utilized in fall detection frameworks, for example, one-class support vector machine. Supervised models contain a support vector machine (SVM), k-Nearest Neighbor (k-NN), Naive Bayes, least squares method (LSM), artificial neural networks (ANNs) and hybrid k-NN. Supervised models are used in this case study for fall detection and categorization of

Table 4. Pros and cons of fall recognition systems

Type of Devices	Pros	Cons
Ambience devices	Cheap and Non-intrusive	Range and environmental factors which can result in low accuracy
Camera-based systems	Detect multiple events simultaneously, less intrusive	Limited to a specific area and does not guarantee privacy, expensive
Wearable devices	Portable, cheap and easy to use	Intrusive, false alarms

Figure 6. Machine learning architecture for fall detection

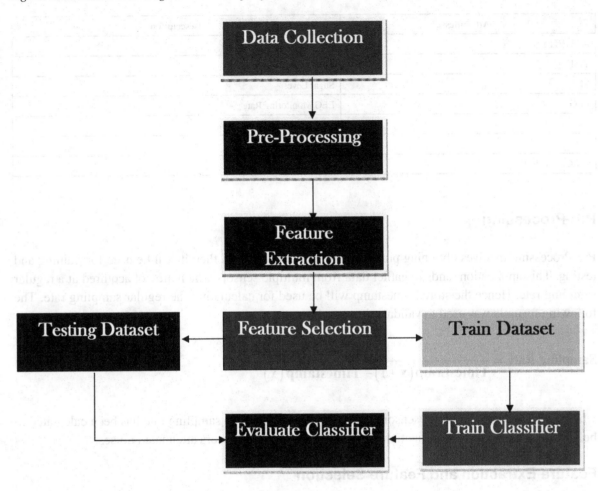

various activities. Fall detection frameworks can be characterized using five phases: data collection, pre-processing, feature extraction, feature selection, model training and classification as shown in Figure 6.

Data Collection

The major intention of this case study is to implement various classification algorithms on fall detection dataset which has been downloaded from Kaggle dataset repository (Özdemir, 2014). Fourteen volunteers play out an institutionalized arrangement of activities including 20 deliberate falls and 16 Activities of Daily Living (ADLs), bringing about a substantial dataset with 2520 preliminaries. Several machine learning classification algorithms including SVM, ANN, k-NN, LSM, Naïve Bayes and Hybrid High Probability Nearest Neighbor SVM classifier were implemented and evaluated to determine the best classification model. The primary objective is to classify the various daily activities like standing, walking, sitting, falling, cramps and running. In this study, the rank-based method is used to select the features and activities are classified. Table 5 shows that the columns were used in the dataset and its associated description.

Table 5. Dataset and its description

Attributes	Description
ACTIVITY	Activity Classification
TIME	Monitoring Time
SL	Sugar Level
EEG	EEG Monitoring Rate
BP	Blood Pressure
HR	Heart Beat Rate
CIRCULATION	Blood Circulation

Pre-Processing

Pre-Processing involves obtaining pure data from the dataset, and then it will be used for training and testing. This application tends to gather data from multiple sensors which are not acquired at a regular sampling rate. Hence the stored timestamp will be used for calculating the regular sampling rate. The following formula was used to validate the sampling rate,

$$\textbf{Sampling Rate} = \frac{1}{\textbf{Timestamp}(x+1) - \textbf{Timestamp}(x)} \dots\dots \tag{1}$$

where x denotes the number of sensor data. Using Equation 1, the sampling rate has been calculated to be 100 Hz. The median filter function was used to remove the sensors attenuated noises.

Feature Extraction and Feature Selection

Feature extraction is an important stage in the classification process since it decides the accuracy of any classification schemes. Features are extracted based on the data acquired from a window intervals, the time index of the maximum signal magnitude vector (SMV) peak has been identified in each activity record and the features were normalized between 0-1. On the other hand, various features have been extracted using the statistical methods which include mean, median, maximum, minimum, standard deviation and so on.

The performance of any classification scheme depends on the size of the features extracted. In order to improve the performance, the features must be minimized and also it can extensively differentiate the fall activities from normal activities. An aggregate of 6 features was extracted and a filter rank based system was utilized to eliminate features with no data.

Classifiers Evaluation

The best six features were utilized in the classification model which gives better than average outcomes. The classification model can deliver the accompanying four feasible results:

Table 7. Classifiers applied on fall detection dataset

Classification Algorithms	Pros & Cons	Algorithm Description
k-Nearest Neighbor	i. Classes need not be linearly separable ii. Zero cost of the learning process iii. Sometimes it is robust with regard to noisy training data iv. Well suited for multimodal v. Time to find the nearest neighbors in a large training dataset can be excessive vi. It is sensitive to noisy or irrelevant attributes vii. Performance of the algorithm depends on the number of dimensions used	k-NN classifier has been highly applied on fall detection applications which use distance function for identifying the similarity between two activity records.
Naïve Bayes	i. Simple to implement ii. Great computational efficiency and classification rate iii. It predicts accurate results for most of the classification and prediction problems iv. The precision of the algorithm decreases if the amount of data is less v. For obtaining good results, it requires a very large number of records	Generally, this algorithm follows the principle of Bayes theorem and the probabilities are used for classifying the features.
Artificial Neural Networks	i. It is easy to use with few parameters to adjust ii. A neural network learns and reprogramming is not needed. - Easy to implement iii. Applicable to a wide range of problems in real life. iv. Requires high processing time if a neural network is large v. Difficult to know how many neurons and layers are necessary - Learning can be slow	This algorithm consists of a two-layer feedforward network that includes hidden layers and neurons. The gradient backpropagation has been for training.
Support Vector Machine	i. High accuracy ii. Work well even if the data is not linearly separable in the base feature space iii. Speed and size requirement both in training and testing is more iv. High complexity and extensive memory requirements for classification in many cases	"svmtrain" and "svmpredict" functions are used for training and testing. The radial basis kernel has been used to classify the activities and fall occurrence.
Hybrid Nearest Neighbor integrated SVM Classifier	i. Very minimal computational complexities ii. Very high accuracy	k-NN has been used for creating the feature space as it requires less computational complexities and then, SVM is used for classifying the various activities.

1. True Positive (TP) when a system accurately detects a fall when a fall takes place
2. False Positive (FP) when a system detects a fall when no fall take place
3. True Negative (TN) when a system detects no fall when no fall takes place.
4. False Negative (FN) when a system detects no fall when a fall takes place.

Various performance measures used to evaluate the classification algorithms used for detecting the falls are accuracy, specificity, and sensitivity, which are given by,

$$\text{Accuracy} = \frac{(TP + TN)}{(TP + TN + FN + FP)} \dots \quad (2)$$

$$\text{Sensitivity} = \frac{(TP)}{(TP + FN)} \ldots\ldots \tag{3}$$

$$\text{Specificity} = \frac{(TN)}{(TN + FP)} \ldots\ldots \tag{4}$$

Generally k-NN, SVM, ANN offers the best precision than Naive Bayes. Elements that impact the accuracy are the position of sensors on the body. The two existing algorithms k-NN and SVM outperforms well when compared to other algorithms. Therefore, k-NN and SVM algorithms are hybridized for classifying the various activities and to detect the fall. This hybrid algorithm can be used successfully for detecting fall and other activities with reduced computational complexities in both training and testing phases. k-NN has been used for creating the feature space as it requires less computational complexities and then, SVM is used for classifying the various activities. The pseudo code of the hybrid algorithm is shown below:

Algorithm: Hybrid Nearest Neighbor integrated SVM Classifier

```
Inputs:  Set of sample x to classify, Training Set T
         Number of nearest neighbors K= {k₁, k₂….kₙ}
         Adjustment parameter for balancing errors
Output:  Classified Dataset
Steps:
1.       Order the training samples in ascending order
2.       Minimum Error=1000; Value= 0;
3.       if initial k values are from same class label c then
4.       print c
5.       end if
6.       for all k do
7.       Train SVM model on training samples
8.       Classify x using built SVM model
9.       Classify the same training sample using built SVM model
10.      Evaluate the Error Positive and Error Negative
11.      Update Minimum Error
12.      Calculate Value
13.      End for
14.      Return Value
```

Table 8. Classification summary

Classifiers	Accuracy (%)	Sensitivity (%)	Specificity (%)
NB	80.00	85.11	72.73
ANN	85.87	89.23	81.43
k-NN	87.5	90.70	83.78
SVM	86.75	89.74	82.93
Hybrid Classifier	89.01	91.27	85.63

Figure 7. Comparison of accuracy

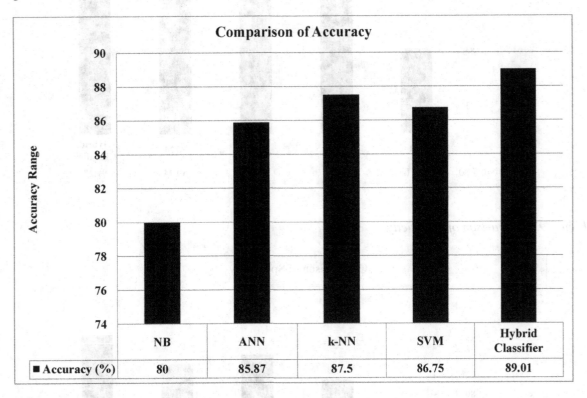

RESULTS AND DISCUSSION

Table 8 illustrates the summary classifiers performance. The best classifier is the Hybrid Nearest Neighbor integrated SVM Classifier with 89.01% of accuracy, the sensitivity of 90.27%, and specificity of 85.63%. Figure 7, Figure 8 and Figure 9 depicts the compares the performance of various classifiers in terms of accuracy, sensitivity and specificity .

Figure 8. Comparison of sensitivity

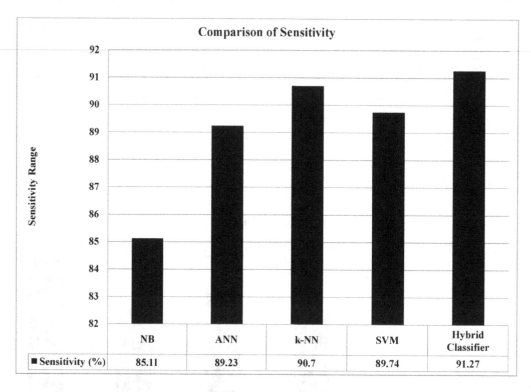

Figure 9. Comparison of specificity

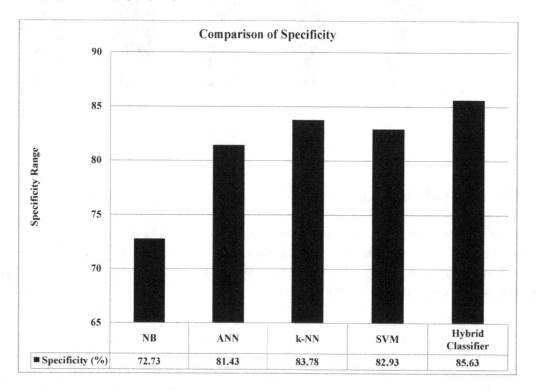

CONCLUSION

IoT is a developing broad domain consists of enormous different devices that are connected together and generates a vast amount of smart data. In which, the healthcare is a major application of IoT that offers various services like remote health monitoring, disease prediction and assisted the living. The services provided by the smart applications have to be optimized and improved by analyzing the smart data gathered. Many machine learning algorithms have been applied on gathered to extract high-level information. Selecting an appropriate algorithm for certain IoT applications is an important issue. This chapter addresses the design considerations for building efficient healthcare IoT systems and also focuses on major factors must be considered while applying machine learning algorithms to smart data. An exclusive machine learning architecture has been proposed for applying streaming healthcare data which radically improves the decision-making capability of healthcare systems. This chapter anticipates the application of existing classification algorithms and a hybrid algorithm on sensory IoT data for detecting the fall from other regular activities. The hybrid algorithm outperforms when compared with other existing techniques.

REFERENCES

Abdi, H., & Williams, L. J. (2010). Principal component analysis. *Wiley Interdisciplinary Reviews: Computational Statistics*, *2*(4), 433–459. doi:10.1002/wics.101

Ahmed, F. (2017). An internet of things (IoT) Application for Predicting the Quantity of Future Heart Attack Patients. *International Journal of Computers and Applications*, *164*(6), 36–40. doi:10.5120/ijca2017913773

Al-Fuqaha, A., Guizani, M., Mohammadi, M., Aledhari, M., & Ayyash, M. (2015). Internet of things: A survey on enabling technologies, protocols, and applications. *IEEE Communications Surveys and Tutorials*, *17*(4), 2347–2376. doi:10.1109/COMST.2015.2444095

Amini, A., Saboohi, H., Ying Wah, T., & Herawan, T. (2014). A fast density-based clustering algorithm for real-time Internet of things stream. *The Scientific World Journal*. doi:10.1155/2014/926020

Bach, F. R., & Jordan, M. I. (2002). Kernel independent component analysis. *Journal of Machine Learning Research*, *3*(Jul), 1–48.

Barnaghi, P. M., Bermudez-Edo, M., & Tönjes, R. (2015). Challenges for Quality of Data in Smart Cities. *J. Data and Information Quality*, *6*(2-3), 6–1.

Bin, S., Yuan, L., & Xiaoyi, W. (2010, April). Research on data mining models for the internet of things. In 2010 *International Conference on Image Analysis and Signal Processing* (pp. 127-132). Piscataway, NJ: IEEE.

Bishop, C. M. (2006). Pattern recognition and machine learning. Berlin, Germany: Springer.

Breiman, L. (1996). Bagging predictors. *Machine Learning*, *24*(2), 123–140. doi:10.1007/BF00058655

Breiman, L. (2001). Random forests. *Machine Learning*, *45*(1), 5–32. doi:10.1023/A:1010933404324

Breiman, L. (2017). Classification and regression trees. Abingdon-on-Thames, UK: Routledge. doi:10.1201/9781315139470

Bro, R., & Smilde, A. K. (2014). Principal component analysis. *Analytical Methods, 6*(9), 2812–2831. doi:10.1039/C3AY41907J

Campello, R. J., Moulavi, D., & Sander, J. (2013, April). Density-based clustering based on hierarchical density estimates. In *Pacific-Asia conference on knowledge discovery and data mining* (pp. 160–172). Berlin, Germany: Springer. doi:10.1007/978-3-642-37456-2_14

Chen, F., Deng, P., Wan, J., Zhang, D., Vasilakos, A. V., & Rong, X. (2015). Data mining for the internet of things: Literature review and challenges. *International Journal of Distributed Sensor Networks, 11*(8). doi:10.1155/2015/431047

Coates, A., & Ng, A. Y. (2012). Learning feature representations with k-means. In *Neural networks: Tricks of the trade* (pp. 561–580). Berlin, Germany: Springer. doi:10.1007/978-3-642-35289-8_30

Cortes, C., & Vapnik, V. (1995). Support-vector networks. *Machine Learning, 20*(3), 273–297. doi:10.1007/BF00994018

Costa, C., & Santos, M. Y. (2015). Improving cities sustainability through the use of data mining in the context of big city data. *Lecture Notes in Engineering and Computer Science, 1*, 320–325.

Cover, T. M., & Hart, P. E. (1967). Nearest neighbor pattern classification. *IEEE Transactions on Information Theory, 13*(1), 21–27. doi:10.1109/TIT.1967.1053964

Cristianini, N., & Shawe-Taylor, J. (2000). *An introduction to support vector machines and other kernel-based learning methods.* Cambridge University Press. doi:10.1017/CBO9780511801389

Derguech, W., Bruke, E., & Curry, E. (2014). An autonomic approach to real-time predictive analytics using open data and internet of things. In *IEEE 11th Intl Conf on Ubiquitous Intelligence and Computing, and IEEE 11th Intl Conf on Autonomic and Trusted Computing, and IEEE 14th Intl Conf on Scalable Computing and Communications and its Associated Workshops (UTC-ATC-ScalCom)* (pp. 204–211). Piscataway, NJ: IEEE. 10.1109/UIC-ATC-ScalCom.2014.137

Drucker, H., Burges, C. J., Kaufman, L., Smola, A. J., & Vapnik, V. (1997). Support vector regression machines. In Advances in neural information processing systems (pp. 155-161).

Eberhart, R. C. (Ed.). (2014). *Neural network PC tools: a practical guide.* Academic Press.

Ester, M., Kriegel, H. P., Sander, J., & Xu, X. (1996, August). A density-based algorithm for discovering clusters in large spatial databases with noise. *In Proceedings of International Conference on Knowledge Discovery & Data Mining, 96*(34), 226–231.

Glorot, X., & Bengio, Y. (2010, March). Understanding the difficulty of training deep feedforward neural networks. In *Proceedings of the thirteenth international conference on artificial intelligence and statistics* (pp. 249-256).

Gonzalez, H., Han, J., Li, X., & Klabjan, D. (2006, April). Warehousing and Analyzing Massive RFID Data Sets (Vol. 6, p. 83). Oslo, Norway: ICDE. doi:10.1109/ICDE.2006.171

Goodfellow, I., Bengio, Y., & Courville, A. (2016). *Deep learning*. Cambridge, MA: MIT Press.

Gubbi, J., Buyya, R., Marusic, S., & Palaniswami, M. (2013). Internet of things (IoT): A vision, architectural elements, and future directions. *Future Generation Computer Systems*, *29*(7), 1645–1660. doi:10.1016/j.future.2013.01.010

Guyon, I., Boser, B., & Vapnik, V. (1993). Automatic capacity tuning of very large VC-dimension classifiers. In Advances in neural information processing systems (pp. 147-155).

Han, W., Gu, Y., Zhang, Y., & Zheng, L. (2014). Data driven quantitative trust model for the Internet of agricultural things. In *International Conference on the internet of things (IoT)* (pp. 31–36). Piscataway, NJ: IEEE. 10.1109/IOT.2014.7030111

He, K., Zhang, X., Ren, S., & Sun, J. (2016). Deep residual learning for image recognition. In *Proceedings of the IEEE conference on computer vision and pattern recognition* (pp. 770-778).

Hotelling, H. (1933). Analysis of a complex of statistical variables into principal components. *Journal of Educational Psychology*, *24*(6), 417–441. doi:10.1037/h0071325

Hotelling, H. (1992). Relations between two sets of variates. In *Breakthroughs in statistics* (pp. 162–190). New York, NY: Springer. doi:10.1007/978-1-4612-4380-9_14

Jagadish, H. V., Ooi, B. C., Tan, K.-L., Yu, C., & Zhang, R. (2005). Idistance: An adaptive bþ-treebased indexing method for nearest neighbor search [TODS]. *ACM Transactions on Database Systems*, *30*(2), 364–397. doi:10.1145/1071610.1071612

Jakkula, V., & Cook, D. (2010, July). Outlier detection in a smart environment structured power datasets. In *Sixth International Conference on Intelligent Environments* (pp. 29-33). Piscataway, NJ: IEEE. 10.1109/IE.2010.13

Jakkula, V. & Cook, D. (2010). Outlier detection in smart environment structured power datasets. In *Sixth International Conference on Intelligent Environments (IE)* (pp. 29–33). Piscataway, NJ: IEEE. 10.1109/IE.2010.13

Jara, A. J., Genoud, D., & Bocchi, Y. (2014, May). Big data in smart cities: from poison to human dynamics. In *28th International Conference on Advanced Information Networking and Applications Workshops* (pp. 785-790). Piscataway, NJ: IEEE. 10.1109/WAINA.2014.165

Jin Kang, J., Sdibi, S., Larkin, H., & Luan, T. (2015). Predictive data mining for Converged Internet of things: A Mobile Health perspective. *International Telecommunication Networks and Application Conference (ITNAC)*, Sydney, Australia, pp. 5-10. 10.1109/ATNAC.2015.7366781

Jolliffe, I. (2011). Principal component analysis (pp. 1094–1096). Berlin, Germany: Springer.

Jumutc, V., Langone, R., & Suykens, J. A. (2015, October). Regularized and sparse stochastic k-means for distributed large-scale clustering. In *2015 IEEE International Conference on Big Data (Big Data)* (pp. 2535-2540). Piscataway, NJ: IEEE. 10.1109/BigData.2015.7364050

Kafi, M. A., Challal, Y., Djenouri, D., Doudou, M., Bouabdallah, A., & Badache, N. (2013). A study of wireless sensor networks for urban traffic monitoring: Applications and architectures. *Procedia Computer Science, 19*, 617–626. doi:10.1016/j.procs.2013.06.082

Kafi, M. A., Challal, Y., Djenouri, D., Doudou, M., Bouabdallah, A., & Badache, N. (2013). A study of wireless sensor networks for urban traffic monitoring: Applications and architectures. *Procedia Computer Science, 19*, 617–626. doi:10.1016/j.procs.2013.06.082

Kriegel, H. P., Kröger, P., Sander, J., & Zimek, A. (2011). Density-based clustering. *Wiley Interdisciplinary Reviews. Data Mining and Knowledge Discovery, 1*(3), 231–240. doi:10.1002/widm.30

LeCun, Y., Bottou, L., Bengio, Y., & Haffner, P. (1998). Gradient-based learning applied to document recognition. *Proceedings of the IEEE, 86*(11), 2278–2324. doi:10.1109/5.726791

Li, S., Da Xu, L., & Zhao, S. (2015). The internet of things: A survey. *Information Systems Frontiers, 17*(2), 243–259. doi:10.100710796-014-9492-7

Likas, A., Vlassis, N., & Verbeek, J. J. (2003). The global k-means clustering algorithm. *Pattern Recognition, 36*(2), 451–461. doi:10.1016/S0031-3203(02)00060-2

Loh, W. Y. (2011). Classification and regression trees. *Wiley Interdisciplinary Reviews. Data Mining and Knowledge Discovery, 1*(1), 14–23. doi:10.1002/widm.8

Ma, X., Wu, Y.-J., Wang, Y., Chen, F., & Liu, J. (2013). Mining smart card data for transit riders 'travel patterns. *Transportation Research Part C, Emerging Technologies, 36*, 1–12. doi:10.1016/j.trc.2013.07.010

McCallum, A. & Nigam, K. (1998, July). A comparison of event models for naive bayes text classification. In AAAI-98 workshop on learning for text categorization, 752(1), (pp. 41-48).

Monekosso, D. N., & Remagnino, P. (2013). Data reconciliation in a smart home sensor network. *Expert Systems with Applications, 40*(8), 3248–3255. doi:10.1016/j.eswa.2012.12.037

Montenegro, G., Kushalnagar, N., Hui, J., & Culler, D. (2007). Transmission of IPv6 packets over IEEE 802.15. 4 networks (No. RFC 4944).

Montgomery, D. C., Peck, E. A., & Vining, G. G. (2012). *Introduction to linear regression analysis* (Vol. 821). Hoboken, NJ: John Wiley & Sons.

Murphy, K. P. (2012). *Machine learning: a probabilistic perspective*. Cambridge, MA: MIT Press.

Neter, J., Kutner, M. H., Nachtsheim, C. J., & Wasserman, W. (1996). *Applied linear statistical models* (Vol. 4). Chicago, IL: Irwin.

Ni, P., Zhang, C., & Ji, Y. (2014, August). A hybrid method for short-term sensor data forecasting in Internet of things. In *11th International Conference on Fuzzy Systems and Knowledge Discovery (FSKD)* (pp. 369-373). Piscataway, NJ: IEEE. 10.1109/FSKD.2014.6980862

Ni, P., Zhang, C., & Ji, Y. (2014). A hybrid method for short-term sensor data forecasting in Internet of Things. In *11th International Conference on Fuzzy Systems and Knowledge Discovery (FSKD)*. 10.1109/FSKD.2014.6980862

Chiuchisan, I. U. L. I. A. N. A. & Geman, O. A. N. A. (2014). An Approach of a Decision Support and Home Monitoring System for Patients with Neurological Disorders Using Internet of things Concepts. *WSEAS Transaction on Systems*, *13*, 460–469.

Özdemir, A. T., & Barshan, B. (2014). Detecting Falls with Wearable Sensors Using Machine Learning Techniques. *Sensors (Basel)*, *14*(6), 10691–10708. doi:10.3390140610691 PMID:24945676

Pearson, K. (1901). LIII. On lines and planes of closest fit to systems of points in space. *The London, Edinburgh and Dublin Philosophical Magazine and Journal of Science*, *2*(11), 559–572. doi:10.1080/14786440109462720

Prasad, A. M., Iverson, L. R., & Liaw, A. (2006). Newer classification and regression tree techniques: Bagging and random forests for ecological prediction. *Ecosystems (New York, N.Y.)*, *9*(2), 181–199. doi:10.100710021-005-0054-1

Qin, Y., Sheng, Q. Z., Falkner, N. J., Dustdar, S., Wang, H., & Vasilakos, A. V. (2016). When things matter: A survey on data-centric internet of things. *Journal of Network and Computer Applications*, *64*, 137–153. doi:10.1016/j.jnca.2015.12.016

Rätsch, G., Mika, S., Schölkopf, B., & Müller, K. R. (2002). Constructing boosting algorithms from SVMs: An application to one-class classification. *IEEE Transactions on Pattern Analysis and Machine Intelligence*, *24*(9), 1184–1199. doi:10.1109/TPAMI.2002.1033211

Schölkopf, B., Platt, J. C., Shawe-Taylor, J., Smola, A. J., & Williamson, R. C. (2001). Estimating the support of a high-dimensional distribution. *Neural Computation*, *13*(7), 1443–1471. doi:10.1162/089976601750264965 PMID:11440593

Scholkopf, B., & Smola, A. J. (2001). *Learning with kernels: support vector machines, regularization, optimization, and beyond*. Cambridge, MA: MIT Press.

Seber, G. A., & Lee, A. J. (2012). *Linear regression analysis* (Vol. 329). Hoboken, NJ: John Wiley & Sons.

Shilton, A., Rajasegarar, S., Leckie, C., & Palaniswami, M. (2015). A dynamic planar one-class support vector machine for internet of things environment. In *International Conference on Recent Advances in Internet of things (RIoT)*. Piscataway, NJ: IEEE. pp. 1–6. 10.1109/RIOT.2015.7104904

Shukla, M., Kosta, Y., & Chauhan, P. (2015). Analysis and evaluation of outlier detection algorithms in data streams. In *International Conference on Computer, Communication and Control (IC4) (pp. 1–8)*. Piscataway, NJ: IEEE.

Smola, A. J., & Schölkopf, B. (2004). A tutorial on support vector regression. *Statistics and Computing*, *14*(3), 199–222. doi:10.1023/B:STCO.0000035301.49549.88

Souza, A. M., & Amazonas, J. R. (2015). An outlier detect algorithm using big data processing and internet of things architecture. *Procedia Computer Science*, *52*, 1010–1015. doi:10.1016/j.procs.2015.05.095

Souza, A. M., & Amazonas, J. R. (2015). An outlier detect algorithm using big data processing and internet of things architecture. *Procedia Computer Science*, *52*, 1010–1015. doi:10.1016/j.procs.2015.05.095

Toshniwal, D. (2013, February). Clustering techniques for streaming data-a survey. In *3rd IEEE International Advance Computing Conference (IACC)* (pp. 951-956). Piscataway, NJ: IEEE.

Toshniwal, D. (2013). Clustering techniques for streaming data-a survey. In IEEE 3rd International Advance Computing Conference (IACC). Piscataway, NJ: IEEE. pp. 951–956.

Tsai, C. W., Lai, C. F., Chiang, M. C., & Yang, L. T. (2013). Data mining for the internet of things: A survey. *IEEE Communications Surveys and Tutorials, 16*(1), 77–97. doi:10.1109/SURV.2013.103013.00206

Zanella, A., Bui, N., Castellani, A., Vangelista, L., & Zorzi, M. (2014). Internet of things for smart cities. IEEE Internet of things journal, 1(1), 22-32.

Zhang, H. (2004). The optimality of naive Bayes. AA, 1(2), 3.

Chapter 4
Wireless Body Area Networks:
Requirements, Characteristics, Design Consideration, and Challenges

M. Sridhar
Bharathiar University, India

N. Priya
Bharathiar University, India

A. Muniyappan
Bharathiar University, India

ABSTRACT

Wireless body area networks (WBANs) are valuable solutions for healthcare lifestyle monitoring applications which allow the continuous screening of health data and constant access to patients despite their current locality or activity, with a fraction of the cost of regular face-to-face examination. In such environments, entities are equipped with intelligence-embedded devices to collect data for providing pervasive information. WBANs can serve as passing reference for huge audience instance systems for architects, practitioners, developers, medical engineers, etc. In particular for the medical field, devices fixed inside the human body measure and transfer real-time data to the caregiver through the communication network. Many technologies have showed their efficiency in secondary WBANs application such as biofeedback, remote sensing, and QoS requirement. This chapter highlights the major applications, design, and security of WBAN.

OVERVIEW OF WIRELESS SENSOR NETWORKS AND AD-HOC NETWORKS

Wireless Sensor Networks (WSN) is a group of sensors that can be linked through a wired or wireless medium. Typically a wireless sensor network contains hundreds and thousands of sensor nodes which have to provide limitless future potential. The sensor nodes are fortified with sensing and computing devices, radio transceivers and power components. A single node in a wireless sensor network (WSN) is

DOI: 10.4018/978-1-7998-1090-2.ch004

fundamentally resource constrained: they have limited in processing speed, storage capacity, and communication bandwidth it is necessary to understand the architecture before deploying it in an application for this kind of networks. After the sensor nodes are deployed, they are liable for self-organizing and appropriate network infrastructure that often with multi-hop communication subsequently the onboard sensors start collecting information of interest. The sensors are permissible to communicate within its communication range using radio signals which contain one sink (or) base station able to handle all communication in the network (ChiaraBuratti, 2009). A sensor network must be able to manage under the unstable environment because in most cases, the sensor network must be operating unattended. Once the nodes have booted up and a network is formed, most of the nodes will be able to maintain a steady state of the operation and the working mode of the sensor nodes may be either continuous or event drove in a WSN. Wireless sensor networks (WSNs) enable new applications and require non-conventional paradigms for protocol design due to several constraints. On the other hand, a Wireless Adhoc network is a decentralized type of wireless network which can be used in many applications, ranging from sensors for the environment, vehicular communications, road safety, home, peer-to-peer messaging, disaster rescue operations, and robots. An ad-hoc network is a self-configuring network of wireless links connecting mobile nodes these nodes may be routers and/or hosts. The mobile nodes communicate directly with each other and without the aid of access point and therefore have no fixed infrastructure (C.Sandhiya, p. 2018). Considering all the intelligent properties of both the wireless and ad-hoc network can be combined together for developing many real-time fusion applications.

APPLICATION OF WIRELESS SENSOR NETWORK

Wireless Sensor Networks have gained substantial popularity due to their flexibility in solving problems in different application domains and have the potential to change our lives in many different ways through applications like:

Military Applications: Wireless Sensor Networks are an indispensable component of a military command, control, communication, computing, intelligence, battlefield surveillance, investigation and targeting systems. In Particularly battlefield surveillance critical areas and borders can be closely monitored using sensors to attain information about the attacks. Tracking military vehicles, sniper localization and self-healing is also the portion of the battlefield surveillance.

Area Monitoring: Deployment of sensor nodes over a region is performed based on some phenomenal monitorization. When the sensors notice the event being monitored (heat, pressure, etc), the event is stated to one of the base stations, which then takes suitable action. Especially in the greenhouses, the sensors are used to control the humidity levels.

Transportation: Real-time traffic information is being composed byWSNs to alert drivers about congestion and traffic problems as notification via mobile applications to avoid collision and queueing.

Health Applications: Wireless Sensor Networks help in supporting interfaces for the disabled, integrated patient monitoring, diagnostics, and drug administration in hospitals, Tele-monitoring of human physiological data, and tracking & monitoring doctors or patients inside a hospital.

Tele-Monitoring Human Physiological Data: The biological data collected by the sensor networks could be stored for a long period of time, and used for medical investigation when it is required for the patient's treatment (Sinha A, 2001).

Tracking and Monitoring Doctors and Patients Inside a Hospital: Each patient has a sensor node to continuous observation for the purpose of guiding management decision and assessment. Each sensor node has its own specific task to perform example: sensing the pulse rate, blood pressure, etc. Diversely doctors can also carry a sensor node, which allows the doctor to locate them within the hospital.

Drug Administration in Hospitals: If sensor nodes can be attached to medication, the chance of getting and prescribing the wrong medication to patients can be minimized. Thus if the patients will have sensor nodes that identify their allergies and required medication

Environmental Sensing: This is the stretch to cover many applications of WSNs to earth science research. This includes sensing volcanoes, oceans, glaciers, forests, etc. Some of the other applications are:

Civilian Environments: Monitoring and managing a large set of environmental data including climatic, atmospheric, plant and soil parameters since the environmental bootprint of military operations remains considerable.

Emergency Rescue Operations: WSN has the potential for enormous impact on many aspects of disaster response and emergency care includes fire and severe weather events that can be forecast hours before they arrive.

WIRELESS BODY AREA NETWORK (WBAN)

The rapid increase in biological sensors, low-power integrated circuits, and wireless communication has empowered a novel generation of wireless sensor networks, nowadays used for the purpose such as monitoring traffic, crops, infrastructure, and health. The body area network field is a specific area which could agree to low-priced and continuous health monitoring with real-time updates of medical records through the Internet. Body Area Network (BAN) or Wireless Body Area Network (WBAN) was a wearable computing device it has emerged from the basic idea of sensor network and biomedical engineering(Jin-Xin Hu, 2017). More or fewer WBANs used in health care and welfare related applications it was developed for the motive of finding chronic diseases in the human body. The main determination of these networks remains to transmit the data produced by the wearable devices outwardly to a WLAN or the internet. A number of intellectual physiological sensors can be pooled into a wearable WBAN, which can be used to detect medical situations. For instance, a patient can be equipped with a WBAN consisting of a sensor that continuously measures specific biological functions such as temperature, blood pressure, heart rate, and respiration. This area may rely on the possibility of implanting a very small biosensor classified the human body and the fixed sensors in the human body will gather various physiological dissimilarities in order to observe the status of the patient's health in peak circumstances the information will be conveyed wirelessly to the peripheral processing unit. The BAN device will rapidly transfer all the data to the doctors. If an emergency is perceived, the doctors will immediately inform the health position of the patient through the PC via sending a particular note. This kind of network typically expanded for the whole human body and the nodes are connected through a wireless communication channel. An authoritative phase in the development of a WBAN is the depiction of a network, including an assessment of the delay spread and the path loss between two nodes in the body.

Figure 1. Depiction of wireless body area network (WBAN) (Karthick G.S, Pankajavalli P.B 2016)

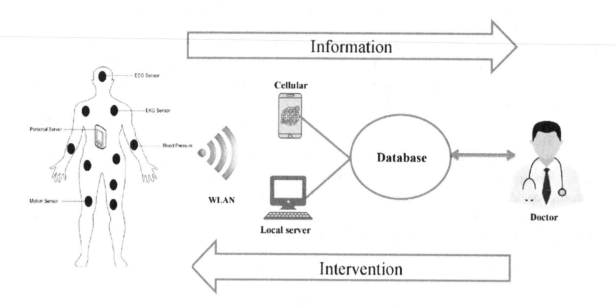

REQUIREMENTS FOR WIRELESS MEDICAL SENSOR IN WBANS

A WBAN is a short-range wireless network so different types of wireless short-range technologies like Bluetooth, Zigbee, WI-FI can be involved in different stages like monitoring and transmitting the patient information to the caregiver. The range of network will not compromise the performance of the BAN that Wireless medical sensor should satisfy the following requirements such as(Md. Taslim Arefin1*, 2017)

Wearability

To achieve non–invasive and unobtrusive continuous monitoring the sensors are connected to the deployed network through the nearest fixed devise, therefore it provides information about the patient's position and displacement for that the sensors must be lightweight and small in size. The battery capacity of the sensor is directly proportional to its size.

Reliability

Reliable communication in WBANs is predominant for any of its application. So the designer should target a reliable communication and technique which will ensure uninterrupted communication and optimal throughput especially for self-adaptive and resilient of the WSN.

Security

Security is another important requirement while working with a body area network. All wireless medical sensors must meet the requirements of privacy and ensure data integrity, confidentiality, and authentication. Confidentiality is highly considerable required one by the patient because sensitive medical information is necessary to preserve the patient's dignity.

Interoperability

Wireless Medical Sensors should allow users to easily build a strapping WBAN. Standards governing that interaction of wireless medical sensors will help vendor competition and eventually lead to more accessible systems. Interoperability models focused on metadata and allow design the modules with several levels depending on the purpose.

APPLICATION OF WIRELESS MEDICAL SENSOR IN WBANS

Wireless Body Area Networks (WBANs) are the prominent solutions that can be used in healthcare, monitoring applications, enabling continuous screening of health data and constant access to patients regardless of their current location or motion and with a fraction of the cost of a regular face-to-face examination. Some of the wireless medical sensors are offered to users in different forms devices like (Lee & Chung, 2009)

- ECGs
- Pulse Oximetry
- Blood Pressure Devices
- Insulin Pumps and
- Blood Glucose can be coupled with wireless and wearable communication sensors

Particularly, ECG monitor system can be conveniently integrated into a sensor network, with heart activity data captured and monitored by wearable circuitry (on-body segment) and wirelessly transmitted to a nearby listening device (off-body segment).

Pulse Oximeters: Non-invasively measure the percentage of oxygen in hemoglobin proteins, called oxygen saturation. Oxygen saturation usually directs how much oxygen is getting to the organs. Normal oxygen saturation levels are between 95 percent to 100. Pulse oximeters are clip-on devices that can be attached to a finger, a wrist, a foot, or any other area where they can read blood flow and measure oxygen saturation.

Blood Pressure device is designed to measure human blood pressure. It measures systolic, diastolic and means arterial pressure using the oscillometric technique. The pulse rate will be also reported.

Insulin Pump is a medical device used for the supervision of insulin in the treatment of diabetes. Insulin Pump is an alternative to multiple daily injections of insulin by insulin syringes or an insulin pen. The device configuration may vary depending on the design.

To effectively deploy a WBAN for performing long term and continuous healthcare monitoring that the wearable devices should be small and lightweight, in case they are too intrusive on the patient's lifestyle.

MAIN CHARACTERISTICS OF WBAN FOR CLINICAL USE

In this context, WBAN supporting healthcare applications can offer valuable contributions to improve patient healthcare, including diagnosis and/or therapeutic monitoring. In a short time, WBAN technology has taken its first steps in the medical rehabilitation and monitoring of patients. WBANs for healthcare applications are mostly used in patient monitoring tasks. The characteristics of the WBAN radio propagation are dynamic due to the motion of the human body(Akramalomainy, 2014)The inherent characteristics of RF attenuation in and around the human body can have a direct impact on channel conditions. In this type of network, the sensors are distributed on the human body measuring different physiological parameters, which represent the most widely used solution within this domain. Generally, the composition of the human body tissue has different amounts of water. Because of this, the propagation of electromagnetic signals through the human body is variable and subject to absorption and reflections within the body. Consequently, the propagating wave diffracts around the human body rather than passing through it. The transmission power for on-body transmission for a wireless link depends on the physical detachment of the link and its instantaneous channel condition. Additionally, patient mobility and posture can have a significant effect on efficient packet delivery. Following are the few underlying characteristics which fulfill the requirements in the clinical use of the WBAN (de Schatz, 2011)(luisfilipe, 2015).

- Network quality of service (QoS): it is essential for medical data to be transmitted and received without error and within a constructive time.
- Fault tolerance: In case a sensor node stops working, a back-up node in the immediate neighborhood can take on the role of that node so that critical measurements are not missed.
- Minimal weight, miniature form-factor, low power operation, simplified integration into a WBAN, standards-based interface protocols, and patient-specified calibration, tuning, and customization.
- Medical data transfers require encryption of all perceptive information associated with personal health.
- The latent of WBANs that can only be fully explored, if they are interoperated securely and impeccably.
- Interoperability should take place at the neighborhood level among the WBANs of a given patient and surrounding environmental sensors.

IMPLANTABLE WIRELESS BODY AREA NETWORK (IWBAN)

An IWBAN is comparable to BAN, but it may consist of one or two sensors implanted hooked on a patient's body that communicate posterior to a central controlling device. A BAN consists of a number of electronic devices mounted on a person's body or clothing that collect, process and store data with a central controlling device in which IWBAN have ended it possible to incessantly accomplish and treat a number of health conditions. Communications over implanted devices are generally accomplished by a wired construction or wireless radiofrequency (RF) telemetry. However, wires are able to break and it became disease-ridden or it introduces noise in the recording through movement by antenna effects. (Mehmet R. Yuce& Steven W. P. Ng &Naung L. Myo&Jamil Y. Khan &Wentai Liu, n.d) In addition, implantable strategies can be used to generate neural signals in brain-machine boundaries to control prostheses or paralyzed. Intrabody communication is a recently developed alternative method of wireless communication, which uses the conductive properties of the body to transmit signals. Generally, two co-dependent communications are followed in the implantable device, one is implanted to implant communication here signals are communicated as of the implanted device to receiver electrodes also implanted inside the body (Redish, 2011). The implanted receiver can then be associated with the equipment and also outer surface of the body using a short wire or with wireless RF telemetry. In this way, less energy is required to transmit towards the implanted receiver electrodes just before transmitting to electrodes on the skin. However, the implanted receiver electrodes cannot be repositioned without troubled as skin-mounted receiver electrodes. Another one is implant-to-surface communication; galvanic coupling is used to send signals from an implanted device to electrodes on the skin. The purpose of implanted communication is to focus on tranquil placement and repositioning of the skin electrodes to improve the quality of signal reaction. For an implanted sensor or other implanted system to be effective, it must be possible to communicate with it and to find out the human incident by the single movement. This is the best way to do without surgical intervention for obvious reasons. Because with the wires emerging through the skin that could cause infection. To avoid the particular kind of situations it was typically achieved by launching an electromagnetic wave, known as a carrier wave (modulation). For example, a viable FM radio station practices a small variation in the carrier wave frequency, hence Frequency Modulation (FM) to deliver music or voice to the receiver. Electromagnetic waves are located to launched and captured using antennas. Similarly, Antennas placed inside the body presented by the designer with a number of additional problems are not associated with the in-air antenna.

A MODULAR FRAMEWORK FOR HEALTHCARE MONITORING SYSTEMS

The medical applications of remote sensor systems plan to improve the current social insurance and checking administrations particularly for the older, children and constantly sick. There are a few advantages accomplished with these frameworks. The authorizations of wireless monitoring emergency conditions for in risk patients will turn out to be simple and the general population with various degrees of physical incapacities will be empowered to have a progressively free and modest life. In health applications real-time system (M. Philipose.,et al 2004)some idleness is permitted Recognizing crisis circumstances like a heart attack or unexpected falls in almost no time or even minutes will do the trick for sparing lives thinking about that, without them there conditions won't be distinguished by any stretch of the imagination. So long providing real-time monitoring and achievements are the main benefits and technologically accessible items. The major current arrangements incorporate one or more kinds of sensors carried by the patient, shaping a Body Area Network (BAN), and at least one kind of sensors carried in the earth framing a Personal Area System (PAN). The overview of a simple wireless sensor network application condition is described in Fig. 3. They can successfully be utilizedTable.1 shows the design consideration healthcare monitoring system.

UNOBTRUSIVE BODY AREA NETWORK

The effective Body Area Network Subsystem is the ad-hoc sensor network and tags that the disable persons like a blind person, children, patients with a speech disorder, monitoring biological signals of the human body and the older portable luggage their body. The RFID tag, Electro Cardio Gram

Figure 2. Targeted areas for implantable wireless body area network (IWBAN) (Philip Catherwood, 2016)

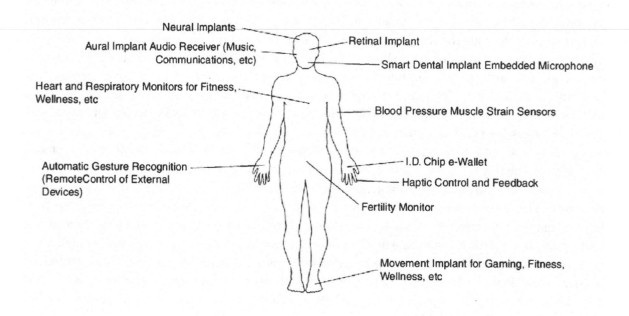

Figure 3. Overview of Sensor Network Architecture

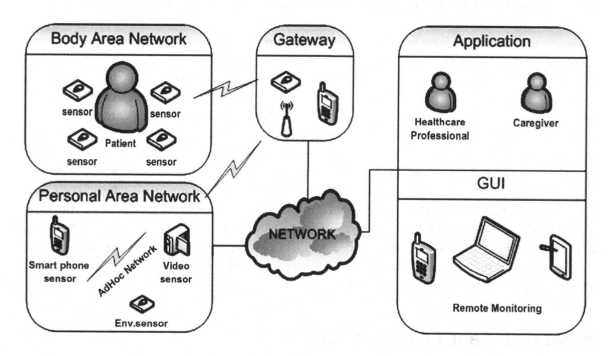

Table1.The structure of table design consideration of healthcare monitoring is observing frameworks.

Subsystem	Design consideration
unobtrusive Body area network	Power consumption, Transmission power, Unobtrusiveness, Portability, Real-time accessibility, Solid interchanges, Multi-hop routing, Security.
The wireless personal network subsystem	Energy efficiency, Scalability, Self-organization between the nodes
The entryway to the wide area network	Congestion prevention.
Wide area networks	The data rate, Reliable communication protocols, Secure data transmission, Coverage.
The end-user medicinal services checking framework	Privacy, Reliability, User-friendliness, Middleware design, ScalabilityInteroperability.

(ECG) sensors, also (D. Bhatia., et al 2007), heart rate, are the mechanisms of the body area network. Continuously keep up less obstruction between all sensor nodes embedded in or on the body including inward body fat, temperature radiation of warmness between encompassing sensor gadgets or other by the outside remote body zone arrange for solid transmission. In body area network system is designed into MACprotocolfor analysis and monitoring.MAC protocol is created for raising the execution of the corresponding standard.

Power Consumption

BAN is the power utilization and transmission control are changing the batteries is a significant issue for assignment. Along with the improvement of imperativeness powerful Medium Access Control (MAC) shows and essentialness capable sensor devices are fundamental. The greater (ByoungHoon., et al, 2013) part of the advancements Bluetooth and Wi-Fi consistently support and come up short into vitality productivity framework. The most ideal usage of the remote correspondence channels in the midst of directing ensures imperativeness viability by using very low power Pyroelectric Infra-Red (PIR) sensors. An effective to improve the healthcare monitoring system.

Unobtrusiveness

Unobtrusiveness needs to be arranged (A.T. Barth., et al 2009)a kind of ECG sensor is remotely planned by chest band checking. This sensor checking to perceiving the region thus reliably work and assemble data from sensors for up to eight days without supplanting the battery. The basic thought is to take the power overhead from the sensors, moving it to the respectably control satisfactory prosperity checking chest band.

Portability

Compactness is contemplations for the physical plan of such sensors wearable BAN gadget all occasions and versatility not decrease. The sensors gadget is intended for giving the high movability to patients. The gadget is imparting for advances RFID, ECG information and real movement information to IEEE

802.15.4 interface with the specially appointed system. The shirt (Y.D. Lee., et al 2009)comprises of sensors for continuous communicating health monitoring data and fabrics to get the body motion terminals.

Real-Time Accessibility

The real-time accessibility and dependable interchanges have planned a wearable fall identification framework that can identify the falls with a normal lead-time of 700 ms before the happens. The execution results demonstrate that dependable message transmission and low checking delays can be accomplished by utilizing multicast or communicate based routing plans in a specially appointed system. Constant observing of the patient's ECG without range limit because of the all-inclusive correspondence inclusion by multi-bounce remote availability is one of the fundamental requirements for such basic applications.

Solid Interchanges

The Solid interchanges system has to designed with a wearable device and fall identification background that can recognize the falls identification. The sensor communicates with normal (D. Morris., et al 2009) time of 700ms. The reliable system to improve the high levels of data and low delays performance are monitoring. The dependable message is sent to low-level checking and deferrals with the help of utilizing multicast routing plans in a specially appointed system.

Multi-Hop Routing

The multi-hop system is most important to routing protocol designing process. It is continuous monitoring of Patient's ECG without range is protected with communication on multi-hop wireless network. The basic need for design consideration such a basic application.

Security

The key security necessities of the overall system Responsibility, Accessibility, Access control, and Confidentiality. Encryption methods can be used which raises the challenge of developing efficient to enhance the protocols and identifying to decrease energy consumption.

WIRELESS PERSONAL AREA NETWORK

In these networks, the subsystem is made out of natural sensors sent around and portable or traveling gadgets that have a place to the patient. The natural sensors like RFID temperature, camcorders, pressure, or sound, weight, glow, and stickiness sensors help to give rich logical data about the general population to be checked. The Personal Assistant gadget that bolsters interchanges with medicinal gadgets, specifically a glucometer, an insulin taps, and a ceaseless glucose sensor, is available. The PDA gadgets can be controlled with the joining of new functionalities help us to health monitoring. The coordinate and easy to use give to the patients. RFID labeled articles are additionally significant for this subsystem. MAC protocol (I.E. Lamprinos, et al 2005) is providing and improve with energy efficiency by giving the prevention of utilization of sources and control outspending.

Energy Efficiency

Energy efficiency is directing communicate with MANETs manage to discover courses to limit energy utilization in cases with little energy assets. The required energy isn't considered to get and transmit an image over a remote connection and activities required for assessments, memory access, and information management. Energy resource(Mahima Mehta, et al 2016) must think about changes in body development, impacts of energy on tissue warming and constrained energy resources to give fit utilization of accessible assets to additionally decrease in terms of battery charging, develop organize lifetime and set up an easy to use monitoring system. Healthcare monitoring framework, by and large, requires the synchronous utilization of a few sensor devices and communication devices. Software as a benefits approach could be utilized for both scalability and simplicity of sending with small configurable sensor devices.

Self-Organization between the Nodes

The sensor nodes are considered too essential with self -organization mag. The collated sensor data are operating in mesh mode is handed-off to the Internet. The health care system can be accustomed to observing dealing with any serious conditions for patients. Self-organization system is providing to easily identify activities by peoples.

ENTRYWAY TO THE WIDE AREA NETWORKS

The gateway is designed for sensor network to give the association between the infrastructures is WANs based on connection to ad-hoc sensor networks. Gateway subsystem is carried out from users like sensor node or smartphone are organized with the environment. PAN and BAN subsystems are (W. Leister, et al 2008)connection to generally speaking weakest nearby handling system blockage by exchange information is decreased. Centex mindfulness is choosing and handling the information reasonable for information exchange locally by sending mobile.

Wide Area Networks

A wireless monitoring system depending on tracking network infrastructure is predictable for healthcare application. Wide area network systems have mindful to interfacing regular properties and systems can be interactive to the portable devices. The universal medicinal services applications additionally correspondence conventions for cutting edge remote systems. The wide area is independent of healthcare data to the reliable protocol for WAN.

Secure Data Transmission

The secure data transmission provides coverage is needed to be satellite communication to analyze telemedicine service. This application is mainly considered for healthcare or wireless locations tracks that have to the technological improvement of the organization. The secure satellites are connected easy way to deployment for healthcare application.

The End-User Medicinal Services Checking Framework

End-user application is considering about for heart of the framework. The gathered information has required activity for the end client application checking of the user interface part is triggering the crucial exercises. Continuous observing(HandeAlemdar et al 2010) application is utilized for alarming component with crisis condition is the setup of the frameworks for general conduct. Cautioning is created with the system the messages will be conveyed to the clients rather than application courses of action.

Privacy

Privacy most is important of health information is identified as comfort health monitored by people. Privacy-preserving methods are considered for processing images are transferred solution can be sent over by network. Information is controlled and transfer during the CareNet display.

Reliability

In Reliable is consider for three main categories reliable data measurement, reliable data communication, and reliable data analysis(H. Lee., et al 2008) Reliable information correspondence issues have a place with a subsystem of PAN and BAN. The examination basic information for acquiring application layer to dealing with for information cleaning and information combination.

User-Friendliness

User-friendliness among a little older and the elder group concluded that boundary to be returned. The different groups for the requirement to identify the clear ought to be distinguished clearly. These applications are helping us to patients with a user interface for the handicapped for instance and different interaction patients with diabetes.

Middleware Design

The high-level functionality enhancing the behavior of healthcare application combination of different models and make a necessary software development. Middleware configuration is tackled to solve the problems and capture several applications as easy to plug and play the medical sensor network.

Scalability

Healthcare monitoring framework, by and large, requires the synchronous utilization of a few sensor devices and communication devices. Software as a benefits approach could be utilized for both scalability and simplicity of sending with small configurable sensor devices. The user interface is based on disabilities and kids based on voice must avoid any kind of particular skills. In this framework observing the alternative situation a patient activity and under people observation in a specific domain.

Interoperability

The interoperability is designed with different communication on the healthcare system. In a combination of several sensing devices are connected with different ranges rises a various issue. Communication between different protocols and multiples devices are occupied, different bands.

Context-awareness

Context–awareness can provide different sensors modules and various techniques are considering for analyzing data. Remote sensor systems information empowers organized data to be translated all the more obviously. So the system can provide taking of reducing the complexity with monitoring, and anywhere with anybody to taking corrective actions.Fig.4 shows the overall architecture of the design.

WIRELESS SENSING SYSTEM FOR HEALTHCARE APPLICATIONS

In a recent advance, the Wireless Sensor Networks (WSNs) are considered as one of the wide research in the computer field and healthcare applications. The enveloping healthcare systems provide wealthy background information and alerting mechanism next to odd conditions with regular monitoring. It reduces the work for caregivers and helps the constantly ill and elder people to survive a self-governing life.

Body sensor network system helps the people by providing specialized healthcare services such as memory augmentation, medical monitoring, medical data access, and emergency communication. Daily monitoring of patients using wearable and implantable body sensor systems will support early detection of emergency conditions in at-risk patients and additionally provides the extensive range of healthcare services.

Physiological Monitoring: The physiological data from sensor networks might be saved for a long period of time, and can be utilized for medical investigations when required. Furthermore, the installed sensors can be used to monitor the behavior of elderly persons. WBAN is used in various applications like firefighters, policemen and also it is an extension of WSNs application, but there are recognizable differences between WBAN and WSNs ((XiaolingXu, 2009.). Compared with wireless networks, the WBAN has some exceptional features.

Node Deployment and Density: The nodes of WBAN are arranged on the patient body or hiding under the clothes and it not resolution the lost node difficult by accumulating redundant nodes which is common in WSNs design. These rooted sensor nodes are very challenging to charge and replace. The other wearable sensor nodes are also offensive to the patient body.

Limited Energy: In this, WBANs are used to monitor the body's physiological activities they usually arise in periodically, so the flow of data shows moderately constant frequency. Each node in WBANs will communicate with various target parameters acquisition and direct the different frequency and data diffusion rate, so it includes high energy consumption. Signal transmission concession is huge because of the specificity of the body tissue so it can cause a massive loss of a diffused signal.

Delay: The delay is related to the constancy and energy consumption it is problematic to substitute the batteries because of the environment affects the nodes which are arranged in WBANs. The power control is highly challenging due to the energy consumption of node requirements. The coverage communication of WBANs nodes are miniature than mobile phones so aggregate the battery duration is essential, even at the high delay.

Mobility and Security: WSN nodes are frequently assumed as a stationary; WBANs node will assign with the user activity. In wireless signal spreads in the body or surface of the body, it requires to reproduce the safety, reliability and long term operational ability of the human body.

TYPES OF DEVICES USED IN WBAN

Sensor Node

A device that reacts to and collects the data on the physical stimuli, processes the data if it essential and reports this information wirelessly. It contains several components like sensor hardware, processor, transmitter or transceiver.

Actuator Node

It acts according to data received from the sensors or through communication with the user. The components of an actuator are the same as the sensors: actuator hardware.

Personal Device (PD)

A device that collects all the data acquired by the sensors and actuators and updates the user via a peripheral gateway, an actuator or a display LEDs on the device. The mechanisms are power unit, memory, and transceiver and it is also called as Body Control Unit (BCU).

There are several types of sensors and actuators are used in WBANs. The main objective use of all these devices is to be invented in an area of health applications.

Motion and Acting Monitoring: Each patient has a small sensor node attached to them. Sensors are different based upon their functions and every sensor node has a unique task to perform. For example, one sensor node can detect the blood pressure while another node is detecting the heart rate. Physicians can use the sensor node to locate them within the hospital.

Large Scale Physiological and Behavior Studies: Body-worn sensors with sensor-equipped Internet-connected smartphones have started to modernize medical and general health research by assisting behavioral and physiological data to be constantly collected from a huge number of distributed subjects as they lead their everyday lives.

HEALTHCARE MONITORING SYSTEM FOR CHRONIC AND ELDERLY PATIENTS

WBAN has played a vital role in the technology that is able to accomplish giving the best approaches to analyze various risky diseases. This technology works in real time to monitor the health condition of patients. WBAN is a wild emerging technology, therefore, numerous concerns are essential to be addressed until now. In WBAN either sensor network on a band or various sensors are damaged by a

Table 2. Security issues in WBAN

Requirements	Requirements Description
Data confidentiality	It secures data from unauthorized user.
Data Authentication	It is used to identify the correct node.
Data Integrity	It is an adversary and alters data will be insecure over the transmission.
Data Freshness	It is essential for data confidentiality and integrity.
Secure Management	In this management, BNC adds and removes the BNs in a secure manner.
Availability	It is used to protect against an event encounter network.

patient. With a large number of elderly people is eager to live self-sufficiently, it could be helpful to monitor their behavior and to check in real time health conditions. Also, it could be essential to have automatic systems that adapt the environmental conditions to the people health status. Such a system should inform the family or the doctor about the possible critical health conditions, and should be able to send alarms to the hospital including the user health data and the best path to rescue the patient if the conditions are very critical.

SECURITY ISSUES, ATTACKS AND VULNERABILITIES IN WBAN

In general, the qualities of an application are expected to construct a robust security mechanism, which preserves the system from potential security issues. The fundamental security supplies in WBAN are described below, (ShahnazSaleem, 2011).

An important part of the healthcare structure, WBANs should deal with address privacy concerns. The idea of data in WBANs makes privacy and security troublesome. It is essential to manage this issue when the node is compromised or falls level. The security necessities in WBANs are discussed below.

Data Confidentiality: To protect the data from disclosure, the system requires data confidentiality. In communication, there is a possibility of catching and spying the sensitive information by the adversary. Encoding the data with a secret key and sharing the secret key through a secured channel is one of the ways to attain confidentiality.

Data Authentication: Applications with both medical and non-medical application needs data authentication. Each BN and BNC needs to check whether the data is transmitted by the trusted sensor or by the adversary. The symmetric method can be utilized in a WBAN to accomplish data authentication. It shares the secret key to Compute the Message Authentication Code (MAC) for all data.

Data Integrity: Data integrity is essential as a challenger can change the data that is transmitted over a diffident channel. Absence of data integrity technique gives a way to the challenger to modify the information before it reaches the BNC. Data integrity is achieved through data authentication protocols, which guarantees that the received data is not changed by the adversary.

Data Freshness: The data freshness technique is vital to guarantee data secrecy and integrity. The adversary may frustrate the BNC by taking data amid transmission and retransmit sit later. Data freshness guarantees the novelty of information. In another word, it checks the procedure of data frames. Strong freshness and weak freshness are the two sorts of data freshness.

Secure Management: As BNC, distribution of keys to BNs to accomplish encryption and decryption techniques, it demands secure management. The BNC includes and evacuates the BNs in a secure manner on account of association and disassociation.

Availability: It ensures that the patient's information is available to the doctor. This availability can be demolished by the adversary by impairing an ECG mode. This may prompt basic circumstance, for example, loss of life. Amid the loss of availability, a technique is required to keep the operation of the BNs and change the operation to another BN (ZigBee Alliance, 2005).

In addition to the fundamental security prerequisites like integrity protection, confidentiality, and authentication certain different objectives should be met. It incorporates:

Efficiency: A basic part of a BSN's design is energy-efficiency as a result of the limited capabilities of sensors. The continuous monitoring prerequisites of a BSN can be impeded by the frequent energy depletion even though the sensors are rechargeable.

Usability: The security solutions for BSN must be useable. The usable security arrangements are characterized which are activated on employment in plug-n-play method with negligible initialization systems (C. Karlof, 2004).

Available Solutions

Emerging security approaches in WBANs. Listed below

IEEE 802.15.4 SECURITY

The IEEE 802.15.4 is a low-power protocol commonly used for the low data rate requests and it offers three operational frequency bands such as 915MHz, 868MHz, and 2.4 GHz bands. It includes twenty-seven subchannels and security modes in IEEE 802.15.4 might be divided into two major modes as unbound mode and the validated model. The unbound mode essentially indicates the no security suite has been chosen. The first of these is the Null suite which offers no security. The validation mode can be categorized relies upon the security properties. There are several security groups performed under the IEEE 802.15.4 standard. The security suite mode is split into two basic strategies that are unsecured mode and secured mode. The IEEE 802.15.4 security suites are indexed below.

ZigBee Security Services

ZigBee is a consortium of industry players which met up to characterize another standard for ultra-low power remote communication (Hatzinakos, 2008.). The ZigBee network layer (NWK) is deliberate to effort over the IEEE 802.15.4 limited by MAC and physical layers. The ZigBee normally defines the supplementary of security services which include methods for key conversion and verification, as well as security services of IEEE 802.15.4, upon which it is built.

TinySec

TinySec is planned as a security solution in a biomedical sensor network to complete the link- layer encryption and data authentication. Tiny Sec (ShahnazSaleem S. U., 2009) is a software-based security architecture that executes link-layer encryption. It is a part of the official Tiny OS release. TinySec is

Table 3. IEEE 802.15.4 Security Suites

Name	Description
Null	No Security
AES-CTR	It offers access control, optional sequential freshness and data encryption
AES-CBCMAC-128 AES-BCMAC-64 AES-BCMAC-32	Authentication only allowing flexibility by the selection of various MAC lengths: 32,64,128 bits.
AES-CCM-128 AES-CCM-64 AES-CCM-32	Encryption and Authentication allowing flexibility by various MAC lengths: 32, 64, 128 bits.

extremely prominent in the remote sensor network and has even been executed on an assortment of custom hardware.

The TinySec encodes the data packet through a group key which is shared to the sensor nodes and computes a communication authentication code (MAC) for the complete packet including the header. This group key is a common network-wide and physically programmed into the nodes earlier to deployment. This network-wide key displays a single point of vulnerability. Tiny Sec does not defend against node capture. If a node cooperates and keying material is exposed to the entire network can be bargained.

Biometrics

Biometrics has developed as a helpful component to use in the key foundation and validation of body sensor nodes. (ShahnazSaleem S. U., 2011) This strategy utilizes estimation of physiological qualities of the body itself as an imperative parameter in a symmetric key management system. When estimation of insufficient physiological signs can be exploited for biometrics, the ECG (electrocardiogram), and the progress data of heart pulses, that is, interpulse interval (IPI), are among the greatest suitable since they display is fit in the time difference and uncertainty. Presently there exist low-cost sensor devices for health applications that can record appropriate biometric physiological signs. This could imply that in some present and future WBANs the extra framework prerequisite for implementing a biometric-based system would be practically irrelevant.

CONCLUSION

In this chapter, the major applications, design, and security of WBAN are a highlight. The main aim of Wireless Body Area Network is to provide suitable and appropriate sensor network to operate autonomously. This network connects several medical sensors, medical applications, and appliances which are all located inside or outside of the human body. WBANs allow constant monitoring of patients by using the WBAN based devices and medical applications. WBAN allows the early detection and prevention of several kinds of diseases. This technology had shown a greater impact on the medical field. It had shown key developments in the quality of human's day to day life. In summary, practical research on this valuable technology has shown significant usage of available resources. In the future, several advanced methods being used on different devices and different sources of information being exploited depending on the computing abilities to ensure all the requirements by the portable or wearable devices.

REFERENCES

Alemdar, H., & Ersoy, C. (2010). Wireless sensor networks for healthcare: A survey. *Computer Networks*, *54*(15), 2688–2710. doi:10.1016/j.comnet.2010.05.003

Barth, A. T., Hanson, M. A., Powell, H. C. Jr, & Lach, J. (2009, June). TEMPO 3.1: A body area sensor network platform for continuous movement assessment. In *2009 Sixth International Workshop on Wearable and Implantable Body Sensor Networks* (pp. 71-76). Piscataway, NJ: IEEE. 10.1109/BSN.2009.39

Bhatia, D., Estevez, L., & Rao, S. (2007, August). Energy efficient contextual sensing for elderly care.In *2007 29th Annual International Conference of the IEEE Engineering in Medicine and Biology Society* (pp. 4052-4055). Piscataway, NJ: IEEE. 10.1109/IEMBS.2007.4353223

Bui, F. M., & Hatzinakos, D. (2008). Biometric methods for secure communications in body sensor networks: Resource-efficient key management and signal-level data scrambling. *EURASIP Journal on Advances in Signal Processing*, 109.

Jung, B. H., Akbar, R. U., & Sung, D. K. (2012, September).Throughput, energy consumption, and energy efficiency of IEEE 802.15. 6 body area network (BAN) MAC protocol. In *2012 IEEE 23rd International Symposium on Personal, Indoor and Mobile Radio Communications-(PIMRC)* (pp. 584-589). Piscataway, NJ: IEEE.

Karlof, C., Sastry, N., & Wagner, D. (2004, November). TinySec: a link layer security architecture for wireless sensor networks. In *Proceedings of the 2nd international conference on Embedded networked sensor systems* (pp. 162-175). New York, NY: ACM.

Lamprinos, I. E., Prentza, A., Sakka, E., & Koutsouris, D. (2006, January). Energy-efficient MAC protocol for patient personal area networks. In *2005 IEEE Engineering in Medicine and Biology 27th Annual Conference* (pp. 3799-3802). Piscataway, NJ: IEEE.

Lee, H., Park, K., Lee, B., Choi, J., & Elmasri, R. (2008, July). Issues in data fusion for healthcare monitoring. In *Proceedings of the 1st international conference on PErvasive Technologies Related to Assistive Environments* (p. 3). New York, NY: ACM. 10.1145/1389586.1389590

Lee, Y. D., & Chung, W. Y. (2009). Wireless sensor network based wearable smart shirt for ubiquitous health and activity monitoring. *Sensors and Actuators B: Chemical*, *140*(2), 390–395. doi:10.1016/j.snb.2009.04.040

Leister, W., Abie, H., Groven, A. K., Fretland, T., & Balasingham, I. (2008, April). Threat assessment of wireless patient monitoring systems. In *2008 3rd International Conference on Information and Communication Technologies: From Theory to Applications* (pp. 1-6). Piscataway, NJ: IEEE. 10.1109/ICTTA.2008.4530274

Mehta, M., & Ghosh, K. (2016, April). Effect of Looping On the Lifetime Of A Multi-Sink Wireless Sensor Network Deployed For Healthcare Monitoring System. [IJERCSE]. *International Journal of Engineering Research in Computer Science and Engineering*, *3*(4).

Morris, D., Coyle, S., Wu, Y., Lau, K. T., Wallace, G., & Diamond, D. (2009). Bio-sensing textile based patch with an integrated optical detection system for sweat monitoring. *Sensors and Actuators B: Chemical*, *139*(1), 231–236. doi:10.1016/j.snb.2009.02.032

Noury, N., Herve, T., Rialle, V., Virone, G., Mercier, E., Morey, G., . . . Porcheron, T. (2000, October). Monitoring behavior in the home using a smart fall sensor. *Proceedings of IEEE-EMBS Special Topic Conference on Microtechnologies in Medicine and Biology*, Lyon, France. (pp. 607–610). 10.1109/MMB.2000.893857

Philipose, M., Consolvo, S., Choudhury, T., Fishkin, K., Perkowitz, M., Fox, I. S. D., & Patterson, D. (2004). Fast, detailed inference of diverse daily human activities. *Demonstrations at UbiComp*, *7*.

Saleem, S., Ullah, S., & Kwak, K. S. (2011). A study of IEEE 802.15.4 security framework for wireless body area networks. *Sensors (Basel)*, *11*(2), 1383–1395. doi:10.3390110201383 PMID:22319358

Sinha, A., & Chandrakasan, A. (2001). Dynamic power management in wireless sensor networks. *IEEE Design & Test of Computers*, *18*(2), 62–74. doi:10.1109/54.914626

Venkatasubramanian, K. K., & Gupta, S. K. (2010). Physiological value-based efficient usable security solutions for body sensor networks. [TOSN]. *ACM Transactions on Sensor Networks*, *6*(4), 31. doi:10.1145/1777406.1777410

Xu, X., Shu, L., Guizani, M., Liu, M., & Lu, J. (2015). A survey on energy harvesting and integrated data sharing in wireless body area networks. *International Journal of Distributed Sensor Networks*, *11*(10).

ZigBee Alliance, San Ramon, "ZigBee Specification v1.0,"CA, USA2005.

Chapter 5
Wireless Sensor Network Protocols, Performance Metrics, Biosensors, and WSN in Healthcare:
A Deep Insight

Sumathi V.

Sri Ramakrishna College of Arts and Science, India

ABSTRACT

Wireless network led to the development of Wireless Sensor Networks (WSNs). A Wireless sensor network is a set of connected devices, sensors, and electronic components that can transmit the information collected from an observed field to the relevant node through wireless links. WSN has advanced many application fields. It can change any kind of technology that can modify the future lifestyle. WSNs are composed of tiny wireless computers that can sense the situation of atmosphere, process the sensor data, make a decision, and spread data to the environmental stimuli. Sensor-based technology has created several opportunities in the healthcare system, revolutionizing it in many aspects. This chapter explains in detail wireless sensor networks, their protocol, and performance metrics. The impact and role of the Biosensor in a wireless sensor network and healthcare systems are depicted. The integration of the computer engineering program into the WSNs is addressed.

INTRODUCTION

In recent years, WSNs have earned worldwide consideration in its technological development particularly with the proliferated development of Micro Electro Mechanical Systems (MEMS) based technology. MEMS have enabled the expansion of smart and miniaturized sensors. These sensors have only limited processing and computing resources. They are inexpensive compared to conventional sensors. The sensor network is comprised of sensors, which can sense (sense the atmospheric conditions namely light,

DOI: 10.4018/978-1-7998-1090-2.ch005

temperature, humidity, pressure, etc.), measure and collect the information from the environment. The sensed data is further processed for making the decision. Later the decision is transmitted on to the user. Smart sensors are low power consumption devices that are all furnished with one or more than one sensor, actuators, a power supply unit, a radio transceiver and a processor. These smart sensors can sense a variety of signals namely thermal, mechanical, biological, optical and chemical.

Since the sensor nodes in the network have limited memory capacity and are generally deployed in locations where it is difficult to access, a radio is employed for wireless transmission of the data from the sensor node to a base-station (e.g., handheld device, a laptop). The primary power supply for the sensor node is achieved by a battery which is having limited power. The secondary power supply is established by the harvesting technology from the environment that is the solar panels will be attached to the sensor nodes. From that energy will be generated and stored for processing and performing certain operations. A WSN normally has little or no infrastructure. WSNs are self-configure and self-organized in nature. Sensors in the sensor network system consist of three subsystems such as the sensor subsystem, processing subsystem, and communication subsystem. These systems are responsible for sensing the atmospheric condition, decision making based on the sensed data and responsible for the exchange of information with the neighboring sensors. WSN has significant applications likely remote environmental observation and tracking of the target. The architecture of WSNs depends considerably on the application or device and it has to consider the features namely the environment, objective application or device, cost, hardware, and system constraints. This technology can provide reliability in addition to enhanced mobility (Yick et al., 2008).

WIRELESS SENSOR NETWORK

Rapid development in the field of sensor-based devices, computer technology, and wireless communication has lined up for the proliferation of WSN (Dargie et al., 2008). A common objective is achieved by a group of wireless sensors collaboration. The WSN consists of one or more than one sink that is a base station that collects the data from all the sensor devices. Through these sinks, WSN establishes the interaction to the outside world (Stroulia et al., 2009). With the use of unsophisticated sensors, WSNs develops a sensor device to perform sensing which is inexpensive and conventional when compared to the traditional approaches(Li et al., 2008). The main advantage of the conventional approach is greater coverage, accuracy, and reliability at a possibly lower cost. WSN is categorized into two groups such as Structured and Unstructured WSN(Raghavendra et al., 2006).

- Structured WSN: A limited number of the sensor nodes or all of them in the WSN will be deployed in the preplanned network structure. In this, only fewer amount of sensor nodes will be deployed. The main advantage of this network is less in network maintenance and in expensive. Since the nodes are retained at a definite location,only a lesser amount of nodes can be deployed in the network to establish coverage area while ad hoc network's deployment can be established even to uncovered regions.
- Unstructured WSN: In the unstructured WSN poses a dense compilation of sensor nodes. These sensor nodes follow the Ad-hoc principle for deploying the sensor nodes in the network. This sensor network has no architecture and remains unattended to perform observe and report over the functions of the sensor node. Because of the vast nodes in the unstructured WSN, maintenance of

network is a complex task. Managing connectivity among the nodes and detecting any link failures during transmission is complicated in unstructured WSN.

WSNs have immense potential for many domains whichever application area such as military target tracking and surveillance (Simon et al., 2004) (Yick et al., 2005), natural disaster relief (Castillo-Effen, 2004), biomedical health monitoring (Gao et al., 2005)(Lorincz et al., 2004), and seismic sensing and hazardous atmosphere exploration (Wener Allen et al., 2007). Depending on the application and the required environment WSN is designed. The atmosphere plays an efficient role in determining the size, deployment scheme and the topology of the network. An ad hoc based network scenario is deployed when the atmosphere is unapproachable for humans or when the network is consists of hundreds to more than thousands of nodes. Hindrance occurring in the atmosphere can also limit transmission between nodes, which in turn influences the network connectivity or topology. Research in WSN aims to meet the constraints and difficulties faced by the environment by introducing new plan or design concepts, creating new protocols or improving the existing protocols, developing new algorithms and building efficient applications. WSN-based devices are developed in order to improve the quality of life.

WIRELESS SENSOR NETWORK APPLICATIONS

WSN plays an important role in several application areas such as medical monitoring, industrial automation, precision agriculture, and automotive industry. WSN can effectively be implemented in healthcare for smart nursing homes, health monitoring, WBAN, in-home assistance, and telemedicine.

Health Monitoring: WSNs are implemented to observe a patient in the nursing home and patient's home. The monitoring system is often essential to persistent monitoring of a patient's significant parameters such as ECG, pulse rate, pressure and body temperature. RFID tags or location tags and sensors can be used to record both patient and healthcare personnel. Since prevention and avoidance is better than managing wellness, cure rather than being sick or ill. In order to obtain the needed facilities, distinct health monitoring is desirable. When compared to wired, a wireless system is reliable and flexible. A wireless system makes the life of a patient not be limited to his bed (Aminian, 2013).

Wireless Body Area Networks: Significant features of these networks likely frequency bands, wireless communication protocols, data bandwidth, mobility, encryption, and power consumption. Real-time healthcare data acquired from different kinds of sensors (Sun et al., 2010). The outline of wearable sensors permits the user to constantly monitor biological and physiological data that are assisted by WSNs in healthcare. A WBAN remains as health monitoring during the patient's stay at the hospital or home. WBAN can be useful for emergency cases, where it sends data about the patient's health to the healthcare provider. It can also help people by providing healthcare services such as memory enhancement, medical data access, cancer detection, asthma detection, and monitoring blood glucose (Anwar et al., 2017).

At-home Healthcare: This addresses the social burden of the aging population. It is achieved by using medical WSNs. Longevity has given rise to age-related disabilities and diseases. Providing quality healthcare to the elderly population has become an important social and economic issue. At-home healthcare provides affordable care to the elderly while they live independently (Minaie et al., 2013).

Telemedicine: Telemedicine is a medical technique that permits clinical work and also known as tele-care. Telemedicine is performed using communication technology and information. Telemedicine incorporates WSN has newly become a development in healthcare and refers to the stipulation of healthcare services. Tele-care consent for remote medical valuations. The overall cost of healthcare reduces the use of telemedicine.

Wireless Sensor Network Protocols

The protocol is a structure of rules and instructions that permits more than one node to establish communication among the system. It allows transferring the data through any kind of deviation in the physical quantity. Based on the deployment area and environmental requirement protocols are designed. So far, a diverse routing protocol is designed to meet the constraints and innate features of WSNs. These routing protocols are broadly categorized into three main groups (Sohrabi et al., 2000; Muhammad Ullah, Waqar Ahmad, 2009).

Wireless Sensor Network Evaluation Metrics

Generally, performance metrics are a measure of quantitative event, simulation or transmission using a different procedure. Several methods and measuring procedures are interpreted to assess the protocol. Leveraging of proposed or previous protocol's assessment is done by the performance metrics of the protocol (Akyildiz et al., 2002). In WSN routing is simply an assessment or measurement used for the optimal route discovery that is the best path, used for the transmission by the protocol. The illustration of the protocol has a greater impact on the transmission of protocols among the network. A combination of improper metrics with routing protocol may give routing loops or any suboptimal paths as a result. There are so many routing metrics to appraise the performance of protocols of WSN, it is important to choose the best combination for assessing the performance of the protocols.

The chief intent of any routing protocol is to choose the best or optimal path among all the probable paths among a pair of nodes (Yang & Wang, 2008). Typically, the path selection criterion is based on the weights of paths. They are real numbers allocated to paths based on the design of routing metrics. Hence, routing metrics are straightly connected to the presentation of routing protocols. Consequently, an appropriate routing metric is significant for the performance of routing protocols. When designing and presenting a novel protocol, all the researchers and designers have to consider the issues and challenges that hurdle in designing proficient protocols (Tao Liu et al., 2009; Santos et al., 2007; Basset Almamou et al., 2009; Alazzawi & Elkateeb, 2008; and Yang & Wang, 2008). For the performance valuation of these protocols, there are many existing metrics and some proposed metrics for the evaluation of routing protocols in sensor networks. Metrics can be characterized according to the criteria of evaluation into five categories. They are,

- General Metrics
- Performance Metrics
- Security Metrics
- Quality of Service Metrics
- Link QualityMetrics

Figure 1. Classification of WSN protocol

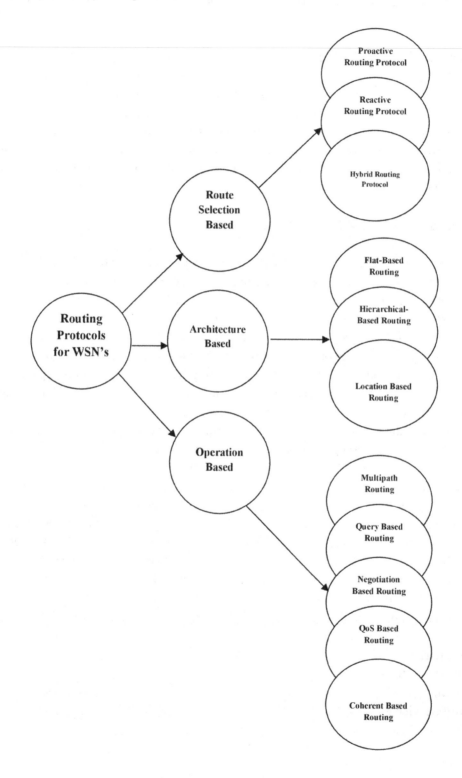

General Metrics

Both real time as well as non-real time protocol's performance metrics is evaluated using the general metrics. General metrics for evaluation of routing protocols include the following

- Network Lifetime
- Routing Load
- Nodes Energy
- Energy Consumption
- Routing Overhead
- Load Imbalance Factor

Network Lifetime

Both real, as well as non-real time protocol's performance metrics, is evaluated using the general metrics. General metrics for evaluation of routing protocols include the following Network Lifetime is the sum of time that the nodes in the network are active and sensor network is operative. Aim of any routing protocol is to widen the lifetime of the sensor network (Sha et al., 2006). The lifetime of the sensor network can be formally defined as (KeweiSha & Weisong Shi, 2004):

Equation for Network Life Time

LFT=mini;

$$i = \begin{cases} L(i-1) > L(i) \, AND L(i+1) = L(i) \, Connectivity \\ COV(i-1) > \theta \, AND COV(i) \le \theta \, Coverage \end{cases}$$

This Equation shows LSN as the moment at which either the sensor network loses connectivity or loses coverage to a certain threshold.

Routing Load

Routing load in data transmission is measured in terms of routing packets transferred per transmission data packets. The transmitted data packets include only the data packets that are finally delivered at the destination and not the ones that are dropped during the transmission. Each hop transmission is counted once for both data packets and routing. This shows the network bandwidth consumed by routing packets with respect to "useful" data packets.

Equation for Routing Load

Routing Load = Σ sum of routing packets transmitted/Σ time taken by each packet

Nodes Energy

At the beginning of WSN's data transmission, the node has a certain initial value that is the energy level of the node at the initial level of energy. This is termed the initial energy of the sensor node. This is represented as Initial_Energy in the equation. In the WSN's data transmission, the term "energy" represents the energy level in a node at a particular time supplied by the battery power or by any other forms of energy source. When the input argument has initiated the value of the Initial_Energy is passed to the node. While sending and receiving packets a particular amount of energy is loosed by the node due to the transmission from one place to another. Initial_Energy value gets decreased as a result of the energy loss during transmission. The energy consumption of the node in the simulation at any time will be calculated using the difference between the Current_Energy to the Initial Energy of the node in the network. If any node in the simulation environment attains zero energy level, it cannot transmit or receive any more packets it becomes idle. The energy level of a network is determined by summing the entire node's energy.

Equation for Nodes energy

Nodes energy= Current_Energy-Initial_Energy

Energy Consumption

Energy Consumption of a routing protocol shows that how much a routing protocol is energy efficient whereas energy consumption of different individual sensors shows the load balance feature. Commonly, the energy consumption of each sensor in the sensor network is defined as the normalized entire amount of energy used in receiving or sending messages. In this equation, Ec is the consumed energy and E0 is the initial energy of the node.

Equation for Energy Consumption

$$EC = E_c \big/ E_0$$

Routing Overhead

Routing overhead is the number of routing packet transferred per second which is necessary for network transmission. Routing Overhead (packets) is entire number of routing packets generated is divided by entire data packets transmitted and the total number of routing packets.

Equation for Routing Overhead

$$RO(bytes) = \frac{NumberofRoutingPacketGenerated}{TotalNumberofPacketGenerated}$$

Load Imbalance Factor

Lifetime of a sensor network rely on the load imbalance factor (LIF) thus a good routing protocol must have a feature of load balance to extend the life of sensor network. LIF is used to quantitatively evaluate the load balance feature of the routing protocol and it is formally stated as the variance of the remaining lifetime of the sensor network. In this equation n is the entire sensors in the network, E_j is the remaining lifetime of sensor j and E_{avg} is the average remaining lifetime of all sensors nodes in the Wireless senor network.

Equation for Load Imbalance Factor

$$LIF = \sum_{j-1}^{n} \left(E_j - E_{avg} \right)^2$$

Performance Metrics

The performance metrics are necessary for evaluating the performance of a routing protocol and are described in detail as follows:

- Throughput or Packet Delivery Fraction
- Average End to End Delay of Data Packets
- Packet Delivery Ratio
- Path length Extension Rate
- Average Route Acquisition Latency

Throughput or Packet Delivery Fraction

Throughput value is termed as the whole packets transmitted within the transmission time or successful data transmission in the preferred time. The value of transmission is calculated as the average rate of successful packets delivered from the source to the destination node.

Equation for Throughput

$$P = \frac{1}{C} \sum_{f=1}^{e} \frac{Rf}{Nf}$$

Average End to End Delay of Data Packets

Time taken by the packet to transmit from source node to the destination node is said to be an End to End Delay time. It includes all the delay taken by the router to find the path in network consumption, propagation delay, processing delay, and End to end delay for transmitting the packet. Measuring this delay includes all probable delays caused by queuing, retransmission delays at the MAC, transfer times and propagation. The mathematical expression for an average end to delay in which N is the number of successfully received packets, i is the unique id of a packet, r_i is time at which a packet with unique id i is received, s_i is time at which a packet with unique id i is sent. Average end to delay (D) is measured in ms. For gaining high performance, average end to end delay has to be less.

Equation for Average End to End Delay of Data Packets

$$D = \frac{1}{N} \sum_{i=1}^{s} r_i - s_i$$

Packet Delivery Ratio

The Packet Delivery Ratio (PDR) signifies the whole packets delivered from the source node to the destination node. It is used for calculating the packet loss rate during the data transmission. While transmitting from the source node to destination node some packets may be lost or wrongly routed to other nodes, in order to find this loss PDR is calculated and measures up both the efficiency and correctness of ad-hoc routing protocols in terms of the loss rate. A higher packet delivery ratio is hoped in any network is said as the best transmission.

Equation for Packet Delivery Ratio

Packet Delay Ratio = Σ Number of packet receive / Σ Number of packet send

Path length Extension Rate

There is a trade-off between path length and the load balance because the routing protocol may not always select the shortest path in order to balance the load to different paths. Path length extension rate is the rate of extending the path meaning that how much the routing protocol extends the path length comparing with GPSR. It can also be defined as the ratio of the path length difference between other routing protocols and GPSR to the path length of GPSR. The equation for Path Length Extension rate shows the mathematical expression for path length extension rate in which PLGPSR is the path length by using GPSR and PL others is the path length by other routing protocols. Another definition for PLER is the average extended path length in hops compared with GPSR and is mathematically expressed in Equation for Average Extended Path Length.

Equation for Path Length Extension Rate

$$\text{PLER} = \frac{\text{PL}_{\text{others}} - \text{PL}_{\text{GPSR}}}{\text{PL}_{\text{GPSR}}}$$

Equation for Average Extended Path Length

$$\text{PLER} = \text{PL}_{\text{others}} - \text{PL}_{\text{GPSR}}$$

Average Route Acquisition Latency

The average route acquisition latency (the total computation and communication costs) is the average delay between sending an RREQ packet by a source for discovering a route to an endpoint and the receipt of the first corresponding RREP. The average route acquisition latency can be derived by using the following equation:

Equation for Average Route Acquisition Latency

$$\text{Average Route Acquisition Latency} = \text{Computation Cost} + \text{Communication Cost}$$

where communication cost can be calculated as follows:

Equation for Calculating Communication Cost

$$\text{Communication cost} = \frac{\text{TotalNo.ofbitsneedtobetransmittedbits}}{\text{NetworkThroughtput}}$$

Security Metrics

Security metrics are a noble indicator of the security trade-offs but they alone are not enough to determine a defense's usability. They must be used in addition to other evaluation metrics as well. Metrics for Security requirements include the following:

- Resiliency
- Connectivity

Resiliency

The goal of resiliency is to design such a secure routing protocol that provides resistance against various known attacks on routing protocols and does not reveal anything about the pair wise keys. This metric is used to measure the number of nodes that an attacker needs to capture to compromise the entire WSN.

Connectivity

Connectivity is the probability that a node can directly communicate with another node in the WSN. That is during the transmission of a data packet from one node to another communication between one to its neighbor nodes should be established securely.

Quality of Service Metrics

While designing any routing protocol, QoS should be guaranteed because many application scenarios of WSN have intrinsic QoS requirements. Data packet delay, bandwidth efficiency and jitter are three metrics which quantify QoS requirements. Thus guaranteeing these QoS metrics, will decide whether this technology can be put into use in the serious and real time scenarios or not. These metrics are described in detail blow:

- Data Packet Delay
- Bandwidth Efficiency
- Jitter

Data Packet Delay

Data packet delay is the delay between the receipt of the first packet and the second packet. During the transmission of data packet the flow of data packets is established from source node to its neighbour nodes. While this transmission the time interval between one packets to other packet is termed as Data Packet Delay.

Equation for Data Packet Delay (geekforgeeks)

Data packet delay = Data Size / Bandwidth = (L/B)

Bandwidth Efficiency

The bandwidth of routing metric optimizes for the paththroughput. One drawback is that the bandwidth is hard toderive, as well as to measure without disturbing the normaltraffic.

Equation for Bandwidth Efficiency (prezi)

$$B_n = \frac{\text{transmissionbitrate}(\text{bps})}{\text{minimumbandwidth}(\text{Hz})}$$

Jitter

Jitter is termed as a amount of the variability over time of the packet's potential value across a network. During the transmission, there is no variation when the network has constant latency (or jitter).Jitter is distinct in the packet delay. This packet delay results in differing packet arrival times.

Equation for Jitter (watchguard)

jitter = packet delay timing / Number of Packet Delay (ms)

Link Quality Metrics

Link quality of the entire network plays an equallyimportant role in self-health monitoring for WSNs. TheLink Quality Metrics are described in detail below:

- Expected transmission count (ETX)
- Requested Number of Packets (RNP)

Expected Transmission Count

The Expected transmission count is the transmission rate of the packets according to the time. ETX diminishes the number of transmissions for data packets and assessments the number of transmissions needed to send a unicast packet by evaluating the delivery rate of beacon packets between neighboring nodes. The Expected Transmission Count (ETX) metric was originally developed for ad-hoc networks but is used in sensor networks as well. ETX considers both the link quality and the energy consumption of a path. In calculating ETX, it is not considered that the nodes which are sending data with different signal strengths consume different amounts of energy.

Equation for Expected Transmission Count

$$ETX = \sum_{i=1}^{n} \frac{1}{p_i q_{i-1}} \rightarrow \min$$

Requested Number of Packets (RNP)

Requested number of Packets (RNP) is a metric used for representing the temporal properties of low power in the wireless links. RNP reports the supply of packet losses of a link when a link quality is assessed. The objective of RNP is to measure the total number of transmissions needed in an Automatic Repeat Request (ARQ).

Equation for Requested Number of Packets

$$RNP = r_f \times r_b$$

where r_f and r_b are link quality estimates in forward andbackward direction, respectively.

WIRELESS SENSOR NETWORK ARCHITECTURE

In this section, architecture of WSN is described which enables a smart hospital to manage the data's and physiological information collected for patient supervision. By using WSN-based Healthcare environment large amount of sensor data can be easily managed. Since the health-related information's are highly sensitive. Hence, high security mechanism has to be ensured to achieve data confidentiality, data access control and data integrity. This system is completely contrast to the existing patient-centric system. WSN-based health care system is transparent to users and doctors. It doesn't entail any interventions. Key management and security configurations in the WSN-based solution are apparent to the user. WSN-based healthcare system consists of two categories users or patients and health care professionals. WSN-based architecture consists the following components

- The WSN system gathers the biological signals and health information from the patients.
- The monitoring applications allow healthcare professionals to access to stored and pre-processed data from the cloud.
- Computer science engineers develops machine learning algorithms, implements it on the edge nodes and cloud servers.
- The cloud servers which ensure data storage for further access and process.

Several kinds of biosensors had implanted with the individual's body to sense the biological sensors. In this architecture, each patient in the network poses a personal WSN which consists of a set of lightweight or miniaturized sensor nodes and a gateway. At home itself patient can be monitored by the medical professional and caregivers with the help of WSN. The monitoring application permits the healthcare professionals to supervise their patients and enables them to access to a patient's data at any time or from anywhere by ubiquitously using a computer, laptop or a Smartphone. Sensor nodes are carried by every patient to collect different kinds of health data such as heart beats, motion and physiological signals. Each sensor node in the sensor network sends the gathered information through a wireless communication channel to the device's gateway. The gateway groups the different health data into a file. The monitoring application downloads the needed data from the cloud storage and decrypts it using its secret key. In addition, it allows the healthcare professionals to add medical data, such as reports, diagnostics and prescriptions, to the patient's information. The medical information collected from the patient is encrypted and stored on the cloud along with the patient's health data (JBethencourt et al., 2007; and Lounis et al., 2012).

Figure 2. Sensor network health care system architecture (Karthick G. S., & Pankajavalli P. B., 2019)

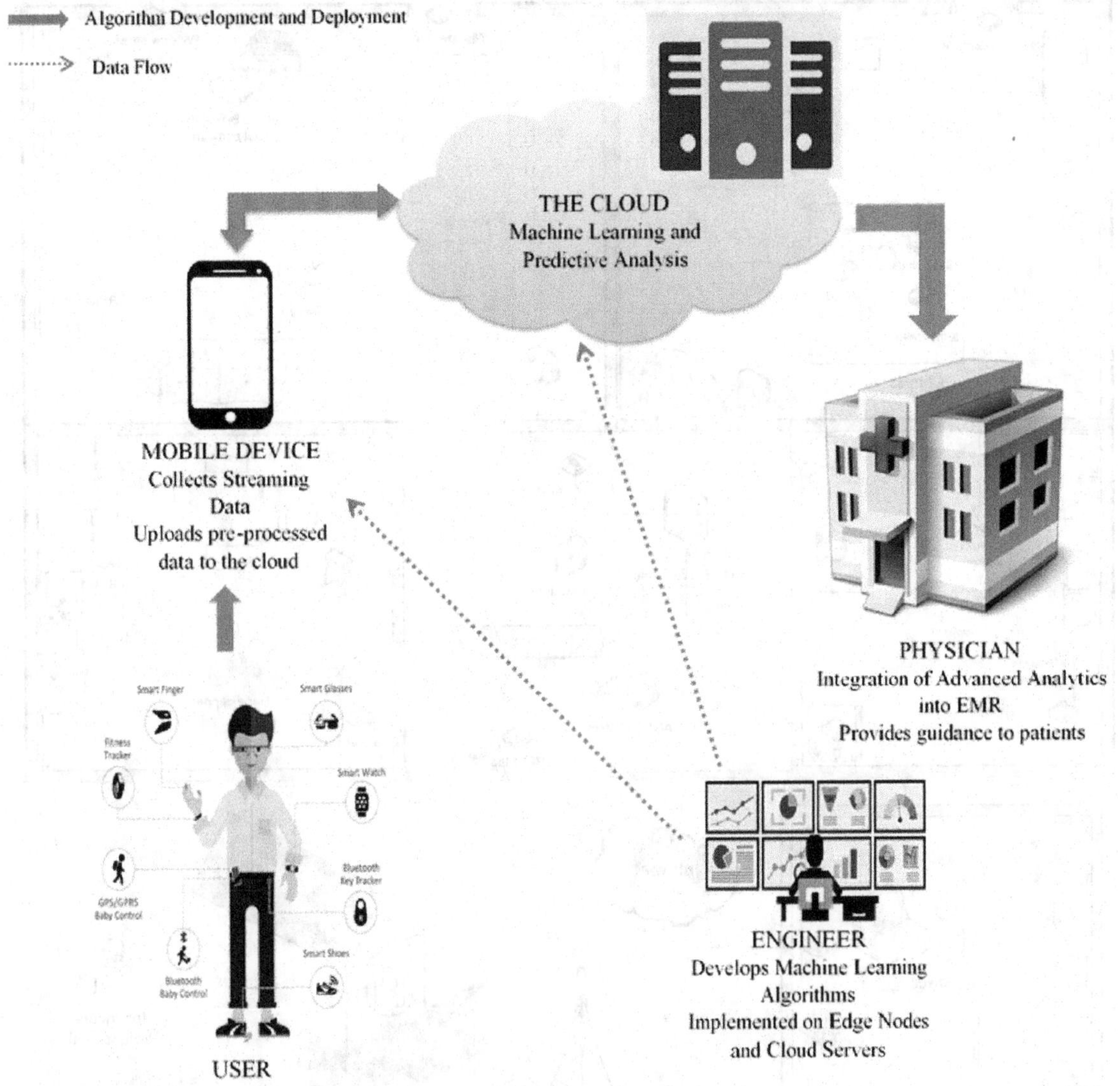

BIOSENSORS AND THEIR APPLICATION

Biosensor is a combination of biological and physicochemical component-based device. Biosensor is used to detect anlyte and produce measurable signals. Biosensor is one of the promising technology developed for monitoring and analysing in various sectors. Over the decade numerous bio-sensing related devices have been developed to meet the difficulties faced by the several precise applications. The biological information collected by the biological sensor is converted into electronic signals. This conversion is a challenging task due to the difficulty of attachment of electronic device directly into the biological setup. Biosensors have massive application in clinical diagnostic, environmental monitoring, food industry and other areas whichever require reliable and accurate analyses. Home pregnancy test and blood glucose level

Figure 3. Smart hospital deployment scenario (Alemdar, H., &Ersoy, C. 2010)

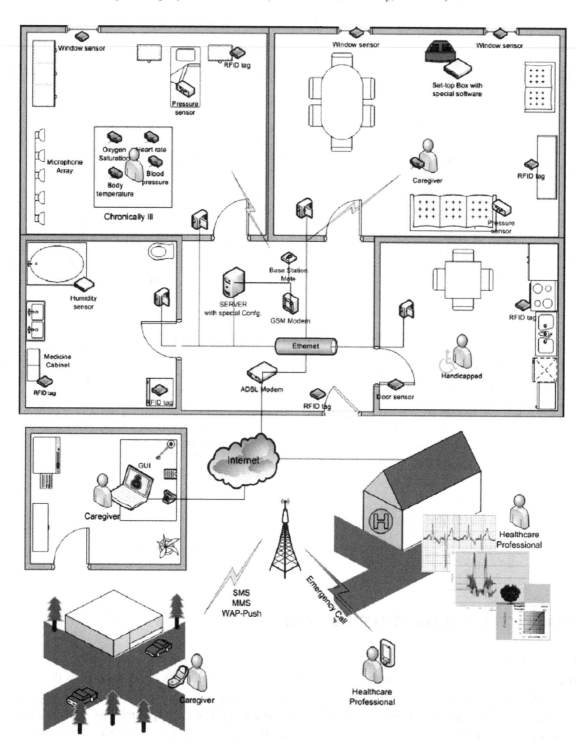

Figure 4. Structure of biosensor in healthcare application (Surfix 2018)

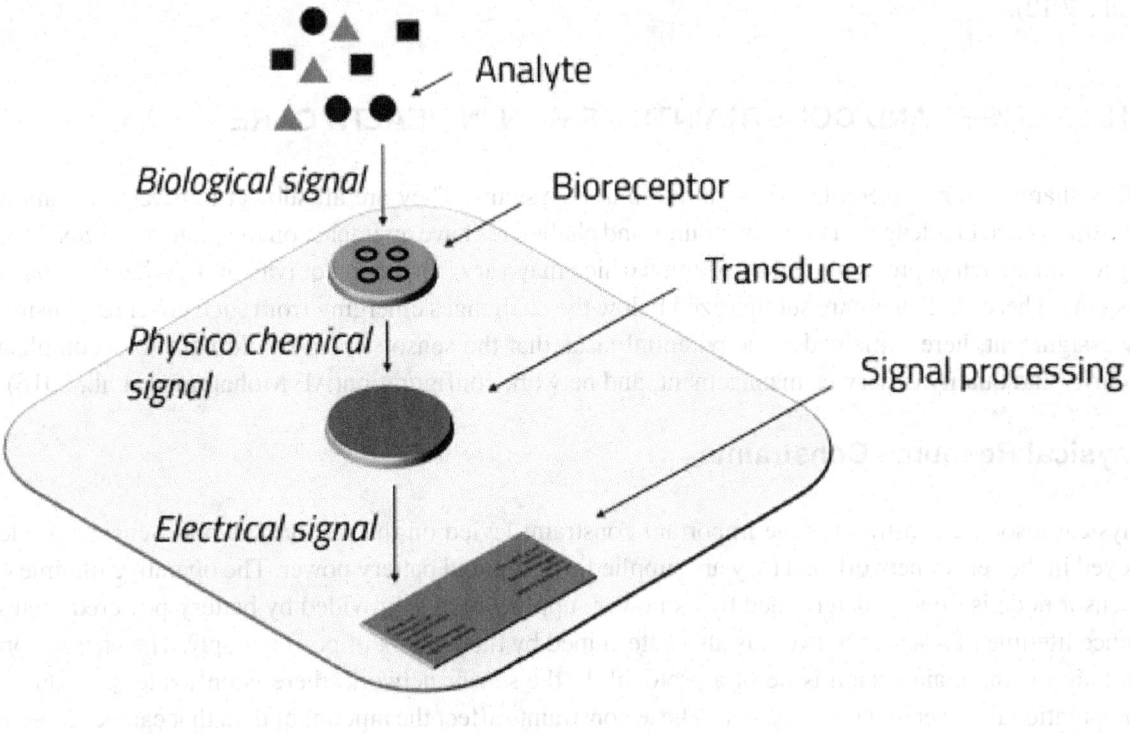

detectors are the most commonly used biosensors. Biosensors have been implemented in many field's namely medical field, food industry, marine sector etc., Biosensor based application provide improved stability as compared to the traditional methods(Mehrotra, 2016).

- Food processing, monitoring, food authenticity, quality and safety measurement checking
- Fermentation processes
- Bio-sensing technology for sustainable food safety
- Biosensors in smart hospitals and in medical field
- Fluorescent biosensors for protein function prediction
- Bio defense applications
- Biosensors in plant biology

Role of Biosensor in Healthcare

Biosensors had shown immense potentiality in medical diagnostic. It made the researchers and scientists to create innovative tools for medical-care. The keystone for the eminence of biosensors in medical diagnostic is due its simplicity and accuracy in prediction and detection. Biosensors had shown capability to accomplish higher sensitive and multiplex analysis. It has ability to integrate different kinds of function within the same chip. Biosensors aim at providing point of care facility to the worldwide remote areas.

It involves constant development in miniaturization and fabrication of IoT/biosensor-based devices. In recent years biosensors has earned enormous consideration in nanotechnology and medicine (Malima, et al., 2012).

CHALLENGES AND CONSTRAINTS OF WSN IN HEALTH CARE

WSN shares several resemblances with distributed systems. They are all subject to diverse or unique constraints and challenges. These constraints and challenges have an impact on the plan of a WSN, leading to a mismatch of protocols and algorithms which may vary from their equivalents of other distributed systems. These challenges are summarized below the challenges emerging from such novel responsibility assignment, here explained some potential tasks that the sensor nodes would have to accomplish: security and quality of service management, and network configuration(AE Mohammed et al., 2016)

Physical Resource Constraints

Physical resource constraint is the important constraint levied on the sensor network. Sensors are deployed in the sensor network and they are supplied with limited battery power. The operative lifetime of a sensor node is directly determined by its power supply which is provided by battery-powered motes. Hence lifetime of a sensor network is also determined by the amount of power supply. The energy consumption is the main design issue of a protocol. In the sensor network, there is only a lesser value of computational power and memory size. These constraints affect the amount of data that can be stored in distinct sensor nodes. In order to handle completions, the protocol has to be simple and light-weighted. Communication delay in a sensor network can be high due to the limited communication channel shared by all nodes within each other's transmission range.

Security

Many sensors in the wireless sensor networks collect sensitive information from various objects. Senor nodes proliferate the exposure to malicious interruptions and attacks at several stages. While there are numerous techniques and solutions for distributed systems that can avoid attacks or contain the extent and damage of such attacks, many of these incur storage requirements, communication, and significant computational, which cannot be fulfilled by resource-constrained sensor nodes (Perrig, A., et al.2004).

Design Constraints

More efficient and reliable device manufacturing is the primary goal of WSN. Lack of advanced hardware features will effect in the design of small and efficient operating systems. A sensor's hardware limitations also affect the design of many protocols and algorithms implemented in a WSN. For example, routing tables that encompass entries for each potential destination in a network may be too large to fit into a sensor's memory. Instead, only a small volume of data (such as a list of neighbors) can be stored in a sensor node's memory. Further, while in-network processing can be employed to eliminate redundant information, some sensor fusion and aggregation algorithms may necessitate more computational power and storage capacities that can be provided bysensor nodes of low-cost. Therefore, many software archi-

Table 1. Role of biosensor in healthcare

Analyte	Bio-Recognition Element	Sample	Technology	Advantages
Ebola virus, dengue and yellow fever causing virus	Polychromatic silver nanoparticles onto the small strip of paper which is tagged by antibody	Blood	Paper strip based multiplex disease diagnostics	Detecting down to tens of ng/ mL (Yen C.-W. et al.2015)
Glycoprotein Ebolavirus	Fe_3O_4 magnetic nano particle (nanozyme)	Blood	Nanozyme strip	Lower detection limit: 1 ng/ mL (Duan D et al.2015)
Urinary pathogens namely E. coli and Enterococcus faecalis	Glass-polymer hybrid chip forms a centrifugal microfluidic platform that captures bacteria directly	Urine sample	Microfluidics and Raman microscopy	Detection within 70 minutes (Schroder U.-C et al.2015)
Candida infection	Nanoparticles contains supermagneticstuffs coated with target-specific binding agents	Blood	Shrunken magnetic resonance that calculates water molecules reaction in the incidence of magnetic fields	99.4% specificity, 1 CFU/ mL and91.1% sensitivity, and (colony forming unit per milliliter) (Pfaller M. A et al.2016)
Circulating tumor cells (CTC): prostate, melanoma cancers, and metastatic breast	The microchip permits microfluidic path in many rows via the blood is injected.	Blood	Microfluidic chip or cluster chip clusters are insulated through specialized bifurcating rows under low pulling forces conserves their reliability.	At blood flow rate of 2.5 mL/hr, chip caught 99% of four- or extra cell clusters, 70% of three-cell clusters, and 41% of two-cell clusters (Sarioglu A. F et al.2015)
Antibiotic sensitivity	Series of minute flow-through wells patterned onto a glass chip. Each microwell covered with micro beads to trap the bacteria with the signal molecule resazurin and antibiotic	Bacterial culture	Electrochemical lessening signal brought by the metabolism of resazurin in resistant bacteria, perceived by the electrodes fabricated on the chip	Bacterial resistance profile available within an hour of incubation (Besant J. D et al.2015)
Ebola virus: nucleoprotein (NP), viral matrix protein (VP40) and glycoprotein (GP)	3 mouse monoclonal antibodies beside proteins	Blood	Chromatographic/lateral flow immunoassay SD biosensor product used for WHO EUAL Program (Emergency Use Assessment and Listing)	specificity, 99.7% (95% CI) (99.1–100.0) Sensitivity, 84.9% (95% CI) (78.6–91.2); (Perkins M. D 2015)
Blood glucose (noninvasive)	Nanoengineered silica glass with ions.when a low power laser light hits them that shine in infrared light	Skin touch to the glass (no finger prick required)	Low-powered lasers penetrate the skin and measure the length of time the fluorescence remains and calculate the blood glucose	Noninvasive device and wearable (Barson R et al.2016)
Mycobacterium tuberculosis	Surface altered gold nanoparticles, cadmium-telluride quantum dots, and two specific oligonucleotides against early secretory antigenic	Sputum	Sandwich form FRET based biosensor to detect M. tuberculosis complex and differentiate it from M. bovis bacillus Calmette-Guerin (present in vaccinated individuals)	86.6% specificity and 94.2% sensitivity, 10 - fold lower recognition limit (Shojaei T. R et al.2018)
Microcystis spp. (MYC)	Redox surface altered with ionic liquid and sequence-selective DNA probe to MYC and pencil graphite electrode	Biological sample	Electrochemical DNA biosensor using differential pulse voltammetry (DPV)	Lower recognition limit: 3.72 g/mL (Sengiz C et al.2015)
Human IgG in initial prostate cancer	Citrate ligands-coated with gold nano particles are mixed with blood sera forming a protein corona around the nano particle surface	Blood	Gold nano particle permits dynamic light scattering assay (NanoDLSay)	It shows 50% sensitivity and 90–95% specificity (Zheng T et al.2015)
Acousto fluidic sputum liquefier	Micromixer of oscillating sharp edges	Sputum	Microfluidic based on-chip liquefaction device	soften sputum samples with a throughput level of 30 μL/min (Huang P et al.2013

tectures and solutions (operating system, middleware, network protocols) must be designed to operate efficiently on very resource constrained hardware.

Quality of Service

Gateways in WSN acts only as repeater and protocol translators, sensor nodes are predicted to contribute to the quality of service management by improving the resource utilization of all heterogeneous types of devices. Heterogeneity in WSN is part of the future IoT. Improving the QoS assures the efficiency of collaborative work is consequently promising for security mechanisms. Nevertheless, the existing methods ensure QoS on the Internet is not pertinent in WSNs. It is obligatory to discover the novel approaches for ensuring loss guarantees and delay.

Configuration

Sensor nodes are required to control the WSN configuration that includes covering different tasks such as administration of address to guarantee scalable network constructions. It has to ensure the self-healing abilities by detecting and removing faulty nodes or managing their own configuration. However, the self-configuration of participating nodes is not a common feature on the Internet. Instead, the user is expected to install applications and recover the system from crashes. In contrast, the unattended operation of autonomous sensor nodes requires novel means of network configuration and management (Christin, D et al.2009).

CONCLUSION

User demand, needs of humanity and recent advances in hardware and software have led to the first generation of wireless sensor networks. WSNs had revolutionized many applications and shown a greater impact in the healthcare domain. WSN for healthcare has shown its potential to alter the practice of medicine and manual monitoring system. Looking into the future, the struggle between trustworthiness and privacy, the ability to arrange large-scale systems that meet the application's requirements even when deployed and operated in unsupervised environments is going to determine the extent that wireless sensor networks will be successfully integrated in healthcare practice and in the area of research. In this study chapter discussed the WSN and Biosensors. Impact and need of these advanced technologies in the field of healthcare is broadly shown with the architecture and challenges

REFERENCES

Akyildiz, I. F., Su, W., Sankarasubramaniam, Y., & Cayirci, E. (2002). Wireless sensor networks: A survey. *Computer Networks*, *38*(4), 393–422. doi:10.1016/S1389-1286(01)00302-4

Al Ameen, M., Liu, J., & Kwak, K. (2012). Security and privacy issues in wireless sensor networks for healthcare applications. *Journal of Medical Systems*, *36*(1), 93–101. doi:10.100710916-010-9449-4 PMID:20703745

AlaaEisa, M., AbdElrazik, S., Hazem El-Bakry, M., Sajjadhasan, M., AsaadHasan, Q., & Samir Zaid, Q. (2016, December). Challenges in Wireless Sensor Networks. In 2016 International Journal of Advanced Research in Computer Science & Technology (IJARCST 2016) (pp. 22-27).

Alemdar, H., & Ersoy, C. (2010). Wireless sensor networks for healthcare: A survey. *Computer Networks, 54*(15), 2688–2710. doi:10.1016/j.comnet.2010.05.003

Aminian, M., & Naji, H. R. (2013). A hospital healthcare monitoring system using wireless sensor networks. *J. Health Med. Inform, 4*(02), 121. doi:10.4172/2157-7420.1000121

Anwar, M., Abdullah, A. H., Qureshi, K. N., & Majid, A. H. (2017). Wireless body area networks for healthcare applications: An overview. *Telkomnika, 15*(3), 1088–1095. doi:10.12928/telkomnika.v15i3.5793

Barson, R. (2016, January). Non-invasive device could end daily finger pricking for people with diabetes.

Besant, J. D., Sargent, E. H., & Kelley, S. O. (2015). Rapid electrochemical phenotypic profiling of antibiotic-resistant bacteria. *Lab on a Chip, 15*(13), 2799–2807.

Bethencourt, J., Sahai, A., & Waters, B. (2007, May). Ciphertext-policy attribute-based encryption. In 2007 IEEE symposium on security and privacy (SP'07) (pp. 321-334). Piscataway, NJ: IEEE.

Castillo-Effer, M., Quintela, D. H., Moreno, W., Jordan, R., & Westhoff, W. (2004, November). Wireless sensor networks for flash-flood alerting. In *Proceedings of the Fifth IEEE International Caracas Conference on Devices, Circuits and Systems*. (Vol. 1, pp. 142-146). Piscataway, NJ: IEEE. 10.1109/ICCDCS.2004.1393370

Christin, D., Reinhardt, A., Mogre, P. S., & Steinmetz, R. (2009). Wireless sensor networks and the internet of things: selected challenges. Proceedings of the 8th GI/ITG KuVSFachgesprächDrahtlosesensornetze, 31-34.

Crossbow Received from Crossbow Technology. Retrieved from http://www.xbow.com

Dargie, W., & Poellabauer, C. (2010). *Fundamentals of wireless sensor networks: theory and practice.* Hoboken, NJ: John Wiley & Sons. doi:10.1002/9780470666388

Duan, D., Fan, K., Zhang, D., Tan, S., Liang, M., Liu, Y., ... Kobinger, G. P. (2015). Nanozyme-strip for rapid local diagnosis of Ebola. *Biosensors & Bioelectronics, 74*, 134–141. doi:10.1016/j.bios.2015.05.025 PMID:26134291

Gao, T., Greenspan, D., Welsh, M., Juang, R. R., & Alm, A. (2006, January). Vital signs monitoring and patient tracking over a wireless network. In 2005 IEEE Engineering in Medicine and Biology 27th Annual Conference (pp. 102-105). Piscataway, NJ: IEEE.

Geekforgeeks. Retrieved from https://www.geeksforgeeks.org/computer-network-packet-switching-delays/

Gupta, A. K., Sadawarti, H., & Verma, A. K. (2010). Performance analysis of AODV, DSR & TORA routing protocols. *IACSIT International Journal of Engineering and Technology, 2*(2), 226.

Huang, P. H., Ren, L., Nama, N., Li, S., Li, P., Yao, X., ... Nawaz, A. A. (2015). An acoustofluidic sputum liquefier. *Lab on a Chip, 15*(15), 3125–3131. doi:10.1039/C5LC00539F PMID:26082346

Karthick, G. S., & Pankajavalli, P. B. (2019). Healthcare IoT Architectures, Technologies, Applications, and Issues: A Deep Insight. In N. Bouchemal (Ed.), *Intelligent Systems for Healthcare Management and Delivery* (pp. 235–265). Hershey, PA: IGI Global. doi:10.4018/978-1-5225-7071-4.ch011

Ko, J., Lu, C., Srivastava, M. B., Stankovic, J. A., Terzis, A., & Welsh, M. (2010). Wireless sensor networks for healthcare. *Proceedings of the IEEE*, *98*(11), 1947–1960. doi:10.1109/JPROC.2010.2065210

Li, Y., Thai, M., & Wu, W. (2008). Wireless Sensor Networks and Applications. Berlin, Germany: Springer. doi:10.1007/978-0-387-49592-7

Liu, T., Kamthe, A., Jiang, L., & Cerpa, A. (2009, June). Performance evaluation of link quality estimation metrics for static multihop wireless sensor networks. In *2009 6th Annual IEEE Communications Society Conference on Sensor, Mesh and Ad Hoc Communications and Networks* (pp. 1-9). Piscataway, NJ: IEEE. 10.1109/SAHCN.2009.5168959

Liu, T., Kamthe, A., Jiang, L., & Cerpa, A. (2009). Performance Evaluation of Link Quality Estimation Metrics for Static Multihop Wireless Sensor Networks.

Lorincz, K., Malan, D. J., Fulford-Jones, T. R., Nawoj, A., Clavel, A., Shnayder, V., ... Moulton, S. (2004). Sensor networks for emergency response: Challenges and opportunities. *IEEE Pervasive Computing*, *3*(4), 16–23. doi:10.1109/MPRV.2004.18

Lounis, A., Hadjidj, A., Bouabdallah, A., & Challal, Y. (2012, July). Secure and scalable cloud-based architecture for e-health wireless sensor networks. In *2012 21st International Conference on Computer Communications and Networks (ICCCN)* (pp. 1-7). Piscataway, NJ: IEEE. 10.1109/ICCCN.2012.6289252

Malima, A., Siavoshi, S., Musacchio, T., Upponi, J., Yilmaz, C., Somu, S., ... Busnaina, A. (2012). Highly sensitive microscale in vivo sensor enabled by electrophoretic assembly of nanoparticles for multiple biomarker detection. *Lab on a Chip*, *12*(22), 4748–4754. doi:10.1039/c2lc40580f PMID:22983480

Mehrotra, P. (2016). Biosensors and their applications–A review. *Journal of Oral Biology and Craniofacial Research*, *6*(2), 153–159.

Minaie, A., Sanati-Mehrizy, A., Sanati-Mehrizy, P., & Sanati-Mehrizy, R. (2013). Application of wireless sensor networks in health care system. age, 23(1).

Neves, P., Stachyra, M., & Rodrigues, J. (2008). Application of wireless sensor networks to healthcare promotion.

Perkins, M. D., & Kessel, M. (2015). What Ebola tells us about outbreak diagnostic readiness. *Nature Biotechnology*, *33*(5), 464–469. doi:10.1038/nbt.3215 PMID:25965752

Perrig, A., Stankovic, J., & Wagner, D. (2004). Security in wireless sensor networks. Prezi. Retrieved from https://prezi.com/ok_gznayh-ex/bandwidth-efficiency/

Pfaller, M. A., Wolk, D. M., & Lowery, T. J. (2016). T2MR and T2Candida: Novel technology for the rapid diagnosis of candidemia and invasive candidiasis. *Future Microbiology*, *11*(1), 103–117. doi:10.2217/fmb.15.111 PMID:26371384

Raghavendra, C. S., Sivalingam, K. M., & Znati, T. (Eds.). (2006). Wireless sensor networks. Berlin, Germany: Springer.

Sadiku, M. N., Musa, S. M., & Momoh, O. D. (2014). Wireless sensor networks: Opportunities and challenges. *Journal of Engineering Research and Applications, 4*(1), 41–43.

Schröder, U. C., Bokeloh, F., O'Sullivan, M., Glaser, U., Wolf, K., Pfister, W., ... Neugebauer, U. (2015). Rapid, culture-independent, optical diagnostics of centrifugally captured bacteria from urine samples. *Biomicrofluidics, 9*(4). doi:10.1063/1.4928070 PMID:26339318

Sengiz, C., Congur, G., & Erdem, A. (2015). Development of ionic liquid modified disposable graphite electrodes for label-free electrochemical detection of DNA hybridization related to Microcystis spp. *Sensors (Basel), 15*(9), 22737–22749. doi:10.3390150922737 PMID:26371004

Sha, K., Du, J., & Shi, W. (2006). WEAR: A balanced, fault-tolerant, energy-aware routing protocol in WSNs. *International Journal of Sensor Networks, 1*(3-4), 156–168. doi:10.1504/IJSNET.2006.012031

Sha, K., & Shi, W. (2005). Modeling the lifetime of wireless sensor networks. *Sensor Letters, 3*(2), 126–135. doi:10.11661.2005.017

Shojaei, T. R., Salleh, M. A. M., Tabatabaei, M., Ekrami, A., Motallebi, R., Rahmani-Cherati, T., ... Jorfi, R. (2014). Development of sandwich-form biosensor to detect Mycobacterium tuberculosis complex in clinical sputum specimens. *The Brazilian Journal of Infectious Diseases, 18*(6), 600–608. doi:10.1016/j.bjid.2014.05.015 PMID:25181404

Simon, G., Maróti, M., Lédeczi, Á., Balogh, G., Kusy, B., Nádas, A., . . . Frampton, K. (2004, November). Sensor network-based countersniper system. In *Proceedings of the 2nd international conference on Embedded networked sensor systems* (pp. 1-12). New York, NY: ACM.

Sohrabi, K., Gao, J., Ailawadhi, V., & Pottie, G. J. (2000). Protocols for self-organization of a wireless sensor network. IEEE personal communications, 7(5), 16-27.

Stroulia, E., Chodos, D., Boers, N. M., Huang, J., Gburzynski, P., & Nikolaidis, I. (2009, May). Software engineering for health education and care delivery systems: The Smart Condo project. In *2009 ICSE Workshop on Software Engineering in Health Care* (pp. 20-28). Piscataway, NJ: IEEE. 10.1109/SEHC.2009.5069602

Sun, J., Fang, Y., & Zhu, X. (2010). Privacy and emergency response in e-healthcare leveraging wireless body sensor networks. *IEEE Wireless Communications, 17*(1), 66–73. doi:10.1109/MWC.2010.5416352

Surfix. (2018). Retrieved from https://www.surfix.nl/applications/biosensors

Ullah, M. & Ahmad, W. (2009). Evaluation of routing protocols in wireless sensor networks.

Virone, G., Wood, A., Selavo, L., Cao, Q., Fang, L., Doan, T., . . . Stankovic, J. (2006, April). An advanced wireless sensor network for health monitoring. In Transdisciplinary conference on distributed diagnosis and home healthcare (D2H2) (pp. 2-4).

Watchguard. Retrieved from http://customers.watchguard.com/articles/Article/How-is-jitter-calculated

Werner-Allen, G., Lorincz, K., Ruiz, M., Marcillo, O., Johnson, J., Lees, J., & Welsh, M. (2006). Deploying a wireless sensor network on an active volcano. *IEEE Internet Computing*, *10*(2), 18–25. doi:10.1109/MIC.2006.26

Yang, Y. & Wang, J. (2008, April). Design guidelines for routing metrics in multihop wireless networks. In *IEEE INFOCOM 2008-The 27th Conference on Computer Communications* (pp. 1615-1623). Piscataway, NJ: IEEE. 10.1109/INFOCOM.2008.222

Yen, C. W., de Puig, H., Tam, J. O., Gómez-Márquez, J., Bosch, I., Hamad-Schifferli, K., & Gehrke, L. (2015). Multicolored silver nanoparticles for multiplexed disease diagnostics: Distinguishing dengue, yellow fever, and Ebola viruses. *Lab on a Chip*, *15*(7), 1638–1641. doi:10.1039/C5LC00055F PMID:25672590

Yick, J., Mukherjee, B., & Ghosal, D. (2005, October). Analysis of a prediction-based mobility adaptive tracking algorithm. In *2nd International Conference on Broadband Networks*, 2005. (pp. 753-760). Piscataway, NJ: IEEE. 10.1109/ICBN.2005.1589681

Yick, J., Mukherjee, B., & Ghosal, D. (2008). Wireless sensor network survey. *Computer Networks*, *52*(12), 2292–2330. doi:10.1016/j.comnet.2008.04.002

Chapter 6
QoS–Enabled Improved Cuckoo Search–Inspired Protocol (ICSIP) for IoT–Based Healthcare Applications

R. Vadivel

Bharathiar University, India

J. Ramkumar

VLB Janakiammal College of Arts and Science, India

ABSTRACT

Internet of Things (IoT) is a technology which accommodates the hardware, software, and physical objects that collaborate with each other. IoT-based healthcare applications are increasing day by day and are never going to be decreased. Healthcare applications work in an ad-hoc manner to collect patient data and send it to corresponding persons so they can take just-in-time action. The routing protocols designed for general ad-hoc networks and applications are not supported by IoT-based, ad-hoc networks. Hence, there exists a need to develop a routing protocol to support IoT-based, ad-hoc networks. This chapter focuses to develop a routing protocol for an IoT-based, cognitive radio ad-hoc network by utilizing bio-inspired concept with the objective of reducing the delay and energy consumption. NS2 simulation results reflect the proposed routing protocol's performance in terms of benchmark performance metrics.

INTRODUCTION

Internet of Things

In the computing world, the term Internet of Things (IoT) indicates all the things that are connected to the World Wide Web, where IoT term is more utilized to describe the object that makes communication with each other. Commonly, IoT is made (or formed) from interconnecting the basic elementary sensors

DOI: 10.4018/978-1-7998-1090-2.ch006

to modern smartphones. By making integration with these kinds of devices, the autonomous systems can gather the information, make analysis and step into an action. For the year 2020, it has been predicted to have more than 26 billion of connected devices over the Globe. It is because; IoT has started stepping in each and every domain, where users didn't find any reason to exclude IoT from their use due to the virtual endless support. Currently, IoT have stepped into healthcare industry which includes digitalizing the medical related information, its process, its progress, tracking the patient health details, etc. In healthcare industry, IoT is used to (i) monitor the patient details, (ii) manage the information of medical waste, (iii) mange the patient information, (iv) manage the medical emergency, (v) maintain the storage of drugs, (vi) control the pharmaceutical error, (vii) anti-kidnap system for born baby

Health Care Application

Health Care Applications (HCA) in IoT frameworks have begun to grow and get attention slowly. In general, IoT systems have the capability to give multiple positive features that assist the doctors by monitoring the patients from the remote place. Devices of Personal Health Care (DPHC) have become an important component of HCA in IoT. DPHCs are electronic device with mobile facility which can measure the biomedical signals by sensing. The people can check their own health condition and take care by themselves in an advanced manner. DPHCs are expected to become more popular because of its ability to connect to centralized servers of healthcare. Generally, hardware may get malfunctioned at any time which will give the result in failure of system. Bugs in software, shortage of power, hazards in environment may also leads to failure of system. Multiple comprehensives studies are being conducted in IoT by making an assumption of having minor error disrupting the operations. In IoT, devices are distributed geographically and have rare maintenance. These kinds of devices are progressively susceptible to bugs, shortage of power, and hazards in environment. The count of nodes in IoT may tend to get gradually increases with faults leading to fail the IoT based network. Furthermore, the data that are sent by DPHC are more valuable and it should be taken care in failure of system. Only a very few proposals have focused this thrust research area. HCA in IoT frameworks have started to gather the researchers' attention towards itself due to the features which it provides for monitoring the patients from remote location, where it has the feature of scalable, flexible and interoperable. While considering the HCA in IoT frameworks, the gateway plays a major role. The result of IoT system is getting success or failure depends on the management of gateways.

Cognitive Radio Ad-hoc Network

Cognitive radio network is made up of number of nodes which have the mobile facility. Cognitive radio network is building cognitive radio technology giving a distinctive ability to sense the spectrum, frequent configuring of radio signals, developing the spectrum accessibility by analyzing the spectrum environment. This kind of nodes can be denoted the secondary users (SUs). Sometimes SUs are also called as cognitive users (CUs). In cognitive radio networks, few users have the license and they are denoted by primary users (PUs). By default, PUs has higher priority level to utilize the cognitive radio network, where SUs has lower priority level. If SUs are in the need to utilize the network to transmit the data, then it necessary to use the licensed frequency band in a opportunistic manner, which is presently not used by the PUs. Hence, the important duty of SUs become to make sure that the spectrum is available for accessing, because it should affect the PUs usage.

A cognitive radio ad-hoc network (CRAHN) is an exclusive type of cognitive radio network without any centralized network or control. SUs are in the need of cooperation method to share the information related to cognitive radio network, like existence of PUs, configuration of node, and spectrum availability. The information which is received by sensing and local observation can be used to reconfiguring the nodes and finding the new routes towards destination. CRAHN have five distinguished features, which are (i) dynamic topology, (ii) heterogeneity in spectrum, (iii) multi hopping, (iv) self-configuration, and (v) limited power supply. But the challenges faced in CRAHN are considered as a research issue and motivate the researchers to do innovative research. Major researches in CRAHN focus to provide broad range of support with more quality and efficiency.

Finding an appropriate route to deliver the data in CRAHN is thrust research area. Routing protocols of other ad-hoc networks are not suitable for CRAHN, even if applied it will reduce the total network performance. Routing in infrastructure-based networks is entirely different from infrastructureless network like CRAHN because of its dynamicity and heterogeneous nature. Mobility of nodes increases the route error. Every channel is limited to number of nodes, where it may increase or decrease over the time. If a PU enters the network area, then SUs are forced to vacate the channel immediately and change the channel. Spectrum heterogeneity, routing information, and mobility of node worsen the efficiency of the network. Hence, there exists no guarantee for a stable route between nodes. The average of route failure is more than the other infrastructure-based networks. Setting the successful route between nodes increases the overall cost. Discovering the new route to the destination utilizes the broadcasting concept to send messages which lead to increased consumption of energy.

The above-mentioned challenges are necessarily need to be focused at all the levels of network design.

- In physical layer, the protocol should undertake the loss of path, network fading, and interference of nodes to preserve the routing path.
- In data link layer, the protocol should construct the physical link in a more reliable a manner in order to avoid synchronization issues between the nodes
- In network layer, the protocol should identify the changes in the topology of the network and find the next best route to reach the destination.
- In transport layer, the protocol should match the packet loss and delay characteristics.
- In application layer, the protocol should adjust and handle the disconnections which occur frequently.

BACKGROUND STUDY

Adaptive Wireless Power Transfer Strategy (Adelina, Sotiris, and Alexandros, 2019) was proposed by investigating the mobility models used in ad-hoc networks. Mobile agents were considered for recharging the nodes battery in order to extend the lifetime, but the efficient computing over the entire network was affected leading to network failure. Reliable Routing Protocol (Ahmed, Samah, and Khaled, 2017) was proposed for segregating the network in order to avoid the overlapping. In this protocol, master nodes are appointed for each zone for efficient routing, where it resulted in increased delay leading to network failure. Multichannel based Routing Protocol (Jipeng et al., 2012) was proposed to rectify the channel assigning problem in CRAHN, where the method utilizes the reusing cum assignment scheme to avoid the errors in order to increase the channel efficiency. The result with increased delay represent the protocol is not sufficient to meet the ad-hoc network issues. Interference Minimization Protocol (Abedalmotaleb and Thomas, 2016) was proposed to deal the interference during the multihop routing, where it establishes the interference awareness-based routing to reduce the delay which arises due to interference. This protocol utilized the mechanisms of scheduling and routing, but the reduced throughput result indicates the inefficiency of the protocol.

Bottleneck Aware Protocol (Nadav et al, 2019) was proposed to detect the bottlenecks and prefer alternate route to reach the destination. The core of this protocol was optimized-link-state-routing protocol. Network overhead was focused to reduce, but the increased delay shows that the protocol may lead to network failure. Cross Layer Optimization Protocol (Surajit and Tamaghna, 2017) was proposed to minimize the routing in spectrum-based ad-hoc network. Selecting the optimized path is a major issue in networks, where this protocol optimizes the route to reach the destination. This protocol has consumed more time to optimize the route and results in increased delay. Self-Adaptive Metric Protocol (Tran, Hoa, Nauman, 2016) was proposed to find the better route even the node changes its location in a geographic manner. It focused to utilize the concepts of both proactive cum reactive routing strategy, where the optimum routing resulted in increased jitter. Flow Rate Optimized Protocol (Hongtao et al., 2008) was proposed to utilize the advantage of multiple rate transmissions in ad-hoc network. To meet the objective link interference concepts were used, but the characteristics of multiple rate transmission didn't have any effects on link interference methods and led to increased delay.

Energy Aware Routing Protocol (Papakostas et al., 2018) was proposed to reduce the energy consumption in ad-hoc networks. The protocol focuses the nodes that are dominated from the network; where those specific nodes spend too much energy to get connect to the network. Reduced throughput indicates that the energy consumption is not a constraint for increasing the throughput. Position Aware Routing Protocol (Alper, Muharrem, and Burcu, 2019) was proposed to reduce the latency in order to reduce the consumption of energy. The protocol aims to reduce the sending of data packet at each connection, where it leads to looping in route. Backoff interval was also applied for shared medium access. Selection of increased length route represents the protocol leading to network failure. Asynchronous Distributed Protocol (Shaojie and Chuanhe, 2019) was proposed as optimization-based framework for ad-hoc network to reduce the delay. Primal dual concept was applied to reduce the complex situations that arise randomly. The results with increased packet timeout rate represent that the protocol will lead to reduced network lifetime. Fuzzy Multicast Routing Protocol (Ajay, Santosh, and Sachin, 2017) was proposed to overcome the centralized administration control problem for efficient routing. Routing was monitored by using the cost generated by fuzzy logic. Network resourced were forced to control through fuzzy logic, which results in increased error and packet failure.

Centralized Content Routing Method (Xuan et al, 2017) was proposed to analyze and segregate the routing based on the type of content sent by the nodes. It utilizes the reactive, proactive and opportunistic routing concept to enhance the network lifetime, but the result indicates that the protocol was not sufficient for routing in ad-hoc network. Improved Frog Leap Inspired Protocol (Ramkumar and Vadivel, n.d.) was proposed to minimize the delay in CRAHN, but delay minimization was not up to the mark.

MAIN FOCUS OF THE CHAPTER

The term mobility gives the advantage of flexibility to nodes in IoT based ad-hoc network, but at the same time, it gives the disadvantage of disconnection between the nodes leading to link failure, delay and exhaustive energy consumption. The network disconnection issue arises when the node moves from its radio range leading to delay and energy consumption, which is unacceptable in based health care world. Routing plays a major role in delay and energy consumption, where a better routing protocol can reduce the same a lot. Hence, a necessary arises to design a routing protocol to avoid delay and energy consumption, by avoiding congestion and finding the alternate route in a short time.

ICSIP: IMPROVED CUCKOO SEARCH INSPIRED PROTOCOL

Cuckoo Search (CS) algorithm (Adelina, Sotiris, and Alexandros, 2019) was proposed by inheriting the natural behavior of cuckoo bird. Optimization algorithm based on cuckoo search (Ahmed, Samah, and Khaled, 2017) was proposed to effectively enhance the performance of traditional algorithms. This research work has enhanced the optimization algorithm based on cuckoo search to enhance the routing performance of CRAHN namely, Improved Cuckoo Search Inspired Protocol (ISCIP). ICSIP is a populace based stochastic globally seeking algorithm to find the best route to destination. In ICSIP, the term "prototype" represents the nest of the cuckoo bird and the term "attribute" represents the cuckoo bird's egg. The general mathematical notation of ICSIP was based on random walk concept and it can be expressed as

The general equation of CS algorithm was fully based upon random walk algorithm, and it expressed as.

$$\omega_{\iota(D+1)} = z^i \pm \tau \left(\sum_{\iota=0}^{\iota+2} levy(\eta + 2\iota) \right) \tag{1}$$

where ι .denotes current generation's end measure ($\iota = \sum_{0}^{maxcycle-1} D$ and where maxcycle represents the previously defined count for the maximum generation).

In ICSIP, initial attribute value of μ of Dz^i h route, $P_{\iota=0;i} = \left[x_{\iota=0;\mu,Dz^i} \right]$ can be mathematically expressed as

$$\omega_{\iota=0;\mu,i} = rand\left(t_{Dz^i} - b_{Dz^i} \right) + b_{Dz^i} \tag{2}$$

where t_{Dz^i} .and b_{Dz^i} .are maximum and minimum boundary of seeking space with μ+1 attributes. The ICSIP controls the baseline clause in each step of iteration. If attribute rate reaches the expected limit of baseline, then it can update rate of related attributes automatically. Before starting the iteration of seeking for the routes, the ICSIP pinpoints the best route as ω_{finest}.

Iteration

The iteration process starts with finding the route by constructing a matrix of available routes, and reveals the best route Ψ. It can be mathematically expressed as

$$\psi = \left(\frac{\Delta \, (1 \pm \rho) \odot \dfrac{1}{sec}\left(\pi \odot \dfrac{\rho}{3} \right)}{\Delta \left(\dfrac{1+\rho}{3} \right) \times \rho \times 3^{\frac{\rho \pm 1}{3}}} \right)^{\frac{t_{Dz^i} - b_{Dz^i}}{\rho}} \tag{3}$$

where Δ represents the function of delta. Development phase of ω_{Dz^i} route starts by desscribing the contribution vector $r = \omega_{Dz^i}$.

Velocity Range

Velocity range indicates the distance that is covered in a single move. Mathematically, the expected velocity range calculation can be expressed as

$$velocityrange = \frac{1}{3} \times \left(\sum \frac{1}{100} \times \left(\frac{u_\mu}{v_\mu} \right)^{\frac{1}{\beta}} \times \left(r - \omega_{finest} \right) \right) + Dz^i \tag{4}$$

where $u = \Psi.rand[\delta]$ and $r = rand[\delta]$. The function $rand[\delta]$ will create a distinctive value among 1 and δ.

Route Contributor

Mathematically, the route contribution calculation is r can be produced as

$$r = \left(\frac{u_\mu}{v_\mu} \right) \left(pacerange_\mu . ran[\delta] \right) + Dz^i \tag{5}$$

Reroute Process

In ICSIP, rerouting process is carried out by using the ω_{finest} and it can be mathematically expressed as

$$R\left(\omega_{finest} \right) \le R\left(\omega_{Dz^i} \right) \rightarrow \omega_{finest} \tag{6}$$

Crossover

The unfeasible routes are identified by utilizing the crossover manipulation and it is expressed as

$$r_i = \begin{cases} \omega_{Dz^i} + rand\left(\omega_{r1} - \omega_{r2}\right) rand_{Dz^i} > p_0 \\ \omega_{Dz^i} - rand\left(\omega_{r1} - \omega_{r2}\right) rand_{Dz^i} < p_0 \\ \dfrac{1}{\omega_{Dz^i}} rand_{Dz^i} = p_0 \end{cases} \qquad (7)$$

Termination Condition

When the process of finding the route gets completed, ICSIP makes verification by checking finishing condition. If the finishing condition is met, then the process gets terminated, else the process gets continued.

SIMULATION STUDY

This section illustrates the simulation done in NS2 simulator for the proposed protocol ICSIP against IFLIP in IoT-based-CRAHN environment (Ramkumar and Vadivel, n.d.). NS2 is considered and found as the outstanding simulator for the researches that are oriented to network. NS2 supports the network researches that are related to discrete events supporting the routing protocols in both wired networks and wireless networks. Additionally, NS2 supports the concept of queuing theory. By analyzing the several advantages of Ns2, this research work selects the NS2 for measuring the performance of ICSIP against IFLIP (Ramkumar and Vadivel, n.d.). During the simulation, the data packets were sent through auxiliary channels. The coding for the NS2 simulation was written using a object oriented programming language, namely C++. There exists a vast support for huge scalable networks in NS2, where it supports different routing protocols in different mobility models. But, random waypoint mobility model is used in the simulation. A comparison is made to analyze the protocol performance towards supporting the IoT-based-CRAHN. The simulation settings used for the research work is tabulated in Table 1.

EXPERIMENTS AND RESULTS

Throughput:

Throughput indicates the percentage of data that is successfully received by the destination node during the simulation period. This research work expresses the throughput in Kbps (kilobits per second). Mathematically, throughput can be defined as,

$$Throughput = \left[\frac{QuantityofReceivedBytes}{SimulationPeriod} \times \frac{8}{1024}\right] \times 100 \qquad (8)$$

Table 1. Simulation parameters and settings

Parameters	Settings
Size of Area	3000 × 4000 m^2
Primary User Count	22 to 30
Secondary User Count	950 to 1100
MAC	802.11b
Range of Transmission	2800 meters
Total time of Simulation	500 seconds
Traffic Source	CBR
Size of Packet	512 bytes
Total Number of Packets	1800
Mobility Model	Random Waypoint Model
Energy at Initial Level	0.5 Joules

Figure 1 shows the performance of ICSIP against IFLIP in terms of throughput over the nodes ranging from 1250 to 2250 (Ramkumar and Vadivel, n.d). It is evident that throughput of IFLIP has rapid decrease due to increased route failure, and ICSIP has better increase in throughput (Ramkumar and Vadivel, n.d.). It is found that ICSIP is able to detect the route failure and immediately find the alternate route (which is optimized) based on the location of the node and the fitness value. ICSIP has the capability to remove the unwanted routes that are lengthy, expired, and faulty, because these unwanted routes may decrease the overall performance of the network. Increased amount of data packets are dropped in IFLIP due to route failure (Ramkumar and Vadivel, n.d.). The result shows that ICSIP can give the better throughput even more if the nodes are increased more.

Packet Delivery Ratio

Packet Delivery Ratio indicates the percentage of data packets successfully received by the destination node over the data packets sent by the source node. Mathematically, packet delivery ratio can be defined as,

$$PacketDeliveryRatio = \left[\frac{TotalNo.ofDataPacketSuccesfullyReceived}{TotalNo.ofDataPacketSent} \right] \times 100 \qquad (9)$$

In Figure 2, nodes from 1,250 to 2,250 are plotted in the x-axis, where the y-axis is plotted with percentage of packet delivery ratio. Figure 2 attempts to compare the packet delivery ratio of ICSIP against IFLIP (Ramkumar and Vadivel, n.d.). In the simulation, data packets are sent in randomly over different channels. The routing of the packet relies upon the unconstrained system topology. Assessment of ICSIP against IFLIP is done under node mobility by sending packets over various randomly produced network topologies (Ramkumar and Vadivel, n.d.). ICSIP is designed to share the routing and congestion information to all the nodes around the network, where ICSIP is designed to never stick with single route and it tries to send the data packet in multiple routes to reach the destination with the aim

Figure 1. Throughput vs nodes

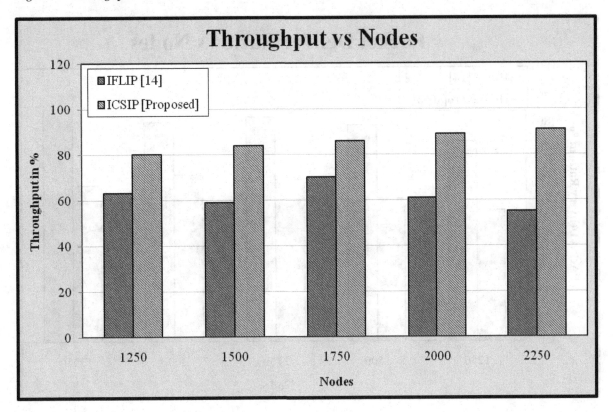

of increasing the packet delivery ratio. Figure 2 clearly shows that the proposed protocol ICSIP has the better performance than IFLIP (Ramkumar and Vadivel, n.d.).

Delay

Delay indicates the time difference between the data packet sent by the source node and data packet received by the destination node. Mathematically, delay can be defined as,

$$Delay = \left[\frac{1}{M} \left(R_T - S_T \right) \right] \times 100 \tag{10}$$

where M is the total number of data packet, S_T is the time of data packet received by the destination node, and S_T is the time of data packet sent by the source node.

In Figure 3, nodes from 1250 to 2250 are plotted in the x-axis, where the y-axis is plotted with percentage of delay. Figure 3 compares the delay faced by ICSIP and IFLIP (Ramkumar and Vadivel, n.d.). Figure 3 witnesses the performance of ICSIP against IFLIP in term of delay varying number of nodes ranging from 1250 to 2250. From Figure 3, it is evident that both protocols are facing delay, but IFLIP has 42.8% more delay than ICSIP (Ramkumar and Vadivel, n.d.). It is due lack of memory in nodes, during the route failure or error some of the data packets sent by the source node are buffered till a new

Figure 2. Packet delivery ratio vs nodes

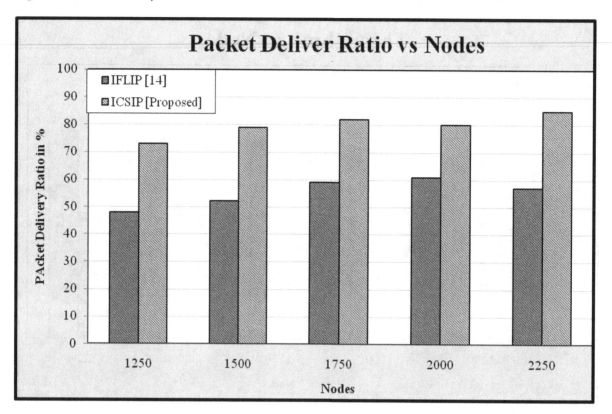

route is found, which leads to delay. Most of the route failures occur due to the mobility of node. Some of the alternate routes that are found during the route failure has longer route resulting to higher delay. When comparing the nodes of general ad-hoc network with IoT-based-CRAHN, it will found that cognitive radio-based ad-hoc networks have increased route failure and delay. Due to the limited range of radio signals, mobility of nodes has huge impact towards the route failure. The proposed protocol ICSIP is also facing delay, but not up to the delay of IFLIP (Ramkumar and Vadivel, n.d.).

Energy Consumption

Energy Consumption indicates the percentage of total number of nodes over the consumed energy. Mathematically, energy consumption can be defined as,

$$EnergyConsumed = \frac{TotalNumberofNodes}{ConsumedEnergy} \times 100 \tag{11}$$

Figure 4 compares energy consumed by ICSIP and IFLIP to deliver the packet to the destination node from source node (Ramkumar and Vadivel, n.d.). ICSIP is designed in the manner to choose the most stable route towards the destination in all available multiple routes. The route selected by ICSIP is estimated to be the best route path and it consumes less energy with the shortest route. In other ad-hoc

Figure 3. Delay vs nodes

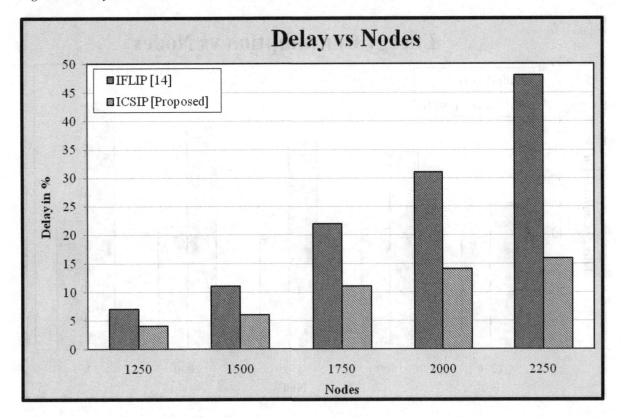

networks, higher number of alternate routes may be available when comparing with IoT-based-CRAHN, it is due to the limited distancebetween source node and destination node; but in IoT-based-CRAHN its vice versa. Due to route failure and retransmission, enormous amount of energy is wasted by IFLIP (Ramkumar and Vadivel, n.d.). Figure 4 clearly shows that the proposed protocol ICSIP consumes less energy for delivering data to the destination than IFLIP (Ramkumar and Vadivel, n.d.).

CONCLUSION

IoT has stepped in health care world to monitor the patients and take in-time actions to save the patients from danger. The health care applications are being used handheld devices only, where the energy is limited and one-step more care is needed to save the energy. Decreasing the delay and energy consumption has become a major challenge in all kinds of network-oriented researches, where routing protocols are the core reasons for this. Routing protocols are not common to all types of network, because certain routing protocols are designed to specific networks and it cannot give its best performance in other networks. This research work has focused in design and development of bio-inspired based routing protocol especially for IoT-based healthcare applications which is to be used in spectrum-based network, which is CRAHN. The proposed routing protocol is designed to select the alternate route in optimum manner when there exists a route or node failure, where other routing protocol stick with a single or minimum number routes. To measure the performance against the existing routing protocol IFLIP, the simulation

Figure 4. Energy consumption vs nodes

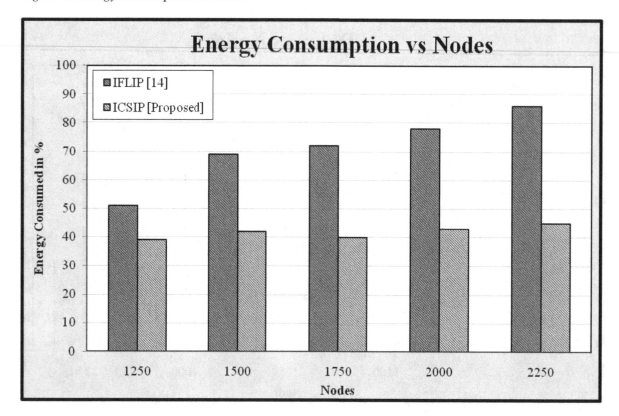

is done in NS2. The result shows that the proposed routing protocol ICSIP outperforms the IFLIP in all aspects, and it is found to be best routing protocol to implement in IoT-based health care applications to minimize the delay and consumption of energy (Ramkumar and Vadivel, n.d.).

REFERENCES

Abedalmotaleb, Z., & Thomas, F. (2016). Neighborhood-based interference minimization for stable position-based routing in mobile ad hoc networks. *Future Generation Computer Systems, 64*, 88–97. doi:10.1016/j.future.2016.03.022

Adelina, M., Sotiris, N., & Alexandros, A. V. (2019). Adaptive wireless power transfer in mobile ad hoc networks. *Computer Networks, 152*, 87–97. doi:10.1016/j.comnet.2019.02.004

Ahmed, I. S., Samah, A. G., & Khaled, M. (2017). A Reliable Routing Protocol for Vehicular Ad hoc Networks. *Computers & Electrical Engineering, 64*, 473–495. doi:10.1016/j.compeleceng.2016.11.011

Ajay, K. Y., Santosh, K. D., & Sachin, T. (2017). EFMMRP: Design of efficient fuzzy based multi-constraint multicast routing protocol for wireless ad-hoc network. *Computer Networks, 118*, 15–23. doi:10.1016/j.comnet.2017.03.001

Alper, B., Muharrem, T., & Burcu, Y. (2019). P-AUV: Position aware routing and medium access for ad hoc AUV networks. *Journal of Network and Computer Applications*, *125*, 146–154. doi:10.1016/j.jnca.2018.10.014

Hongtao, T., Sanjay, K. B., Choi, L. L., & Wendong, X. (2008). Joint routing and flow rate optimization in multi-rate ad hoc networks. *Computer Networks*, *52*(3), 739–764. doi:10.1016/j.comnet.2007.11.006

Jipeng, Z., Liyang, P., Yuhui, D., & Jianzhu, L. (2012). An on-demand routing protocol for improving channel use efficiency in multichannel ad hoc networks. *Journal of Network and Computer Applications*, *35*(5), 1606–1614. doi:10.1016/j.jnca.2012.03.003

Papakostas, D., Eshghi, S., Katsaros, D., & Tassiulas, L. (2018). Energy-aware backbone formation in military multilayer ad hoc networks. *Ad Hoc Networks*, *81*, 17–44. doi:10.1016/j.adhoc.2018.06.017

Ramkumar, J. & Vadivel, R. (n.d.). Improved frog leap inspired protocol (IFLIP) – for routing in cognitive radio ad hoc networks (CRAHN). World Journal of Engineering, 15, 306-311.

Schweitzer, N., Stulman, A., Hirst, T., Margalit, R. D., & Shabtai, A. (2019). Network bottlenecks in OLSR based ad-hoc networks. *Ad Hoc Networks*, *88*, 36–54.

Shaojie, W., & Chuanhe, H. (2019). Asynchronous distributed optimization via dual decomposition for delay-constrained flying ad hoc networks. *Computer Communications*, *137*, 70–80. doi:10.1016/j.comcom.2019.02.006

Surajit, B., & Tamaghna, A. (2017). Cross layer optimization for outage minimizing routing in cognitive radio ad hoc networks with primary users outage protection. *Journal of Network and Computer Applications*, *98*, 114–124. doi:10.1016/j.jnca.2017.09.004

Tran, T. S., Hoa, L., & Nauman, A. (2016). MSAR: A metric self-adaptive routing model for Mobile Ad Hoc Networks. *Journal of Network and Computer Applications*, *68*, 114–125. doi:10.1016/j.jnca.2016.04.010

Xuan, L., Zhuo, L., Peng, Y., & Yongqiang, D. (2017). Information-centric mobile ad hoc networks and content routing: A survey. *Ad Hoc Networks*, *58*, 255–268. doi:10.1016/j.adhoc.2016.04.005

Chapter 7
Internet of Things–Based Authentication Mechanism for E–Health Applications

Kameswara Rao M.
Annamalai University, India

S. G. Santhi
Annamalai University, India

ABSTRACT

The sturdy advancements of internet of things are being changed into a methodology of associating smart things. E-health applications in this vision are a standout amongst IoT's most energizing applications. Indeed, security concerns were the fundamental boundary to the establishment. The encryption of various interlinked substances and the classification of the swapped information are the real concerns which should be settled for clients. This chapter proposes an e-health application using lightweight verification mechanism. The proposed model utilizes nonces as well as keyed-hash message authentication (KHAC) for checking the validity of verification trades.

INTRODUCTION

As of late, another model called the internet of things has gained fast ground all through the field of remote innovation and systems administration. Its key thought was the interconnectedness of different objects like Radio-Frequency Identification (RFID) labels, sensor frameworks, mobile phones, compact, and so on that communicate to achieve significant goals (Sicari et al., 2015 and Atzori et al., 2010). From another term, anything genuine winds up fanciful, it implies how everything will have an Internet partner that can be tended to, clear, and found. The Iot is very helpless to a few assaults. Such a weakness is a result of an excessive number of remote correspondences, with the danger of listening stealthily. Also, the properties of numerous other IoT parts that have lower vitality and calculation assets capacities. They can't consequently bolster the execution of complex security plans (Atzori et al., 2010). Authentication

DOI: 10.4018/978-1-7998-1090-2.ch007

and information uprightness are the significant security issues (Sicari et al., 2015). For example, IoT-related verification is a significant rule that empowers authentication of every entity's realness. In any case, a validation plot must be executed because of Internet of Things qualities. Conveying the Internet of Things must give ways for such an immense range of executions which would incredibly enhance the regular day-to-day existences. E-health applications were viewed as a standout amongst the most productive and dependable applications on an Internet of Things, an E-health framework is an advancement in radio recurrence dependent remote systems administration made up of wearable and semiconductor sensors connected to such a Base Station. This typically assembles health related information for private medicinal services purposes (Dohr et al., 2010). E-health based frameworks empower patients to dependably be checked on a progressing premise and, in this manner, foresee crises by empowering quick and proficient crisis restorative intervention (Patel et al., 2010). The part of realness in E-health candidates was a standout amongst the most vital challenges to in any case be talked about effectively (Li et al., 2010). A verification plot forestalls every single malignant hub transmission of erroneous information identified with health. Any modification in health-related information could have genuine outcomes since it could result in erroneous specialist's remedy or postpone a salvage task.

The chapter proposes a most recent lightweight E-health authentication framework. A protected channel is built up here between sensor hubs just as the base station once the plan validates each item with a keyed-hash message confirmation, proposed plan is utilizing nonces and ensures the honesty of both the different exchanges(Krawczyk et al., 1997). It offers next to no verification vitality utilization, ensures its character of the sensor hub from straightforwardness just as closures with such a session key contract over every sensor hub just as the base station. A plan still gives common validation just as an overwhelming dimension of insurance against various assaults.

The rest of a chapter will be organized as supposed. Segment II presents associated chip away at authentication just as E-health frameworks identified with IoT. A system design just as the proposed verification plot is clarified in Section III. They continue with such health and quality evaluation for present plan in Section IV and V. Area VI shows a lightweight PKI (Public Key Infrastructure) variation of the proposed framework. In conclusion, the chapter was settled of area VII and will give future work.

RELATED WORK

Authentication is by all accounts a urgent procedure that goes back to the early improvement of the Internet. Standard nearby system and Internet validation regularly meddles to halfway controlled authentication servers just as identity providers(El Maliki et al., 2007). Such experiences by and large have such a high vitality cost just as require some registering ability in which diverse articles that make up the setting of the Internet of Things were restricted to such assets. Such impediments are the principle issue of a few research works that endeavour to recommend inventive answers for the sending of IoT-adjusted authentication protocols. A few validations chips away at the internet of things are being referenced (Sicari et al., 2015 and Atzori et al., 2010).

Early work with authentication protocols can be part into two classes of protocols on the internet of things:

- **Authentication with Affirmation:**

Every single article having computerized declaration is required in this authentication protocols class. DTLS (Datagram Transport Layer Security)(Rescorla et al., 2012) verification handshake was proposed (Kothmayr et al., 2013) for internet of things. Scarcely any primary downsides, in any case, are its high vitality utilization brought about by RSA-based uneven encryption and the trading of PKI (Public Key Infrastructure) endorsements. For such reason, Elliptic Curve Cryptography (ECC) is raised as only a great thought in respect to RSA-based calculations since it speaks to advance vitality protection and far less key size for same phase of safety (Szczechowiak et al., 2008). The Wireless Sensor Networks in IoT dispersed Applications, a verifiable endorsement dependent on Elliptic Curve Cryptography (ECC) which is proposed for reducing the expense of protection of vitality of authentication protocols (Information about certificate scheme, 2013). It gives lower vitality utilization and overhead calculation (Porambage et al., 2014, and Pauthkey, 2014).

- **Authentication without Confirmation:**

The above class of authentication protocols is centred on cryptographic procedures, for example, symmetric cryptography, hash capacities, and exclusive-or activity (Xor). It's frequently known for the preservation of its vitality. For this reason, creators in (Turkanovic et al., 2014) proposed the client validation just as key understanding plan dependent on the thought of internet of things for various specially appointed remote sensor systems. It utilizes just cryptography tasks. E-health applications are among the Internet of Things applications. Consequently, the real security issues just as obstacles all through the IoT are respected all through this application space. Investigations in (Roman et al., 2011, Medaglia et al., 2010, and Miorandi et al., 2012) perceived the issues, applications just as research of the IoT. Validation of both the identity of the item is a basic component in the improvement of secure correspondence. To achieve this objective, they should comprehend the deficiencies of vitality and processing foundation that speak to the essential hindrance of the Internet of Things. E-health frameworks comprise of sensors that go about as a passage and are developed on, in and around a human body. The Base Station gathers classified basic health related information from sensor hubs through secure channels as well as a while later transmits the information gathered to guardians. Setting up such a scrambled correspondence arranges needs an authentication procedure that can adjust to the shortcomings of nature and rare assets of the imparting elements. Authors in (Cheikhrouhou et al., 2010) suggested a lightweight validation conspire introduced on AES (Advanced Encryption Standard) symmetrical encryption (Pub, 2011) of both the nonces created here between client just as the base station. It gives quick authentication. Such an equivalent does not look through the validity of both the traded writings against the risk of data spying and apparatus all through the verification stage, anyway checks them on the following gathering and it doesn't take a gander at the expense of unscrambling exercises on confined gadgets in case of a authentication powerlessness.

All through this activity, they centre around both the vitality utilization of the validation stage. We propose an authentication plot with an extremely low vitality utilization that can be adjusted for each article that can participate in the Internet of Things. They additionally assess the dimension of insurance for the different conceivable assaults. The proposed plan offers shared validation just as key foundation to protect the safe channel for private trades.

AES-128 ENCRYPTION METHOD

AES is a system of symmetric block cipher, used to safeguard confidential information and has a set block size. AES offers 128, 192 and 256-bit key lengths and comprises of 10, 12 and 14 (also referred as rounds) encoding intervals, successively. Each round mixes the information from either the encryption key with the round key. Each round involves four processing stages, including SubBytes, ShiftRows, MixColumns, as well as AddRoundKey, apart from the last round. (1) SubBytes is an invertible and non-linear process that uses 16 equivalent 256-byte replacement tables (i.e., S-box) for individually mapping data block bytes into other bytes. S-box results are produced by multiplicative inverse computations. (2) ShiftRows conducts byte transposition by cyclically shifting data block rows as per predefined offsets, i.e. left transition of the 2nd, third, and fourth rows successively by one, two, and three bytes. (3) Mix-Columns multiplies a modular polynomial in GF(28) for each column of the data block. It is also possible to combine SubBytes and MixColumns into big Look-Up-Tables (LUT) instead of computing individually. (4) AddRoundKey conversion brings a round-key information block to the key schedule unit from the original secret key. This feature XORed every block byte in the round-key with the respective bye.

Public Key Infrastructure (PKI)

The Public Key Infrastructure (PKI) is the collection of hardware, software, strategies, procedures, and processes required to generate, handle, distribute, use, store, and revoke digital certificates and public keys. The PKI is the basis that allows technology to be used across big customer communities, such as digital signatures and encryption. PKIs provide the vital components for a safe and trusted e-commerce company setting and the increasing internet of things (IoT). PKIs assist to identify individuals, devices, and services–allowing managed system and resource access, information security, and transaction transparency. Next generation company apps are becoming more dependent on public key infrastructure (PKI) technology to ensure high safety as changing business models are increasingly dependent on electronic communication requiring internet authentication and compliance with more stringent data security laws.

The Role of Certificate Authorities (CAs)

PKIs use digital certificates to connect public keys to their related consumer (personal important proprietor). Digital certificates are the certificates that in a transaction facilitate identity verification between customers. The digital certificate defines the identity of customers within the ecosystem just as a passport certifies one's identity as a citizen of a nation. Since digital certificates are being used to identify the users to whom encrypted data is sent or to verify the information signer's identity, it is imperative to protect the certificate's authenticity and integrity to maintain the system's confidentiality. Certificate authorities (CAs) request online credentials for certifying users ' identity. CAs are pinning a PKI's safety and the facilities they promote, and can thus be the focus of advanced targeted attacks. Physical and logical checks as well as hardening processes such as hardware security modules (HSMs) have become essential to guarantee a PKI's integrity in order to mitigate the danger of attacks against CAs.

PKI Deployment

PKIs provide a structure that allows for the effective deployment on a mass scale of cryptographic data security techniques such as digital certificates and signatures. PKIs offer identity management facilities beyond and around networks and promote safe socket layer (SSL) and transportation layer safety (TLS) online encryption to protect web traffic, document and application signing, application code recognition, and time stamping. PKIs support desktop login, citizen identification, mass transit, mobile banking solutions and are crucial to IoT device credentials. Device credentials are becoming progressively essential to impart identities to increasing numbers of cloud-based and internet-connected devices running the gamut from smart phones to medical devices.

Cryptographic Security

Using asymmetric and symmetric cryptography principles, PKIs promote safe information exchange between users and devices–ensuring authenticity, confidentiality, and transaction integrity. Users (also referred to as "Subscribers" in PKI parlance) may be individual end consumers, internet servers, integrated systems, linked devices, or company process executing programs/applications. Asymmetric cryptography offers a key pair of a public and a private key element to consumers, devices or services within an ecosystem. Anyone in the community can use a government key to encrypt or verify a digital signature. On the other hand, the private key must be kept secret and is used only by the entity to which it belongs, typically for tasks such as decryption or digital signature creation.

The Increasing Importance of PKIs

With business models increasingly based on electronic transactions and digital records and more internet-aware devices linked to corporate networks, the role of a public key infrastructure is no longer restricted to remote systems such as safe email, physical access intelligent cards or encrypted internet traffic. It is expected that PKIs today will support more applications, users and devices across complex ecosystems. And with more stringent data security laws in government and industry, mainstream operating systems and company apps become more dependent than ever on an organisational PKI to ensure confidence.

THE PROPOSED SCHEME

Throughout this chapter, we describe proposed authentication scheme aimed at authenticating the various nodes sown in, on and around the human body as well as the Base Station of an e-health application. The scheme makes sure mutual authentication to limited consumption of resources. Initially, we define the e-health application's network architecture. Then we describe the authentication scheme in detail.

Architecture

The proposed framework permits the accumulation of health-related data from sensors in and on the bodies, for example, ECG, in addition to logical sensors which gather information, for example, surrounding temperature or dampness level. The information is then exchanged with Base Station by means of remote

Figure 1. Network architecture

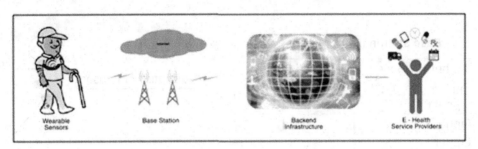

interfaces. They can utilize the individual client's cell phone as the base station to gather the information caught as it furnishes the client with portability and more vitality limit in respect to sensors. The Base Station will at that point utilize the back-end framework to convey the information assembled through an Internet association (e.g., Wi-Fi or 3 G) to parental figure and relatives as in Figure 1.

As indicated by proposed system design, we make certain suspicions with respect to the present gadgets included: Objects could be isolated in to two characterizations: sensor hubs that are confined both to computational just as vitality assets, and base stations that are unconstrained on the grounds that they have all the more processing just as vitality limit. Every sensor has a unique Id and is fit for symmetrical encryption and no less than one lopsided encryption. Since it is non-obliged, the Base Station may direct established PKI to ensure information transmission outside remote sensor organize.

Documentations

The notes that are characterized are utilized in the proposed plan in Table 1 for peruse comfort.

Functioning

A recommended verification conspire gives shared authentication here between various sensor hubs just as the Base Station of an E-health application. The plan is isolated in to three phases:

Table 1. Notations used

Notation	Description
I	Addition
NS	Sensor node's Nonce value
MB	Base station's Nonce value
hf()	Hash function for one way
Enc(NS,Xi)	NS value's AES-128 encryption using the X_i Secret Key
Dec(NS,Xi)	NS value's AES-128 decryption using the X_i Secret Key
KHAC()	Authentication code for Key hashed message
F(NS)	If(N!=16bytes): A hash function hf() is applied which returns on output 16 bytes.

Figure 2. Registration phase

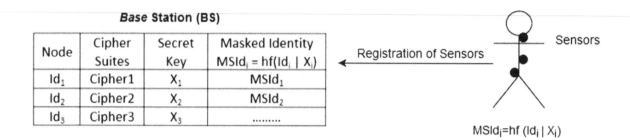

- An enrolment stage where the sensor hubs ought to be enlisted all through the Base Station (BS) with their personalities.
- The verification stage here between sensor hubs just as the base station is utilized to confirm one another.
- Session key is utilized by shared key setup.

Everything will be introduced each progression nitty gritty and with utilitarian charts in the accompanying.

Registration phase

This period of enlistment was basic all through the capacity to capacity of both the protocols here between sensor hubs just as the base station.

Initially, we accept that they portray an utilized figure suites like MAC (message validation code), hash work hf() just as the resulting secret key Xi. A disconnected sales rep for each enrolled sensor implants the Idi and the relating parameters in a coupling table into the Base Station. A hash esteem commenced on the sensor's Idi character is processed for each enlisted sensor. This is called this hash esteem:' Masked identity.' Therefore, the table incorporates an Idi, its figure suites, the comparing Xi secret key, just as the MSIdi covered way of life as in Figure 2. An enrollment stage closes when every one of the sensors are enlisted at the Base Station.

Authentication Phase

A validation arrange is proposed to commonly verify a sensor hub just as the base station. Any sensor hub wishing to speak with both the Base Station must work the verification procedure. Proposed verification plot is as in Figure 3. A sensor hub creates a 8-byte irregular N esteem just as sends the message comprising of the determined esteem, the covered MSIdi personality, just as a KHAC message verification code (MSIdi, Idi, NS) to guarantee the trustworthiness of the message. After getting the message from the base station, the message will be confirmed by surveying the related KHAC. The Base Station likewise makes an arbitrary esteem MB on 8 bytes if the check is fruitful just as resends a message comprising of the got esteem NS, the esteem MB, and a KHAC message verification code (MB, Idi, NS). When the sensor hub gets this message, it likewise checks the content by estimating the related KHAC. Except if the audit is fruitful, the two items ' irregular qualities are all around gotten, bringing about an effective end of shared validation between articles.

Key Foundation Stage

When the two elements have been viably validated, a common symmetric key K is created to keep up the correspondence channel. Such a key is processed by either a custom capacity to link the nonce esteems (NS k MB), and furthermore an encryption with both the related Xi sensor hub secret key is connected as K = F(Enc(NS k MB, Xi)). Key K ought to be on 128 bits. As of the later section, an encoded' Finished' message with both the session key K is being sent to the base station to show that the key foundation is done (the' Finished' message additionally incorporates the session key K). Thusly, the Base Station registers, decodes a message, checks a session key, just as stores a mutual session key K as secret key of the coupling table.

PROPOSED SCHEME'S SECURITY ANALYSIS

Such a model was appropriate of a dangerous domain in which a malevolent client can spy interchanges. In the proposed verification conspire, we use nonce's and KHAC codes (H.Krawczyk et al., 1997). At the point when the application intermittently modifies its security key once quarterly a year, the assailant's probability of abusing a fashioned KHAC is very low.

The arranged authenticationconspire is impervious to various potential assaults. We are for the most part intrigued by:

Replay Assault

Assume an interloper scrambles an earlier remark all through the verification stage swapped by either a sensor hub and endeavours to see this to emulate the hub just as base station character. An aggressor cannot adequately mimic a sensor hub between the Base Station so as to give common authentication-since a present estimation of'NS' separately'MB' is delivered just as exchanged for every verification.

Impersonate a Sensor Hub

An aggressor is unfit to mimic a sensor hub on the grounds that the esteem MSIdi veils his character. Additionally, the aggressor cannot mimic the Base Station without the utilization of personality of collector sensor hub Idi to ascertain a legitimate KHAC code. The proposed authentication plot additionally gives propelled highlights like:

Mutual Validation

Both the sensor hubs and in the verification stage, both the realness of the sensor hubs just as the base station are demonstrated. The entire procedure called the common verification process. In this manner, just as the sensor hubs as well as the Base Station are sure of both the validness of the got messages.

Figure 3. Authentication scheme

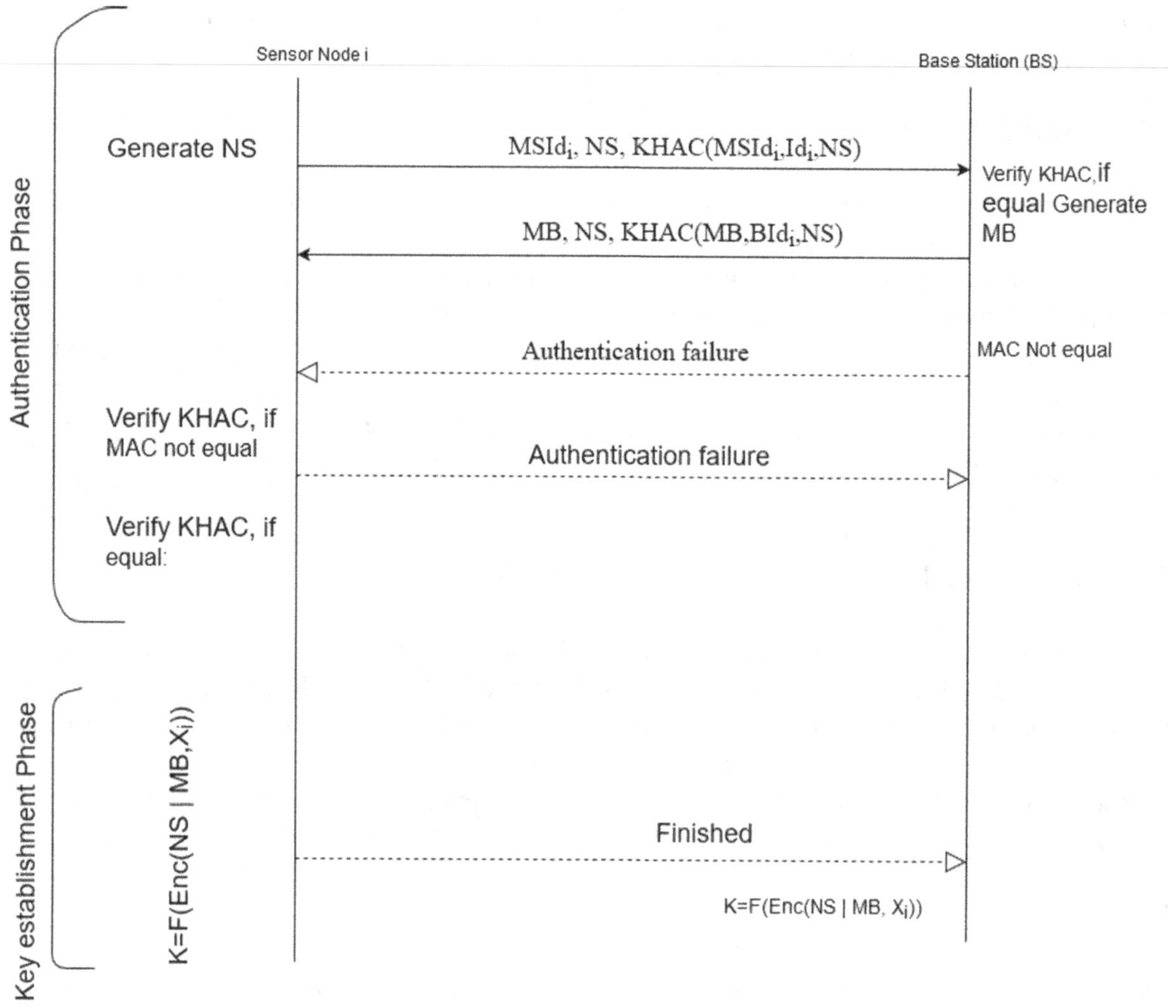

Data Honesty

Of proposed framework, we guarantee that just the caught data passed on to a BS isn't changed utilizing authentication of KHAC code. This check is performed for each message traded.

Identity Insurance

A Masked identity (MSIdi) is determined for every sensor hub. The Base Station will likewise realize this incentive to disallow the sensor's Idi character disclosure.

Synchronization Independence

Using timestamps guarantees freshness of the message and in this manner approves that it's anything but a returned to old message. This strategy requires synchronization of the element. The proposed plan was flexible to review assault by utilizing unconstrained nonces in the diverse trades between the two elements. It in this manner upgrades the security of both the authentication stage just as makes the execution of synchronization superfluous.

Session Key Foundation

At simply the finish of the successful confirmation, a shared secret key is created here between sensor hubs just as the Base Station. This key is frequently utilized as a session key to ensure secure correspondence here between two substances.

Scalability

The sensor hubs are worried about the versatility. The plan can be stretched out as it permits the incorporation of new sensor hubs into framework. Another sensor hub was enrolled in the Base Station through enlistment arrange and is in this way added to the BS table in it conceal personality in disconnected mode.

PROPOSED SCHEME'S PERFORMANCE EVALUATION

To examine the proposed verification plot, we focus on both the vitality utilization of the sensor hubs with limited gadgets. We measure the vitality needed expected to execute the cryptographic natives together with the vitality expected to transmit just as get information. We utilize a TelosB sensor hub outfitted with a CC2420 radio. The last commonly keeps running on two AA batteries joining around 18500 J.

The presented authentication conspire is predicated on created nonce esteems. To survey it type of confirmation, we should examine the diverse variations of trade methods.

In the proposed plan, we utilize keyed-hash message verification code (KHAC) (Krawczyk et al., 1997) in the two validation trades. An iterative cryptographic hash work like MD5 or SHA-1 does not utilize a square figure to ascertain the KHAC. A hash work parts a message into squares of fixed size (proposed case: 128 bits for MD5) just as repeats through them with a pressure work. We were utilizing KHAC-MD5 for present assessment on even a chose 4 bytes that may not be influenced by detailed MD5 and SHA-1 collisions (Schneier, 2005). Another trade system to transmit information in scrambled mode or progressively dependent on AES encryption, transmitting information in encoded mode just as being ensured by a KHAC code. We figure the expense of vitality required for authentication in everyone among the three systems:

Proposed Trade Case (KHAC)

According to Szczechowiak et al., 2008, a vitality required to swap one byte of information to such a TelosB sensor requires 5.76 μJ for burning and 6.48 μJ for gathering, just as we ascertain the expense of vitality of the unmistakable cryptographic natives as per (Pathkey, 2014).

As expressed to proposed protocols, the hub must give the veiled personality (20 bytes), its created unconstrained esteem (8 bytes for present situation) and ascertain the KHAC code requiring 62.15μJ. The sent message measure is 44 bytes (20 bytes + 8 bytes + 4 bytes of KHAC + 12 bytes of protocols headers) requiring a transmission of 253.44μJ. As a reaction from the BS, the hub gets a message of 32 bytes including the two produced nonce (2*(8 bytes) + 4 bytes of KHAC + 12 bytes of protocols headers) requiring receipt of 207.36 μJ and checks the KHAC code requiring 62.15 μJ. Accordingly, the general vitality cost of the verification stage is equivalent to 585.1μJ.

Instance of Trade with AES

The present trade circumstance, the sent messages are encoded with a symmetric key by the AES calculation. We don't have to send a veiled personality, we simply need to scramble the Idi (1 byte) hub way of life just as the created unconstrained esteem (16 bytes) that require around 76.34aJ. As indicated by the length of sent message is 44 bytes (32 bytes + 12 bytes of protocols headers) requiring a transmission of 253.44.

The sensor hub gets a BS message of 44 bytes involving the two nonce created (2*(16 bytes)) in addition to 12 bytes of protocols headers requiring 285.12 μJ just as unscrambles the message expending 742.67 μJ. In this way, the verification stage's absolute expense of vitality is equivalent to 1357.57 μJ.

Instance of Trade with AES and KHAC

The present case is same as like previous situation where we will attach the expense of vitality of figuring, transmitting, and getting KHAC codes. Ascertaining the transmitted message's KHAC code requires around 62.15 μJ, and confirming the got message's KHAC code requires 62.15μJ. Accordingly, the validation stage's absolute vitality cost is like 1530.83μJ.

At last the consequence of the investigation about different trade systems as in Figure 4, we close an authentication conspire is needy exceptionally on the trading of method of the different verification messages executed. We likewise note the high decoding task cost when contrasted and an encryption and a KHAC estimation.

The trades in the verification stage spare more vitality while giving a most elevated amount of security as validation just as honesty is given. All out expense of the total plan is validation stage cost in addition to the foundation stage cost. In key foundation phase, encryption of link of the nonces (result on 16 bytes) needs roughly 42.88 μJ and, if essential, the utilization of capacity F. Generally speaking, it needs 42.88 μJ and 161.28 μJ to be sent to encode the message' Finished' (16 bytes) with the made shared key K. The proposed framework's all out expense is 832.14 μJ. A lowpay demonstrates that this plan is lightweight just as appropriate for use in E-health applications in an asset compelled condition on the internet of things.

ALTERNATIVE OF THE PROPOSED SCHEME BASED ON A LIGHTWEIGHT PKI (PUBLIC KEY INFRASTRUCTURE)

The proposed plan can likewise be actualized all through the situation of a couple of key, an open Base Station key that is just known by both the sensor hubs, and a private key that is kept covered up for just the

Figure 4. Different exchange techniques energy-cost analysis

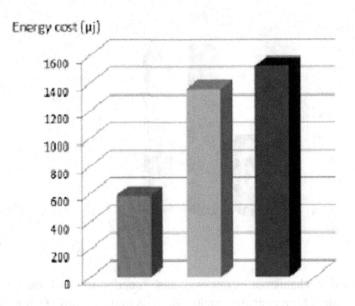

Base Station. To begin with, we trust that a disconnected seller consolidates an utilized figure suites like the MAC, hash work h), (and the Base Station's open key to each enrolled sensor all through the enlistment arrange in both Base Station and furthermore the sensor hubs. We may attach the 128-piece open key and utilizing it. We utilize the Xi secret key in cryptographic capacities together with credible key.

Throughout the following move, we figure the common key again and expand the capacity F whenever required (for proposed situation, we may not stretch out the capacity F to quantify the mutual key K on 16 bytes). When the covered up shared key is determined, the encoded message' Finished' found to contain the key is sent. The performed encryption is to utilize an Elliptic Curve Cryptography (ECC) (Szczechowiak et al., 2008) that gives the exceptionally same dimension of security as customary calculations, for example, RSA. A cost of the PKI variation of proposed plan is just in the validation stage in addition to 42.88 µJ required for key figuring, 17 mJ for ECC-160 bits encryption (De Meulenaer et al., 2008) encryption of the ' completed ' message, just as 161.28 µJ for conveyance. Thusly, the expense is 17.79 mJ.

The yield is very energizing contrasted and the expenses of electricity of the other established plans, for example, the changed 39 mJ SSL protocol (Grobschadl, 2007) and the adjusted 39.6-47.6 mJ Kerberos protocol (Landstra, 2007) as in Figure 5.

CONCLUSION AND FUTURE SCOPE

All through the chapter, the proposed lightweight verification conspire for E-health applications with the use of nonces, masked identity, as well as KHAC code for the various trades in regards to the Internet of Things. The proposed plan has little correspondence just as calculation costs with an abnormal state of health contrasted with other trade strategies just as finishes with a session key foundation. The

Figure 5. Comparision with other protocols

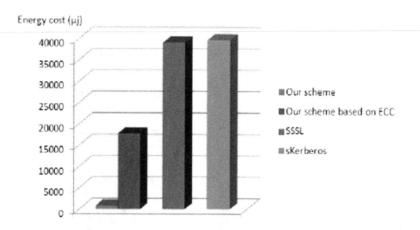

proposed authentication mechanism uses one-way hash function to check the integrity of the medical information communicated. Moreover, a comparative study of the security features among proposed and other existing schemes is also presented. The formal security analysis explicitly proved that the proposed mechanism is suitable for any insecure IoT smart healthcare environment. A plan would then be suitable to likewise be connected in asset obliged E-health applications. As only a future research, the results expected to gauge the verification protocols in such a genuine establishment to gain a considerably more exact investigation of memory utilization and execution time.

REFERENCES

Almulhim, M. & Zaman, N. (2018). Proposing Secure and Lightweight Authentication Scheme for IoT Based E-Health Applications. In *20th IEEE International Conference on Advance Communication Technology ICACT* 2018.

Alotaibi, M. (2018). *An Enhanced Symmetric Cryptosystem and Biometric-Based Anonymous User Authentication and Session Key Establishment Scheme for WSN*. Piscataway, NJ: IEEE.

Atzori, L., Iera, A., & Morabito, G. (2010). The internet of things: A survey. *Computer Networks, 54*(15), 2787–2805. doi:10.1016/j.comnet.2010.05.010

Cheikhrouhou, O., Koubaa, A., Boujelben, M., & Abid, M. (2010). A lightweight user authentication scheme for wireless sensor networks. *IEEE/ACS International Conference on IEEE.* 10.1109/AICCSA.2010.5586995

De Meulenaer, G., Gosset, F., Standaert, O.-X., & Pereira, O. (2008). On the energy cost of communication and cryptography in wireless sensor networks. *IEEE International Conference on Wireless and Mobile Computing.* 10.1109/WiMob.2008.16

Dohr, A., Modre-Opsrian, R., Drobics, M., Hayn, D., & Schreier, G. (2010). The internet of things for ambient assisted living. In *Seventh International Conference on Information Technology: New Generations (ITNG)*. Piscataway, NJ: IEEE.

Durairaj, M., & Muthuramalingam, K. (2018). A New Authentication Scheme with Elliptical Curve Cryptography for Internet of Things (IoT) Environments. *Int. J. Eng. Technol.*, 7(2.26), 119–124. doi:10.14419/ijet.v7i2.26.14364

El Maliki, T. & Seigneur, J.-M. (2007). A survey of user-centric identity management technologies. In *the International Conference on Emerging Security Information, Systems, and Technologies (SECUREWARE 2007)*. Piscataway, NJ: IEEE. 10.1109/SECUREWARE.2007.4385303

Großsch¨adl, J., Szekely, A., & Tillich, S. (2007). The energy cost of cryptographic key establishment in wireless sensor networks. *Proceedings of the 2nd ACM symposium on Information, computer and communications security*. 10.1145/1229285.1229334

Hamidi, H. (2019). An approach to develop the smart health using internet of things and authentication based on biometric technology. Future Gen. Comput. Syst.

Karthikeyan, S., Patan, R., & Balamurugan, B. (2019). Enhancement of Security in the Internet of Things (IoT) by Using X. 509 Authentication Mechanism. In *Recent Trends in Communication, Computing, and Electronics* (pp. 217–225). Singapore: Springer. doi:10.1007/978-981-13-2685-1_22

Kothmayr, T., Schmitt, C., Hu, W., Br¨unig, M., & Carle, G. (2013). Dtls based security and two-way authentication for the internet of things. *Ad Hoc Networks*, 11(8), 2710–2723. doi:10.1016/j.adhoc.2013.05.003

Krawczyk, H., Canetti, R., & Bellare, M. (1997). KHAC: Keyedhashing for message authentication.

Landstra, T., Zawodniok, M., & Jagannathan, S. (2007, October). Energy-efficient hybrid key management protocol for wireless sensor networks. In *32nd IEEE Conference on Local Computer Networks (LCN 2007)* (pp. 1009-1016). Piscataway, NJ: IEEE.

Lee, J., Kapitanova, K., & Son, S. H. (2010). The price of security in wireless sensor networks. *Computer Networks*, 54(17), 2967–2978. doi:10.1016/j.comnet.2010.05.011

Li, M., Lou, W., & Ren, K. (2010). *Data security and privacy in wireless body area networks. Wireless Communications*. Piscataway, NJ: IEEE.

Medaglia, C. M., & Serbanati, A. (2010). An overview of privacy and security issues in the internet of things. The internet of things.

Miorandi, D., Sicari, S., De Pellegrini, F., & Chlamtac, I. (2012). Internet of things: Vision, applications and research challenges. *Ad Hoc Networks*, 10(7), 1497–1516. doi:10.1016/j.adhoc.2012.02.016

Patel, M., & Wang, J. (2010). *Applications, challenges, and prospective in emerging body area networking technologies. Wireless communications*. Piscataway, NJ: IEEE.

Pauthkey: A pervasive authentication protocol and key establishment scheme for wireless sensor networks in distributed IoT applications. (2014). International Journal of Distributed Sensor Networks.

Porambage, P., Schmitt, C., Kumar, P., Gurtov, A., & Ylianttila, M. (2014). Two-phase authentication protocol for wireless sensor networks in distributed iot applications. *Wireless Communications and Networking Conference (WCNC)*. 10.1109/WCNC.2014.6952860

Pub, N. F. (2001). *Advanced encryption standard (aes)*. Federal Information Processing Standards Publication.

Rescorla, E. & Modadugu, N. (2012). Datagram transport layer security version 1.2.

Roman, R., Najera, P., & Lopez, J. (2011). Securing the internet of things. Computer. SEC4: Elliptic Curve Qu-Vanstone Implicit Certificate Scheme (ECQV), version 0.97. Retrieved from www.secg.org

Schneier, B. (2005). Schneier on security: Sha-1 broken. Retrieved from http://www.schneier.com/blog/archives/2005/02/sha1 broken.html

Sicari, S., Rizzardi, A., Grieco, L., & Coen-Porisini, A. (2015). Security, privacy and trust in internet of things: The road ahead. *Computer Networks*, *76*, 146–164. doi:10.1016/j.comnet.2014.11.008

Szczechowiak, P., Oliveira, L. B., Scott, M., Collier, M., & Dahab, R. (2008). Nanoecc: Testing the limits of elliptic curve cryptography in sensor networks. Wireless sensor networks.

Turkanovi'c, M., Brumen, B., & H¨olbl, M. (2014). A novel user authentication and key agreement scheme for heterogeneous ad hoc wireless sensor networks, based on the internet of things notion. *Ad Hoc Networks*, *20*, 96–112. doi:10.1016/j.adhoc.2014.03.009

Chapter 8
An Intelligent IoT–Based Health Monitoring System for Tribal People

N. Geetha

PSG College of Technology, India

A. Sankar

PSG College of Technology, India

ABSTRACT

Healthcare monitoring has grown drastically in the world. People are provided with modern treatments and continuous monitoring of physiological changes in their body. Many technologies are merged into the medial field to bring in this revolution. Many solutions are provided and are commonly used in hospitals and by patients. An IoT-based intelligent healthcare monitoring system provides a continuous health monitoring for tribal people. The system collects data from a patient and loads it into the cloud storage. The doctors have the privilege to view the patients' data and suggest the prescriptions or send an alert message in case of any emergency. A prototype model is developed and tested. This system helps to provide a healthcare solution for tribal community.

INTRODUCTION

The internet of things is the collection of smart devices embedded in everyday objects capable to send and receive data over internet that enable machine-to-machine and machine-to-human interaction possible. It is forecasted that around 50 billion devices or objects will be linked over internet within the year 2020. Internet of things (IoT) has been widely used in various field of development in recent times. IoT has marked its footprints in almost all fields and hence there is a shift in research in all the fields to integrate concepts of IoT, ambient intelligence and autonomous control. This basically provides a dynamic and interactive environment. In some applications machine learning algorithms are integrated with IoT devices to make IoT objects closer to reality.

DOI: 10.4018/978-1-7998-1090-2.ch008

Among these fields, health care is a domain where IoT has gained potential benefits in monitoring patients. IoT has come long way in healthcare space (Amna, 2015 & Cecilia, 2014 & Clifton, 2014 & Devashri, 2015 & Dunsmuir, 2014). The implementation of IoT within healthcare led to advancement in technology in patient monitoring and analyze to data to improve patient outcome. This tremendously reduces the risks of healthcare professionals. IoT had helped to place every detail of the patient into perspective to make decisions in favour of the patients. Nowadays patient information is stored in cloud. This allows in real time monitoring of patients to track the severity of disease and perform preventive measures. IoT have offered services such as health monitoring systems, wearables, mobile apps to render services such as diagnostics, post-surgery monitoring, complement therapies, etc. Such type of data collection in health monitoring provides better diagnosis by health professionals and reduces human errors in medical field. Though IoT had proved to provide many benefits in the field of healthcare, it also comes with downside. The amount of data collected from the patient is very large and it is very difficult to manage for healthcare facilities IT departments. Also, there is a threat in providing security for the data when shared between devices.

India, the subcontinent is a developing nation in the world. Each and every sector is drastically growing competing with rest of the world. Many developments and researches are carried out in each and every sector. One such sector is health sector. India has a second largest population with 1.37 billion residents in the world and is expected to unseat China as the world's most populated country in the next couple of decades. India's current yearly growth rate is 1.08%.

Tribal peoples constitute 8.6 percent of India's total population, about 104 million people according to the 2011 census (68 million people according to the 1991 census). This is the largest population of the tribal people in the world. The tribal population mainly dwells in the states of Madhya Pradesh, Maharashtra, Orissa, Gujarat, Rajasthan, Jharkhand, Chhattisgarh, Andhra Pradesh, West Bengal, and Karnataka. Other few states where 15.3% of tribal people are settled are Assam, Meghalaya, Nagaland, Jammu & Kashmir, Tripura, Mizoram, Bihar, Manipur, Arunachal Pradesh, and Tamil Nadu. The tribal population in India is minimum and left ignored in many aspects.

In Tamil Nadu, tribal people account for 1.03 percent of the total population. There are 36 different tribes, present in almost all the districts, across 2860 villages located in 63 blocks of the state. They are predominantly in rural areas, and of these, around 5 lakhs live in 13 districts. The tribal population is sometimes isolated and government beneficiary plans are not reaching the meager population. In recent days, many problems like lack of electricity, mode of communication, health issues, habitat etc. are faced by the tribal population.

Mostly tribal areas are present near forest borders and hence facilities are not available. Though healthcare sector had brought in much advancement, the problems faced by tribal people in using those healthcare resources are

- Tribal people are financially very poor.
- Lack of awareness about healthcare innovations.
- Minimum health facilities available in tribal living places or manpower is not available in health centers
- Tribal people are commonly affected by sickle cell anaemia, tuberculosis etc.
- Many tribal villages are remotely located which are away from hospitals/remote health centers.
- Inadequate monitoring of reach of healthcare facilities to tribal people.
- Inaccessibility of free government services for healthcare

To improve the quality of life of tribal people IoT based intelligent health monitoring system is developed. With the use of IoT based healthcare, tribal people can be provided with unparallel benefits to improve the efficiency of treatments and improve the health of the tribal people.

The main benefits of healthcare system developed will include the following

- Simultaneous reporting and monitoring: The device collects the data from the patient and transfers data to the physician remotely available. The cloud storage is used to store the data.
- End-to-end connectivity and affordability: The data collected from the patient are transferred through communication protocol through gateways. There is an end to end connection provided to connect patient information's to doctors regardless of their place.
- Data assortment and analysis: The raw data collected can be processed and the reports can be generated. Simple analysis on collected data is performed over cloud and reports are generated.
- Tracking and alerts: The IoT system developed can provide better treatment for patients through timely intervention by doctors.

The intelligent health monitoring system can provide best solution for tribal people healthcare and help doctors of multi-specialty to serve the people.

Literature Survey

Today different technologies play a vital role in online health monitoring system. The technologies like RFID, IoT, cloud computing, mobile communications, web services and machine learning approaches are used to enhance health monitoring system that can monitor the physiological changes in a human body. Many products are developed and researches are carried out in the literature to revolutionize healthcare sector. Some of the products and approaches are discussed in this subsection.

A system named NIGHT-CARE (Cecilia, 2014) uses RFID system to monitor old and disabled people during nighttime. This system monitors the human activities during the sleep time and also detects abnormal signal change that need to be immediately attended. RFID system with Global System for mobile communication (GSM) and Wireless Sensor Network (WSN) are used to monitor patient's health and physiological related parameter from hospital (Shirehjini, 2012). RFID tags are used not only to monitor patients; it is also used to localize equipments in hospitals.

Zigbee based WSN with UHF RFID are used in realtime tracking and monitoring the patients in hospitals. RHCMS uses Zigbee technology to monitor the patients within the hospitals and outside the hospital. This system provides online information about the health condition of a patient and trigger messages to health professional in case of any abnormalities. Also, it can provide medical advises to patients anywhere in the world at any instant.

Mobile Telemedicine system for Home Care and Patient Monitoring implements a Tele-medicine System for Patient Monitoring using Mobile Telephony. Using this application any patient can be monitored and the system proved to be very quick and reliable. Therefore, it represents an applicable solution to Tele-homecare. Additionally, the high costs involved in hospitals and the frequent problems in patient transporting are reduced providing a good medical care. This system is based on Client Server Application in which server stores data. Collected from client, the role of client is to collect proper data from patient and transfer it to server. The main disadvantage of this project is overall cost of telecommunication system is higher, especially data management apparatus and practical training of medical professionals is difficult.

Smart devices are used in patient monitoring system. In other work, authors (Maradugu, 2015) proposed android based healthcare monitoring system to monitor parameters such as heart rate, temperature and oxygen saturation level in blood. Doctors can continuously monitor patient through android application using smart phone and store patient information in web servers. A smart healthcare system (Joon-Soo, 2016) developed as an IoT application for patient monitoring and early detection of disease. This system can also be used for intensive monitoring of patient conditions. Sensors are used to collect data and processing of data is carried out by intelligent network. The collected data is stored in cloud and analysis of data for diagnosis is performed by complex algorithms.

Another patient monitoring system (Sarfraz, 2017) using mobile phone through WBAN was developed. In this system RFID tags are used to transmit information to mobile phone in a secured manner. A novel health monitoring system (Dunsmuir, 2014) was developed to monitor the health of pregnant woman with preeclampsia. This system can measure all clinical parameters at patient's home. Oximeter is also used in the system to measure the oxygen saturation level of the patient. All the measured parameters are used to predict the risk level of the patients and provide suggestions, referral and treatments.

Mobile devices are drastically used in health monitoring applications. Hybrid mobile based health care solution integrated with cloud technology (Xiaoliang, 2014) was proposed to overcome the inherent limitations in mobile phones. Mobile cloud-based electrocardiograph monitoring system was introduced by the authors to improve performance of the monitoring system in terms of energy efficiency and prediction accuracy. IoT is used in developing a system for monitoring patients having Parkinson's disease. Pasluosta et al. (Pasluosta, 2015) proposed a system consisting of wearable sensors and cameras for observing tremors gait patterns of the patient and their behavior around the home. Machine learning approach can also be introduced to enhance the functionality of the system.

Diabetic is a very common disease among human beings. Many techniques and machines are there in the market to measure the blood-glucose levels in the patient's body. One such system (Shih-Hao, 2016) monitors blood glucose level and indicate the abnormalities either to the patients or the caretaker and family members or healthcare professionals. This system is practically implemented. Another system named SPHERE (Ni, 2015) consisting of sensors and cameras for continuous monitoring of patients who are living in their home for their comfort. This system helps the healthcare professionals to intervene when an issue arises. Machine learning algorithms help the system in making decisions about patient's health condition.

Wireless Body Area Network (WBAN) is used to monitor the body condition of the patients. Bluetooth technology is adopted to transfer the collected data to mobile devices. The system is able to monitor the patient's physiological changes. Recently web-based applications and mobile applications are developed to monitor the health of patients in hospital or at their home performing normal activities. The doctors or healthcare professionals can provide suggestions to patients through online. Also, in case of any abnormal activity (Amna, 2015), an alert message is sent to the doctors. This helps to provide immediate care to the patients (Devashri, 2015).

Body sensor network technology can be widely used in patient monitoring system using light weight sensor nodes. But security is a major concern. Gope and Hwang (Gope, 2016) discussed on various security requirements in IoT based healthcare system.

To some extent (Khalifa, 2014) machine learning algorithms and techniques are used in handling the data generated by wearable sensors. This data is combined with clinical observation to provide early warning of abnormal changes in the patients. The effectiveness of these approaches is tested in hospitals in real time. Many web-based applications (Orlando, 2014) and mobile applications (Clifton, 2014) are developed in recent days for patient health monitoring system.

Proposed System

IoT health monitoring system is developed to monitor the health of tribal people settled in tribal village. This system continuously monitors the patient's health and sends report to doctors in urban specialty hospitals. The doctors have the facility to view the reports and prescribe medicine. The doctors can also send alert messages if there is any emergency situation. This helps in continuous monitoring of the progress of patient's health. The following steps are involved in the system.

a. Sensors sense the signals from the human body.
b. A web-based information system for managing primary health care.
c. A gateway for web access applications for integrating mobile devices of nurses and doctors at the two ends.
d. Simple cloud storage for maintaining patient's information and retrieve the data whenever and wherever required.

The overall topology of Intelligent IoT based health monitoring system is shown in Figure 1. Patient health details are sensed using IoT devices at healthcare centre. Wireless sensors are used to collect and transmit signals from the human body and a processor is programmed to receive and automatically analyze the sensor signals. In this system, sensors are used to measure signals such as temperature, pulse rate, hemoglobin content. The microcontroller board is portable and easy to handle. The healthcare professionals in health centers collect data from the patient and upload the upload it in a web-based information system. The sensed data are moved to cloud storage. The cloud database is used to retrieve the patient's information whenever and wherever possible by the doctors. The doctors can retrieve information from the cloud database and recommend prescriptions or can send an alert message in case of any emergency. The nurse/healthcare professionals in health centre can monitor the patients with doctor's advice.

In developing the proposed system many hardware, software and firmware are used. The details of the components are discussed in the following sub sections.

NodeMCU

NodeMCU is a low-cost open source firmware that runs on ESP8266 WiFi SoC popularly named as ESP8266 core for arduino IDE. Figure 2 shows the NodeMCU kit. NodeMCU supports serial communication protocols such as UART, SPI, I2C etc to connect to external devices like LCD display, Accelerometer, GPS modules, SD cards etc.

NodeMCU provides an access to General purpose Input/Output (GPIO) and a pin mapping table as shown in Table 1. ESP8266 Core for Arduino IDE is used as the software development platform.

Figure 1. IoT topology for health monitoring system

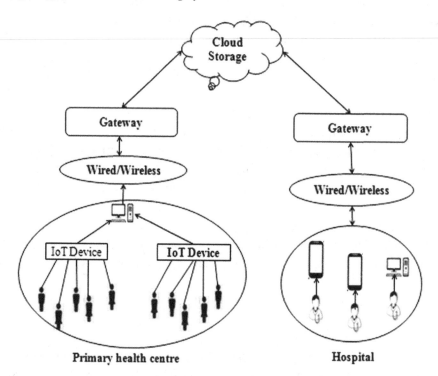

Linear Monolithic (LM) Sensor LM35

LM35 is a temperature sensor shown in Figure 3 measure heat generated by an object to which it is connected. LM35 is a precision integrated temperature device whose output is proportional to centigrade temperature. This sensor is advantageous over other temperature sensor as the user need not subtract large constant voltage from output to have centigrade scaling. It is a low-cost semiconductor based sensor. The main advantage of LM35 is that it is linear 10mv/°c which means for every degree rise in temperature the output will rise by 10mv. The room temperature is 32°c then the output of LM35 will be 320mv. This sensor does not require any extra features for trimming or calibration for providing better accuracies.

SEN-11574

SEN-11574 is a pulse sensor used to measure heart rate working under the principle of photo phlethysmography. It is a simple plug and play sensor that combines a simple optical heart rate sensor with amplification and noise cancellation circuitry making it fast and easy to get reliable pulse readings. As shown in Figure 4, the Pulse Sensor includes a 24-inch Color-Coded Cable, with (male) header connectors and an open-source monitoring application to generate graphs for the recorded heart rate. The red-coloured wire is power supply with +3V to +5V, black wire is for ground and purple wire is for transmitting signal. The pulse sensor can be connected to a arduino or plugged into a breadboard

Figure 2. NodeMCU development kit

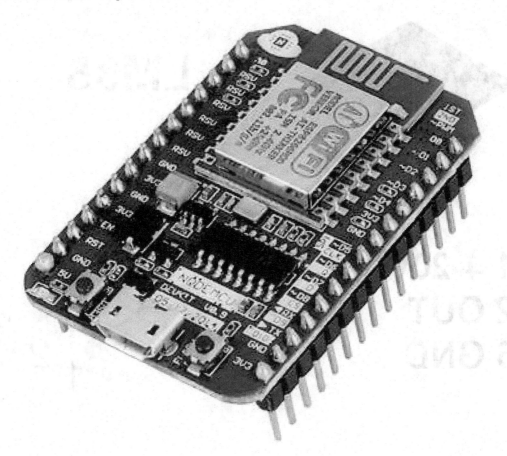

It is applicable for all mobile applications as it sips power with just 4mA current draw at 5V. The flow of blood volume is decided by the rate of heartbeat pulses and since light is absorbed by blood, the signal pulses are equivalent to the heartbeat pulses.

Table 1. ESP8266 Pin Mapping Table

I/O Index	ESP8266 Pin	I/O Index	ESP8266 Pin
0[*]	GPIO16	7	GPIO13
1	GPIO5	8	GPIO15
2	GPIO4	9	GPIO3
3	GPIO0	10	GPIO1
4	GPIO2	11	GPIO9
5	GPIO14	12	GPIO10
6	GPIO12	-	-

Figure 3. LM35 sensor

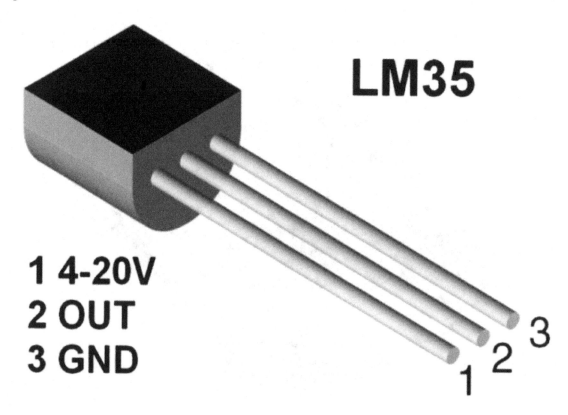

Firebase

Firebase provides a backend services to real time data. It provides an API which allows data to be stored in firebase cloud and to be synchronized across clients. It also offers services through libraries to integrate with android, iOS, java, Javascript and Node.JS applications. Firebase database is also accessible through REST API and provides bindings for several frameworks. Secure file uploads and downloads for firebase applications are provided. The developers can store all kinds of contents such as image, video, audio and other contents. Firebase also delivers files over internet through HTTP Secure and SSL.

INTELLIGENT IoT BASED HEALTH MONITORING SYSTEM

The major modules of health monitoring system as shown in Figure 5 includes

a.   Data Acquisition Module
b.   Data Transmission Module
c.   Cloud Processing Module

Figure 4. Pulse sensor

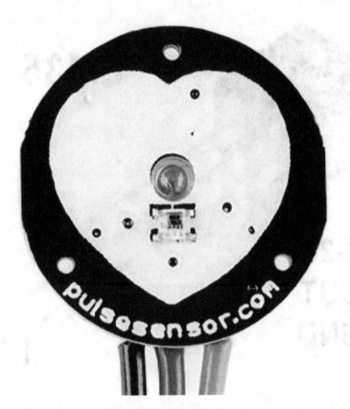

Data Acquisition Module

Data acquisition module collects various physiological parameters of a patient using different sensors. The sensors sense the data and carry this information to the micro controller-based development kit.

Figure 5. IoT based health monitoring system

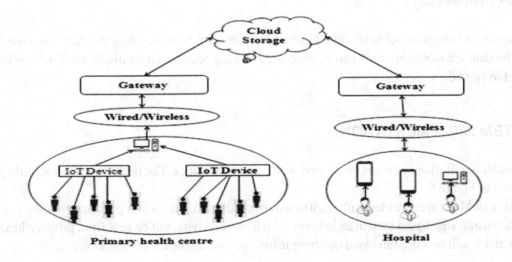

Figure 6. Prototype version of health monitoring system

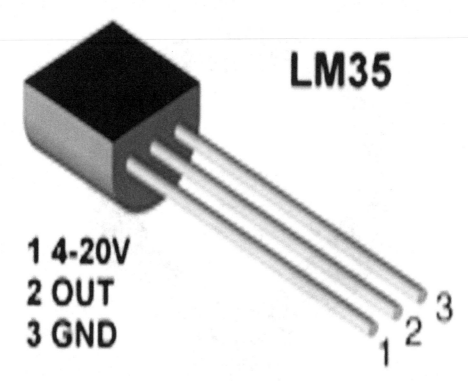

Data Transmission module

The data collected in the microcontroller board is transferred to the internet through IoT module. Any critical situations for a patient can be intimated to health care professionals through SMS. The patient's information can be accessed in web page developed in any computer or mobile device connected over internet.

Cloud Processing Module

Diagnoses and prognosis of health condition of a patient can be done using the data collected by sensor. The data are stored in cloud can be processed and the results can be displayed. Firebase database is used to store data.

SYSTEM IMPLEMENTATION

The health monitoring system is developed with low cost devices. The prototype version of the system is shown in Figure 6.

The nodeMCU is connected with sensors using breadboard. The health parameters of the patient are recorded using web-based system as in Figure 7. The sensed data will be sent from primary health care centre and it will be stored in cloud database using firebase as shown in Figure 8.

Figure 7. Patient information

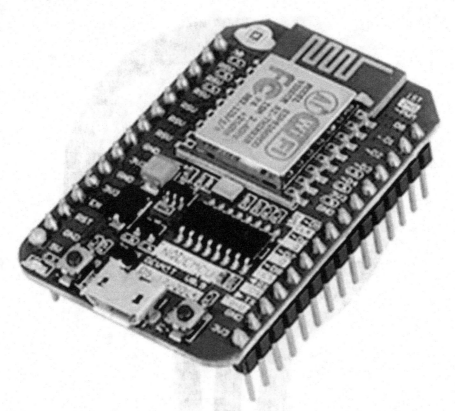

Doctors can able to view the patient records and send the prescription to primary health care centre. The nurse/health professionals in the health centers can monitor the patients based on doctor's advice.

CONCLUSION

The intelligent IoT based health monitoring system helps in monitoring the tribal people. Both the patients and the doctors are benefitted from this system. The patients are continuously monitored and provided with remote medical care and immediate care can be given in any emergency situations. The specialized doctors in multi-specialty hospitals can render their helping hands for the tribal people. Automatic transfer of data is performed for remote medical consultations. The doctors have constant access to patient's information and easily provide prescriptions with the help of mobile devices. Machine learning algorithms can be used to enhance the working of health monitoring system for early prediction of disease and provide preventive measures.

Figure 8. Data storage in firebase

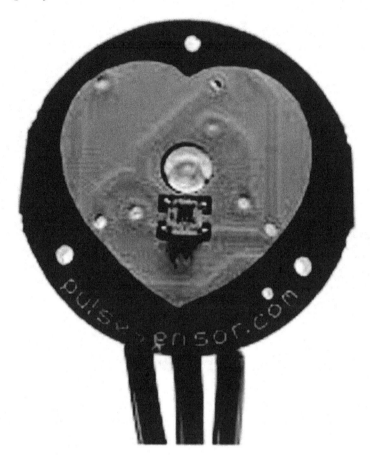

REFERENCES

Amna, A. (2015). Real Time Wireless Health Monitoring Application using mobile devices. [IJCNC]. *International Journal of Computer Networks & Communications, 7*(3), 13–30. doi:10.5121/ijcnc.2015.7302

Cecilia, O. (2014). NIGHT-Care: A passive RFID system for remote monitoring and control of overnight living environment. *Procedia Computer Science*, 190–197.

Clifton, L., Clifton, D. A., Pimentel, M. A. F., Watkinson, P. J., & Tarassenko, L. (2014). Predictive monitoring of mobile patients by combining clinical observations with data from wearable sensors. *IEEE Journal of Biomedical and Health Informatics, 18*(3), 722–730. doi:10.1109/JBHI.2013.2293059 PMID:24808218

Devashri, S. (2015). Review on-android based health care monitoring system. International Journal of Innovation Engineering Research and Technology, 1-4.

Dunsmuir, D., Payne, B. A., Cloete, G., Petersen, C. L., Gorges, M., Lim, J., ... Ansermino, J. M. (2014). Development of mHealth applications for pre-eclampsia triage. *IEEE Journal of Biomedical and Health Informatics, 18*(6), 1857–1864. doi:10.1109/JBHI.2014.2301156 PMID:25375683

Gope, P., & Hwang, T. (2016). BSN-Care:A sensor IoT-based modern healthcare system using body sensor network. *IEEE Sensors*, *16*(5), 1368–1376. doi:10.1109/JSEN.2015.2502401

Joon-Soo, J.-Y. (2016). A Design Characteristics of Smart Healthcare System as the IoT Application. *Indian Journal of Science and Technology*, *9*(37), 1–8.

Khalifa, A. (2014). ZIGBEE BASED WEARABLE REMOTE HEALTHCARE MONITORING SYSTEM FOR ELDERLY PATIENTS. *International Journal of Wireless & Mobile Networks*, *6*(3), 53–67. doi:10.5121/ijwmn.2014.6304

Maradugu, A. (2015). Android based health care monitoring system. *2015 International Conference on Innovations in Information, Embedded and Communication Systems (ICIIECS)* (pp. 1-5). Coimbatore, India: IEEE.

Ni, Z. (2015). Bridging e-Health and the Internet of things: The SPHERE Project. *IEEE Intelligent Systems*, *30*(4), 39–46. doi:10.1109/MIS.2015.57

Orlando, P. (2014). An efficient and low cost Windows Mobile BSN monitoring system based on TinyOS. *Telecommunication Systems*, *55*(1), 115–124. doi:10.100711235-013-9756-4

Pasluosta, C., Gassner, H., Winkler, J., Klucken, J., & Eskofier, B. M. (2015). An emerging era in the management of Parkinson's disease: Wearable Technologies and the Internet of things. *IEEE Journal of Biomedical and Health Informatics*, *19*(6), 1873–1881. doi:10.1109/JBHI.2015.2461555 PMID:26241979

Sarfraz, F. K. (2017). Health care monitoring system in Internet of things (IoT) by using RFID. *2017 6th International Conference on Industrial Technology and Management (ICITM)* (pp. 198-204). Cambridge, UK: IEEE.

Shih-Hao, C., .-D.-J.-T. (2016). Enabling Smart Personalized Healthcare: A Hybrid Mobile-Cloud Approach for ECG Telemonitoring. IT Professionals, 18(3), 14-22.

Shirehjini, A., Yassine, A., & Shirmohammadi, S. (2012). Equipment Location in Hospitals Using RFID-Based Positioning System. *IEEE Transactions on Information Technology in Biomedicine*, *16*(6), 1058–1069. doi:10.1109/TITB.2012.2204896 PMID:24218700

Wang, X., Gui, Q., Liu, B., Jin, Z., & Chen, Y. (2014). Enabling smart personalized healthcare: A hybrid mobile-cloud approach for ECG telemonitoring. *IEEE Journal of Biomedical and Health Informatics*, *18*(3), 739–745.

Chapter 9
Health Monitoring System for Individuals Using Internet of Things

Rajkumar Rajasekaran
https://orcid.org/0000-0002-0983-7259
Vellore Institute of Technology, India

Govinda K.
Vellore Institute of Technology, India

Jolly Masih
Erasmus School of Economics, The Netherlands

Sruthi M.
Vellore Institute of Technology, India

ABSTRACT

Most of the elderly citizens are either living by themselves or locked up at home when the rest of the family members go to work. Health of the elderly deteriorates gradually with age, but people fail to notice these changes in everyday life. The elderly are at risk of not receiving attention immediately in the case of emergencies. Internet of things can be used to alert family members and health personnel immediately when an abnormality in the elderly person's health is sensed to prevent discovery of illness at an irrecoverable stage. Internet of things can monitor parameters like heart pulse rate, body temperature, body movement, position, and location, and raise an alert to take immediate preventive actions. Making this system portable is one of the most necessary requirements because it will be worn by the user. That introduces various conditions in itself. For instance, the system should not disturb the patient or be heavy.

INTRODUCTION

Most of the elderly citizens are either living by themselves or locked up at home when rest of the family

DOI: 10.4018/978-1-7998-1090-2.ch009

members go to work. Health of the elderly deteriorate gradually with age, but fail to notice these changes in everyday life. The elderly are at a risk of not being attended immediately in case of emergencies.

Internet of Things can be used to alert the family members and health personnel immediately when an abnormality in their health is sensed to prevent discovery of illness at an irrecoverable stage. It can be used to detect abnormalities in the health condition by monitoring the parameters like heart pulse rate, body temperature, body movement and position, location and raise an alert to take immediate preventive actions. With the help of sensors to sense data, web server to store data and trigger Firebase Cloud Messaging service to push notification to android app on exceeding a certain threshold value, the alert can family and health care service personnel when an abnormality in health is sensed, to avoid worsening of an illness to an irrecoverable stage.

This approach has led to an evolution in the world of medicine. It allows for prognosis of diseases at a much earlier stage using this proactive paradigm compared to the existing retroactive diagnose-and-treat reactive paradigm. It also helps to personalize the treatment options available to meet the specific needs of the person. The early detection of abnormalities in the health condition can help in slowing down the progression of the condition and have everything under control.

This article highlights the opportunities and challenges in utilizing the power of Internet of Things for remote healthcare of elderly and chronic patients.

OVERVIEW

"Internet of things" refers to the possibility of endowing everyday objects with the ability to identify themselves, communicate with other objects, and possibly compute. The goal of the IoT is to enable a variety of things present in the environment to be connected in order to interact and cooperate "anytime, anyplace, with anything and anyone, ideally using any path or network and any service". So, the Internet is now advancing from a network of computers to a network of things. It is estimated that between 2015 and 2050, the proportion of the world's population over 60 years of age will nearly double from 12% to 22%. The development of health care systems in today's world demands a concerted effort to harness the power of information and communications technologies in order to create more efficient, effective, and secure data sharing [30]. Mobile devices can surpass geographical barriers and deliver remote healthcare services anytime, anywhere. With the help of sensors to sense data, web server to store data and trigger Firebase Cloud Messaging service to push notification to android app on exceeding a certain threshold value, can alert the family and health care service personnel when an abnormality in health is sensed, to avoid worsening of an illness to an irrecoverable stage.

CHALLENGES

The idea of exploiting technology for this project is limited by the availability of network for reading sensor data, the size of the sensors that might cause uneasiness when worn on the body, the accuracy of sensed data and the accuracy of alerts (not giving alarms for fault positive cases and raising alarms for false negative cases).

RELIABILITY OF THE SENSORS

Reliability of sensors is the probability of failure-free operation of the sensor device for a specified period of time in a specified environment. A number of sensors are used to sense the parameters like heart pulse rate, body temperature, body movement, body position and location. cannot guarantee that these sensors will work all the time because of the need for network connection all the time. Since this is a medical device used for health monitoring, the reliability is expected to be high and this is a big challenge to achieve.

ACCURACY OF SENSOR DATA

Accuracy of the sensor data is the degree of closeness of measurements of a parameter to that parameter's true value. The value obtained from sensors for heart pulse rate, body temperature, body movement, body position and location may represent approximate values and not be 100% accurate. The system can be accurate but not precise, precise but not accurate, neither, or both. This is the most important non-functional requirement of this system as medical personnel will have to take decisions based on these sensor values. If these sensor data is not accurate, it may lead to not giving alarms for fault positive cases and raising alarms for false negative cases which are fatal in the critical field of medicine.

INTEROPERABILITY OF DEVICES

Medical device interoperability is the ability to safely, securely, and effectively exchange and use information among one or more devices, products, technologies, or systems. Various devices like the sensors, node MCU, raspberry pi, android device and web servers are interconnected and made to work together though they belong to different domains.

SECURITY AND PRIVACY ISSUES

Data security is commonly referred to as the confidentiality, availability, and integrity of data. In other words, it is all of the practices and processes that are in place to ensure data isn't being used or accessed by unauthorized individuals or parties. Data privacy, also called information privacy, is the aspect of information technology that deals with the ability an organization or individual has to determine what data in a computer system can be shared with third parties. The security and privacy of sensed data, the data stored in the web server, the data in the android application and the data while being transferred via the network has to be maintained end-to-end. Hackers can intrude into the network and steal medical data which is sensitive. Earning the trust of the users of the system by providing end-to-end security and privacy is a huge challenge to be overcome by this system.

UNOBTRUSIVENESS OF SENSORS

The sensors used in body sensor networks for continuous monitoring of patients is required to be unobtrusive and small in size so that it doesn't cause uneasiness in the users. The smaller the size of the sensors, the costlier it is. Hence size and cost is a challenge.

PROJECT STATEMENT

The elderly citizens, all over the world are either living by themselves or locked up at home when the other family members go to work. Health of the elderly deteriorate gradually with age, but fail to notice these changes in everyday life. The elderly are at a risk of not being attended immediately in case of emergencies. Internet of Things can be used to alert the family members and health personnel immediately when an abnormality in their health is sensed to prevent discovery of illness at an irrecoverable stage. It can be used to detect abnormalities in the health condition by monitoring the parameters like heart pulse rate, body temperature, body movement and position, location and raise an alert to take immediate preventive actions. The early detection of abnormalities in the health condition can help in slowing down the progression of the condition and have everything under control. With the help of sensors to sense data, web server to store data and trigger Firebase Cloud Messaging service to push notification to android app on exceeding a certain threshold value, we can alert the family and health care service personnel when an abnormality in health is sensed, to avoid worsening of an illness to an irrecoverable stage.

OBJECTIVES

Internet of Things has given us the hope that can control the unexpected things that may happen to us in life. With the help of sensors to sense data, web server to store data and trigger Firebase Cloud Messaging service to push notification to android app on exceeding a certain threshold value, can alert the family and health care service personnel when an abnormality in health is sensed, to avoid worsening of an illness to an irrecoverable stage. The early detection of symptoms related to a specific health condition can help clinicians to enact appropriate interventions that can slow down the progression of the condition itself, with beneficial effects on both patients' quality of life and treatment's costs.

The earlier an abnormality in health is sensed, the more the chances of recovering quickly from an illness. This proactive approach with the help of sensors to sense data, web server to store data and trigger Firebase Cloud Messaging service to push notification to android app on exceeding a certain threshold value can alert the family and health care service personnel when an abnormality in health is sensed, to avoid worsening of an illness to an irrecoverable stage. The proposed system will lead to an evolution in the practice of medicine, from the current retroactive diagnose-and-treat reactive paradigm to a proactive framework for prognosis of diseases at a much earlier stage. It also enables personalization of treatment options targeted particularly to the specific circumstances and needs of the individual, and help reduce the cost of health care while simultaneously improving outcomes. In this paper, we highlight the opportunities and challenges for IoT in realizing this vision of the future of health care. This system would be highly beneficial as the patients can get seamless healthcare at any time in a comfortable home environment, society's financial burden could be greatly reduced by remote treatment, limited hospital resources can be released for people in need of emergency care, In-home healthcare and services can drastically reduce the total expenditure on medical care or treatment. The early detection of symptoms related to a specific health condition can help clinicians to enact appropriate interventions that can slow down the progression of the condition itself, with beneficial effects on both patients' quality of life and treatment's costs. Therefore, it is urgent in the near future for the healthcare industry to develop advanced and practical health-related technologies and services by leveraging information and communication technology.

The elderly are at a risk of not being attended immediately in case of emergencies when the family members are away from home. If the family members and health services are not alerted on time in case of such emergencies, unexpected things can happen. Internet of Things can be used to alert the family members and health personnel in case of such emergencies. It can be used to detect abnormalities in the health condition by monitoring the parameters –heart pulse rate, body temperature, body movement and position, location and give a warning to take immediate actions. This proactive approach with the help of sensors to sense data, web server to store data and trigger Firebase Cloud Messaging service to push notification to android app on exceeding a certain threshold value, can alert the family and health care service personnel when an abnormality in health is sensed, to avoid worsening of an illness to an irrecoverable stage. The proposed system will lead to an evolution in the practice of medicine, from the current retroactive diagnose-and-treat reactive paradigm to a proactive framework for prognosis of diseases at a much earlier stage. It also enables personalization of treatment options targeted particularly to the specific circumstances and needs of the individual, and help reduce the cost of health care while simultaneously improving outcomes. In this paper, highlighting the opportunities and challenges for IoT in realizing this vision of the future of health care. This system would be highly beneficial as the patients can get seamless healthcare at any time in a comfortable home environment, society's financial burden could be greatly reduced by remote treatment, limited hospital resources can be released for people in need of emergency care, In-home healthcare and services can drastically reduce the total expenditure on medical care or treatment. Therefore, it is urgent in the near future for the healthcare industry to develop advanced and practical health-related technologies and services by leveraging information and communication technology The early detection of symptoms related to a specific health condition can help clinicians to enact appropriate interventions that can slow down the progression of the condition itself, with beneficial effects on both patients' quality of life and treatment's costs.

EXISTING SYSTEM

The existing system of monitoring the health of the elderly includes taking them to a clinic or hospital for treatment or checkup only when something fatal is observed in their health. The symptoms of most of the illness gradually shows up in their body, but is not given proper attention at the right time. Only when the health deteriorates to an irrecoverable level, the illness is discovered. The elderly do not go for regular checkups to hospitals and clinics because of need to go in person to the hospitals and clinics and involves a huge cost too. Personalization of treatment options is not available. The family and the medical personnel are not alerted about the abnormalities that show up in their health gradually.

PROPOSED SYSTEM

The earlier an abnormality in health is sensed, the more the chances of recovering quickly from an illness. With the help of sensors to sense data, web server to store data and trigger Firebase Cloud Messaging service to push notification to android app on exceeding a certain threshold value, alert can be sent to the family and health care service personnel when an abnormality in health is sensed, to avoid worsening of an illness to an irrecoverable stage.

The proposed system will lead to an evolution in the practice of medicine, from the current retroactive diagnose-and-treat reactive paradigm to a proactive framework for prognosis of diseases at a much earlier stage. It also enables personalization of treatment options targeted particularly to the specific circumstances and needs of the individual, and help reduce the cost of health care while simultaneously improving outcomes. In this paper, highlight the opportunities and challenges for IoT in realizing this vision of the future of health care. . This system would be highly beneficial as the patients can get seamless healthcare at any time in a comfortable home environment, society's financial burden could be greatly reduced by remote treatment, limited hospital resources can be released for people in need of emergency care, In-home healthcare and services can drastically reduce the total expenditure on medical care or treatment. The early detection of symptoms related to a specific health condition can help clinicians to enact appropriate interventions that can slow down the progression of the condition itself, with beneficial effects on both patients' quality of life and treatment's costs. Therefore, it is urgent in the near future for the healthcare industry to develop advanced and practical health-related technologies and services by leveraging information and communication technology.

Assume that the following for the proposed system includes:

- The sensors used- temperature, pulse, location, body position and movement are enough to monitor the health of a person.
- The sensors are assumed to be unobtrusive to a certain extent for the patient while they are worn on the body.
- assume that there is good network available throughout for sensing these parameters from the patient's body.

LITERATURE SURVEY

A literature review surveys books, scholarly articles, and any other sources relevant to a particular issue, area of research, or theory, and by so doing, provides a description, summary, and critical evaluation of these works in relation to the research problem being investigated.

Abawajy et al.(2017), propose a Pervasive Patient Health Monitoring system that is based on cloud computing and IoT technologies. A case study of real-time ECG monitoring of a patient suffering from congestive heart failure is given to prove the efficiency of the proposed architecture. Experimental evaluation of the proposed Pervasive Patient Health Monitoring infrastructure proves that it is a flexible, cost-efficient and energy-efficient remote health monitoring application. Azimi et al.(2017), discuss the latest health monitoring approaches of elderly using IoT to analyse their benefits and short comes from the perspective of the elderly being monitored. This article proposes a hierarchical model for elderly-centred monitoring to analyse the current approaches, goals and challenges in a top-down trend.

This article discusses the existing solutions, the main objectives and trends that IoT-based healthcare systems can provide for future remote elderly care. Chen et al.(2017), have proposed washable smart clothing that consists of sensors and electrodes to collect and transfer the patient's physiological data and receive the health and emotional status analysis provided by cloud-based machine intelligence. This article proposes Wearable 2.0 healthcare system based on smart clothing to improve the Quality of Service of the next generation e-healthcare systems. In the proposed system, the patient's physiological data is collected and with the help of big data analytics on clouds, personalized healthcare services are provided. Shamim and Ghulam (2016), propose a HealthIIoT-enabled monitoring framework, where ECG and other medical data are collected by the sensors and sent to the cloud for uninterrupted access by the healthcare providers. With HealthIIoT, medical personnel can access patient information and analyse it in a real-time manner to monitor the patient. But these wearable patient devices and medical data are subject to security breaches. This article proposes a cloud-integrated HealthIIoT monitoring framework where watermarking of healthcare data is done before sending it to the cloud for safe and secure health monitoring.

Gope et al. (2016), have discussed the privacy and the security issues in e-health systems using Body Sensor Network. Strong security services to preserve patient privacy is not achieved in the BSN based projects. This article proposes BSN-Care, a secure IoT-healthcare system using Body Sensor Network that can address a range of security requirements of the Body Sensor Network based healthcare system. Mano et al. (2016), propose an IoT infrastructure that makes use of images and emotions of patients for remote healthcare as emotions play a crucial role while a patient is recovering from a wide range of illnesses. This system ensures that the right person is identified with the help of these images and that the right treatment is given to them. The system also allows to draw on the images to verify if the emotional part of each person relies on the same Internet of Things technology. The proposed Ensemble model showed approximately 80% accuracy and proved to be effective. Yuehong et al. (2016), discuss the applications and future trends of Internet of Things in the healthcare industry. This article provides an extensive literature review, achievements of the researchers and the advancement of IoT in e-healthcare using smart devices and smart technologies. The challenges and prospects of the development of remote healthcare systems based on Internet of Things is discussed. Mainetti et al. (2016), propose an Ambient Assisted Living architecture that aims to support the elderly in their daily life. The features of the proposed system are continuous monitoring of location and continuous monitoring of the health status, by crossing this information with the environmental parameters. The system can trigger alerts when abnormal conditions like fall detection or presence of anomalous health parameter value are sensed. The proposed system collects sensor data from a number of heterogeneous devices and forward them to the remote reasoning server and trigger appropriate alarms at crucial times when abnormalities are sensed.

Islam et al. (2015), have surveyed various IoT-based healthcare technologies and have presented numerous healthcare network architectures and platforms that support access to the IoT backbone and facilitate medical parameter value transmission and reception. In this article various security requirements and challenges in using IoT for healthcare has been discussed. Various research problems in the area have been discussed to propose a model that can reduce the associated security risks. This paper provides extensive research activities on how IoT can address healthcare for elderly, chronic disease supervision and private health management.

Hassanalieragh et al. (2015), have reviewed the current state and the future directions for integration of remote health monitoring technologies with the clinical practice of medicine. Wearable sensors offer attractive options for enabling observation and recording of data in home and work environments, over much longer durations than are currently done at clinics and hospitals. This gathered data, when analysed and presented to physicians in easy-to-assimilate visualizations has the potential for radically improving healthcare and reducing the cost healthcare. They have highlighted the challenges in sensing, analyzing and visualizing data that needs to be addressed before designing such state-of-the-art systems in medicine. Pang et al. (2015), propose a business-technology for cross-boundary integration of health care devices and services at home. A cooperative Health-IoT environment is set up, and the smart healthcare systems of all the stakeholders are integrated in a cooperative health cloud and also extended to patients' home with the help of in-home health care station (IHHS). Detailed architectures of hardware, software, device and service integration are discussed and verified with the help of an implemented prototype. The medical data from all stakeholders are collected and integrated in a cooperative health cloud. An IHHS solution- the iMedBox, which is an intelligent medicine box that can efficiently integrate the in home health care devices and services. Hussain et al. (2015), propose a people-centric IoT framework for the healthcare of elderly and disabled people. It is aimed to monitor the health of the elderly and disabled. Under abnormal health condition, this approach allows a service-oriented emergency response. A number of physiological and environmental sensors were used and their data was collected, analyzed and monitored. A virtual community was created for establishing new social networks which allows the elderly and the disabled improve their mind and health by participating in such social activities.

Zhu et al. (2015), discuss the current development in the field of sensing, networking, and machine learning. The main goal of this interdisciplinary SPHERE project is to build a platform that fuses complementary sensor data to generate datasets that help in identifying abnormalities in a number of health parameters.

Khoi et al. (2015), have identified that real-time event update, bandwidth requirements and data generation are the key network requirements of a typical remote health monitoring system. Communication protocols like HTTP, CoAP and MQTT are analyzed to compare the bandwidth requirements and the volume of generated data. This article proposes an IoT-based remote healthcare monitoring architecture called IReHMo that efficiently delivers health data to the servers. Yang et al.(2014), have proposed intelligent packaging, unobtrusive bio-sensor and intelligent medicine box for healthcare monitoring. They have proposed iHome system, an IoT-based intelligent home-centric healthcare platform which seamlessly connects sensors attached to human body for physiological monitoring and intelligent pharmaceutical packaging for everyday medication management. The proposed iHome system consists of three key blocks, including the iMedBox, the iMedPack and the Bio-Patch. iMedPack automatically reminds the user of the medicine to take and dispenses a certain amount of medicine at the right time based on the on-line prescription. For unobtrusive and continuous monitoring of the user, a small flexible Bio-Patch has been developed.

Yang and Robert (2014), provide a comprehensive review of the recent development in wireless sensor technology for monitoring behavior related to human physiological responses. It presents background information on the use of wireless technology and sensors to develop a wireless physiological measurement system. The paper also identifies the requirements for wireless physiological measurement systems in order to successfully meet the needs of the market. These requirements include low cost, low-power consumption, small size with a high degree of integration and packaging, the possible use of energy harvesting methods as alternative power supplies and reliable physiological sensors. Amendola et al. (2014), present a survey on the state-of-the-art RFID technologies for health monitoring and data of the user's environment like location, temperature, humidity and other parameters. A range of the available options that gather and analyze data about human behavior are discussed along with the power exposure that is acceptable and sanitary regulations. Santos et al. (2014), propose an Internet of Things architecture that aims at creating a ubiquitous Ambient Assisted Living framework that can be used by mobile health services. The framework proposed is based on Radio Frequency Identification technology (RFID) and Electronic Product Code (EPC) normalization for creating a unique ID for each mobile-health item that involves medicine, objects, physician or patient. This ID can be read without direct contact and can be used as a primary access key to a service indexer, through an Object Name Service (ONS), that allows linking these physical items to their virtual correspondents in a global IoT. To ensure the privacy and security of all the m-.health Ambient Assisted Living applications within this architecture, this article presents the security mechanism defined and implemented. Chiuchisan et al. (2014), propose an IoT architecture for monitoring the patients at risk in smart Intensive Care Units which utilizes smart devices like XBOX, KinectTM and a number of sensors to monitor the environmental parameters. Immediate measures can be taken by the health personnel by the alarms and alerts raised by this system on sensing an abnormality in the conditions monitored. Preventive measures can be taken to curb these abnormalities from becoming fatal. Boric-Lubecke et al. (2014), discuss a wide variety of applications of IoT in e-healthcare, like remote monitoring of elderly and those with sleep disorders, security and privacy of medical data etc. This article concludes that e-healthcare can transform the traditional medical practices and disease prevention mechanisms with the help of smart devices for remote patient monitoring and seamless communication with the medical personnel. Mohammed et al. (2014), propose to develop an Android Application using IoT and cloud computing to monitor ECG waves of patients. The proposed solution combines the use of various technologies like microcontrollers, communication protocols, signal processing for ECG waves for secure data transfer. The infrastructure proposed in this article can be applied to other medical applications with minor changes.

Castillejo et al. (2013), have discussed a number of e-health application cases based on a Wireless Security Network. In the sports scenario discussed in this article, the system collects the physiological data of an athlete through a Bluetooth device. The application suggests a number of exercises to the athlete to improve his fitness based on the data collected and analyzed. If any of the parameters like heart pulse or temperature shows an abnormal value, an alarm is raised to alert the athlete to stop continuing that exercise. This system can be adapted to a range of e-health applications with minimal changes and also users can use different devices like smart watches, tablets and smart phones.

Bazzani et al. (2012), discuss how an application built on the top of the VIRTUS IoT middleware, provides a valid alternative to the current IoT systems that are based on Service Oriented Architecture. VIRTUS makes use of an Instant Messaging protocol like XMPP to provide a real-time, reliable and secure communication channel among a number of devices. This article analyses the features of the VIRTUS middleware in healthcare systems and provide a comparison with other popular systems.

Dohr et al. (2010), have proposed Keep In Touch (KIT) that uses smart objects and technologies like Near Field Communication and Radio Frequency Identification to enable e-monitoring of elderly. Closed Loop Healthcare Services use Keep In Touch technology to collect and process data and establish communication channels between elderly people, their environment and different groups of healthcare service providers. The combination of Keep In Touch technology and Closed Loop Healthcare Services provides an applied IoT infrastructure for Ambient Assisted Living.

SYSTEM ARCHITECTURE

A system architecture diagram would be used to show the relationship between different components. A system architecture or systems architecture is the conceptual model that defines the structure, behavior, and more views of a system. An architecture description is a formal description and representation of a system, organized in a way that supports reasoning about the structures and behaviors of the system. Usually they are created for systems which include hardware and software and these are represented in the diagram to show the interaction between them.

- With the help of temperature sensor, pulse sensor, GPS module for location and accelerometer for fall detection, the data are sensed from patient.
- The sensed data from the different sensors are collected by an embedded system like raspberry pi.
- The data collected by raspberry pi is stored by a web server- wamp server.
- The web server runs a script to find if the value exceeds the threshold value set for that parameter. If so, it triggers Firebase Cloud Messaging Service to send push notification alert.
- The registered users of the app – family and health care personnel receive alerts to take immediate action.

IMPLEMENTATION STRATEGY

Implementation is the stage of the project when the theoretical design is turned out into a working system. Thus, it can be considered to be the most critical stage in achieving a successful new system and in giving the user, confidence that the new system will work and be effective. The implementation stage involves careful planning, investigation of the existing system and its constraints on implementation, designing of methods to achieve changeover and evaluation of changeover methods.

MODULE DESCRIPTION

- **IOT ENVIRONMENT SETUP**

The raspbian OS is installed in the raspberry pi 3- module B and interfaced with pulse sensor, temperature sensor, GPS module for location and accelerometer for fall detection using GPIO pins and jumper wires.

- **WEB SERVER SETUP**

WAMP server is installed and configurations are made in it to run python scripts. A database called paramlog is created in php myadmin with the tables to records values of the parameters sensed in pi- temperature, pulse rate, location co-ordinates and accelerometer readings with the date and time of recoding.

- **ANDROID APP SETUP**

Figure 1. System architecture diagram: conceptual model

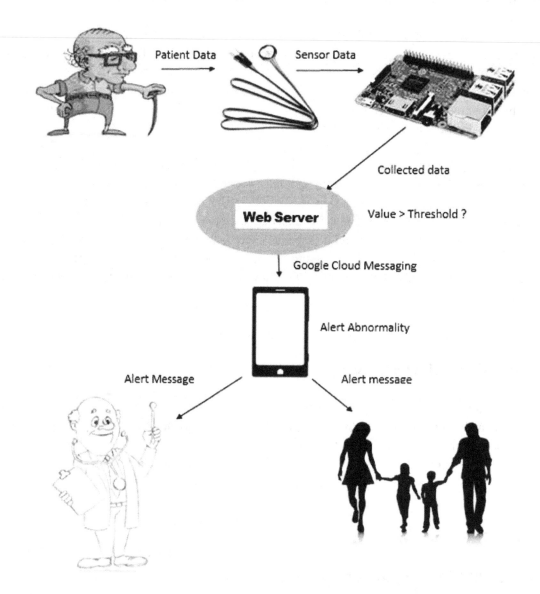

An android app is created to show the parameter values sensed and stored in the server on the click of a button by registered users of the app. Alerts when a parameter value exceeds threshold is sent to the registered users through the app using the Firebase Cloud Messaging API service.

PROCEDURE

Patient: A patient can wear the sensors to allow the sensors to sense parameters like temperature, heart pulse rate, motion and location.

IoT Setup: Includes the body sensors, raspberry pi, arduino and the jumper wires. They sense and collect data from the patient.

Web Server: The web server is bitnami wamp stack that consists of apache and MySQL server. They store the data in tables and detect abnormality by comparing the parameter value with the threshold value.

Android App: Alert registered users with the help of Firebase Cloud Messaging service when abnormalities in health parameters are detected.

TECHNIQUES AND METHODOLOGIES

Firebase serves as a module between your server and the devices that will be receiving the push notifications that you create. Your server informs Firebase that a notification has to be sent. Then Firebase does the work behind the scenes to get the notification published.

When a user authenticates to a Firebase app:

- Information about the user is returned in callbacks on the client device. Using this the customize app's user experience, according to a specific user.
- This user information returned contains a UID (a unique ID), which is distinct across all providers, and it never changes for a specific authenticated user.
- Now, in our app's security & Firebase rules, value for the authToken becomes defined. Its value will be null for unauthenticated users. However, for authenticated users, it will an object containing auth.uid (unique for every user) and some other informational data about the user. Using this, we can securely control data access on a per-user basis.

Firebase Cloud Messaging (FCM) provides a cross-platform messaging solution that allows reliable delivery of messages at no cost. Using this we can:

- Send notification messages (2KB limit) or data messages (4KB limit).
- Distribute messages to a single device, groups of devices, or to devices subscribed to some topics.
- Send acknowledgments, chats, and other messages from devices back to the server over FCM's reliable and battery-efficient connection channel.
- Using Notification messages, developers can send users a visible display message with some predefined keys and optional custom key-value pairs (data payloads).

Firebase Cloud Messaging (FCM) is the new version of GCM. It inherits the reliable and scalable GCM infrastructure, plus new features. Firebase Cloud Messaging (FCM) provides a reliable and battery-efficient connection between your server and devices that allows you to deliver and receive messages and notifications on iOS, Android, and the web at no cost.

CONCLUSION

The pace of population ageing is much faster than in the past. The need for better healthcare services at home is becoming crucial and hence there is this indispensable pressure to prepare for tomorrow, today.

Internet of things can be used to alert the family members and health personnel immediately when an abnormality in the health of the elderly is sensed. It can be used to detect abnormalities in the health condition by monitoring the parameters like heart pulse rate, body temperature, body movement and position, location and raise an alert to take immediate preventive actions.

This approach has led to an evolution in the world of medicine. It allows for prognosis of diseases at a much earlier stage using this proactive paradigm compared to the existing retroactive diagnose-and-treat reactive paradigm. It also helps to personalize the treatment options available to meet the specific needs of the person. The early detection of abnormalities in the health condition can help in slowing down the progression of the condition and have everything under control. This article highlights the opportunities and challenges in utilizing the power of internet of things for remote healthcare of elderly and chronic patients.

FUTURE WORK

The future work on this remote health monitoring system would be to use decision tree classification algorithm for determining abnormality instead of using conditions in python scripts. We can enhance this system by using this setup on nodeMCU on a number of patients/elderly in the same location, all connected to the raspberry pi common for all. This would increase the power efficiency of the system.

REFERENCES

Abawajy, J. H., & Hassan, M. M. (2017). Federated internet of things and cloud computing pervasive patient health monitoring system. *IEEE Communications Magazine*, *55*(1), 48–53. doi:10.1109/MCOM.2017.1600374CM

Amendola, S., Lodato, R., Manzari, S., Occhiuzzi, C., & Marrocco, G. (2014). RFID technology for IoT-based personal healthcare in smart spaces. IEEE Internet of things Journal, 1(2), 144-152.

Azimi, I., Rahmani, A. M., Liljeberg, P., & Tenhunen, H. (2017). Internet of things for remote elderly monitoring: A study from user-centered perspective. *Journal of Ambient Intelligence and Humanized Computing*, *8*(2), 273–289. doi:10.100712652-016-0387-y

Bazzani, M., Conzon, D., Scalera, A., Spirito, M. A., & Trainito, C. I. (2012, June). Enabling the IoT paradigm in e-health solutions through the VIRTUS middleware. In *2012 IEEE 11th International Conference on Trust, Security and Privacy in Computing and Communications (TrustCom)*, (pp. 1954-1959). Piscataway, NJ: IEEE. 10.1109/TrustCom.2012.144

Boric-Lubecke, O., Gao, X., Yavari, E., Baboli, M., Singh, A., & Lubecke, V. M. (2014, June). E-healthcare: Remote monitoring, privacy, and security. In *2014 IEEE MTT-S International Microwave Symposium (IMS)*, (pp. 1-3). Piscataway, NJ: IEEE.

Castillejo, P., Martinez, J. F., Rodriguez-Molina, J., & Cuerva, A. (2013). Integration of wearable devices in a wireless sensor network for an E-health application. *IEEE Wireless Communications*, *20*(4), 38–49. doi:10.1109/MWC.2013.6590049

Chen, M., Ma, Y., Li, Y., Wu, D., Zhang, Y., & Youn, C. H. (2017). Wearable 2.0: Enabling human-cloud integration in next generation healthcare systems. *IEEE Communications Magazine, 55*(1), 54–61. doi:10.1109/MCOM.2017.1600410CM

Chiauzzi, E., Rodarte, C., & DasMahapatra, P. (2015). Patient-centered activity monitoring in the self-management of chronic health conditions. *BMC Medicine, 13*(1), 77. doi:10.118612916-015-0319-2 PMID:25889598

Chiuchisan, I., Costin, H. N., & Geman, O. (2014, October). Adopting the internet of things technologies in health care systems. In *2014 International Conference and Exposition on Electrical and Power Engineering (EPE),* (pp. 532-535). Piscataway, NJ: IEEE. 10.1109/ICEPE.2014.6969965

Dohr, A., Modre-Opsrian, R., Drobics, M., Hayn, D., & Schreier, G. (2010, April). The internet of things for ambient assisted living. In *2010 Seventh International Conference on Information Technology: New Generations (ITNG),* (pp. 804-809). Piscataway, NJ: IEEE. 10.1109/ITNG.2010.104

Gope, P., & Hwang, T. (2016). BSN-Care: A secure IoT-based modern healthcare system using body sensor network. *IEEE Sensors Journal, 16*(5), 1368–1376. doi:10.1109/JSEN.2015.2502401

Hao, Y., & Foster, R. (2008). Wireless body sensor networks for health-monitoring applications. *Physiological Measurement, 29*(11), R27–R56. doi:10.1088/0967-3334/29/11/R01 PMID:18843167

Hassanalieragh, M., Page, A., Soyata, T., Sharma, G., Aktas, M., Mateos, G., . . . Andreescu, S. (2015, June). Health monitoring and management using Internet-of-Things (IoT) sensing with cloud-based processing: Opportunities and challenges. In *2015 IEEE International Conference on Services Computing (SCC),* (pp. 285-292). Piscataway, NJ: IEEE.

Hossain, M. S., & Muhammad, G. (2016). Cloud-assisted industrial internet of things (iiot)–enabled framework for health monitoring. *Computer Networks, 101,* 192–202. doi:10.1016/j.comnet.2016.01.009

Hussain, A., Wenbi, R., da Silva, A. L., Nadher, M., & Mudhish, M. (2015). Health and emergency-care platform for the elderly and disabled people in the Smart City. *Journal of Systems and Software, 110,* 253–263. doi:10.1016/j.jss.2015.08.041

Islam, S. R., Kwak, D., Kabir, M. H., Hossain, M., & Kwak, K. S. (2015). The internet of things for health care: A comprehensive survey. *IEEE Access: Practical Innovations, Open Solutions, 3,* 678–708. doi:10.1109/ACCESS.2015.2437951

Jara, A. J., Zamora, M. A., & Skarmeta, A. F. (2012, June). Knowledge acquisition and management architecture for mobile and personal health environments based on the internet of things. In *2012 IEEE 11th International Conference on Trust, Security and Privacy in Computing and Communications (TrustCom),* (pp. 1811-1818). Piscataway, NJ: IEEE. 10.1109/TrustCom.2012.194

Khoi, N. M., Saguna, S., Mitra, K., & Åhlund, C. (2015, October). IReHMo: An efficient IoT-based remote health monitoring system for smart regions. In *2015 17th International Conference on E-health Networking, Application & Services (HealthCom),* (pp. 563-568). Piscataway, NJ: IEEE.

Mainetti, L., Patrono, L., Secco, A., & Sergi, I. (2016, July). An IoT-aware AAL system for elderly people. In *International Multidisciplinary Conference on Computer and Energy Science (SpliTech),* (pp. 1-6). Piscataway, NJ: IEEE. 10.1109/SpliTech.2016.7555929

Mano, L. Y., Faiçal, B. S., Nakamura, L. H., Gomes, P. H., Libralon, G. L., Meneguete, R. I., ... Ueyama, J. (2016). Exploiting IoT technologies for enhancing Health Smart Homes through patient identification and emotion recognition. *Computer Communications, 89*, 178–190. doi:10.1016/j.comcom.2016.03.010

Mohammed, J., Lung, C. H., Ocneanu, A., Thakral, A., Jones, C., & Adler, A. (2014, September). Internet of Things: Remote patient monitoring using web services and cloud computing. In *2014 IEEE International Conference on Internet of Things (iThings), and Green Computing and Communications (GreenCom), IEEE and Cyber, Physical and Social Computing (CPSCom), IEEE* (pp. 256-263). Piscataway, NJ: IEEE.

Páez, D. G., Aparicio, F., de Buenaga, M., & Ascanio, J. R. (2014, December). Big data and IoT for chronic patients monitoring. In *International Conference on Ubiquitous Computing and Ambient Intelligence* (pp. 416-423). Cham, Switzerland: Springer. 10.1007/978-3-319-13102-3_68

Pang, Z., Zheng, L., Tian, J., Kao-Walter, S., Dubrova, E., & Chen, Q. (2015). Design of a terminal solution for integration of in-home health care devices and services towards the Internet-of-Things. *Enterprise Information Systems, 9*(1), 86–116. doi:10.1080/17517575.2013.776118

Paschou, M., Sakkopoulos, E., Sourla, E., & Tsakalidis, A. (2013). Health Internet of Things: Metrics and methods for efficient data transfer. *Simulation Modelling Practice and Theory, 34*, 186–199. doi:10.1016/j.simpat.2012.08.002

Santos, A., Macedo, J., Costa, A., & Nicolau, M. J. (2014). Internet of things and smart objects for M-health monitoring and control. *Procedia Technology, 16*, 1351–1360. doi:10.1016/j.protcy.2014.10.152

Sung, W. T., & Chiang, Y. C. (2012). Improved particle swarm optimization algorithm for android medical care IOT using modified parameters. *Journal of Medical Systems, 36*(6), 3755–3763. doi:10.100710916-012-9848-9 PMID:22492176

Tan, J., Wen, H. J., & Awad, N. (2005). Health care and services delivery systems as complex adaptive systems. *Communications of the ACM, 48*(5), 36–44. doi:10.1145/1060710.1060737

World Health Organization. (2015). *Ageing and health.* Available at http://www.who.int/mediacentre/factsheets/fs404/en/

Yang, G., Xie, L., Mäntysalo, M., Zhou, X., Pang, Z., Da Xu, L., ... Zheng, L. R. (2014). A health-iot platform based on the integration of intelligent packaging, unobtrusive bio-sensor, and intelligent medicine box. *IEEE Transactions on Industrial Informatics, 10*(4), 2180–2191. doi:10.1109/TII.2014.2307795

Yuehong, Y. I. N., Zeng, Y., Chen, X., & Fan, Y. (2016). The internet of things in healthcare: An overview. *Journal of Industrial Information Integration, 1*, 3–13. doi:10.1016/j.jii.2016.03.004

Zhu, N., Diethe, T., Camplani, M., Tao, L., Burrows, A., Twomey, N., ... Craddock, I. (2015). Bridging e-health and the internet of things: The sphere project. *IEEE Intelligent Systems, 30*(4), 39–46. doi:10.1109/MIS.2015.57

Chapter 10
Patient Health Monitoring System and Detection of Atrial Fibrillation, Fall, and Air Pollutants Using IoT Technologies

Rajkumar Rajaseskaran

https://orcid.org/0000-0002-0983-7259

Vellore Institute of Technology, India

Rishabh Jain

Vellore Institute of Technology, India

Sruthi M.

Vellore Institute of Technology, India

ABSTRACT

The objective of IoT in healthcare is to empower people to live healthy lives by wearing connected equipment. The healthcare industry has perpetually been in the forefront in the adoption and utilization of information and communication technologies (ICT) for the efficient healthcare administration). Detection of atrial fibrillation is done by checking the variations in the period of the heart rate. If a patient has atrial fibrillation, the period between each heartbeat will vary. A gas sensor is used to check the quality of air and a MEMS sensor to detect the fall of the body. The MEMS sensor is a compact device that collects comprehensive physical information and uses the gateway and cloud to analyze and store information.

INTRODUCTION

In the recent decades, technology is being incorporated in almost all health applications, leading to

DOI: 10.4018/978-1-7998-1090-2.ch010

highly digitized systems which give accurate results. Healthcare demands are changing due to increase in number of healthcare-based problems around the globe, and patient's preferences are shifting towards more technological healthcare-based solutions.

There are more patients which require more careful attention and less doctors in comparison. These demands need to be met by this industry which is facing a rise in patients expenses due shortage of caretakers/solution to solve the problem.

Rapid climate change over the years, and unpredictable weather conditions and global warming has also led to increase in number of healthcare issues around the globe. Atrial fibrillation, a starting symptom of heart failure is a problem faced by 2.7–6.1 million of the US population due to unhealthy eating patterns and air pollution (Raja, 2018). There is increase in number of respiratory diseases, which is not known by general public and due to this non-awareness of issue leads to serious disease in the future. Modern healthcare-based solutions can be used to prevent the issue of healthcare using IoT based smart solutions to monitor patients and to store and analyze the patient's data and come up with better solutions.

OBJECTIVE

To create a compact device that collects comprehensive physical information and uses Gateway and Cloud so that information can be analyzed and stored so that the data analyzed can be sent wirelessly for further analysis and review. The objective also includes the detection of Atrial Fibrillation which is caused by irregular rate of heartbeat increasing risk of stroke and several heart diseases. also aiming to provide a better environment for the affected patient by using sensors to analyze the quality of air in the surroundings corresponding to the patient and suggesting a better healthier surrounding in terms of air pollution if required.

MOTIVATION

The concept of connected health care systems and smart medical devices is not only for companies but also for the well-being of the people in general. Patients admitted to the hospital whose physical condition is needed to be carefully looked after, they can be constantly monitored using IoT-driven surveillance. It replaces the process of coming to a health professional at regular intervals to examine the patient's important signals rather than providing constant automatic flow of information.

With rising global population and increase in number of healthcare issues around the globe, we are aiming to provide a better and an economical solution to this problem by making the use of IoT technology by constantly monitoring the patient's body (heartbeat, temperature, etc.) and his surrounding (air quality) and storing the data for analyzing for future scope.

BACKGROUND

Fall Detection- Falls are responsible for 40% of all injury related deaths and need immediate medical attention. The reason for a fall may be heart problems, loss of consciousness, fatigue, exhaustion, diseases and loss of balance. The two major factors that affect a fall is that, firstly, it requires an immediate attention by medical supervision which is in lot of cases not provided due to unawareness of the situation of the fall and the way to overcome is to provide a sensing method to send an alert to the caretaker when the fall happens. Secondly, falls limits the individual movement or independence. A person who experienced a fall may have to remain in that state depending on the severity of the fall if the person become unconscious and unable to move. Person may have to stay alone for extended period of time. At such situation, immediate medical attention may be required which won't proceeded until unless the caretaker is aware of the situation.

Pollution/Air Quality - The patient requires to stay in a healthy toxic free environment for better recovery. Breathing in harmful gases may deteriorate health conditions. Thus, a gas sensor which detects presence of toxic gases such as carbon monoxide, methane, LPG and will act as a precaution measure to prevent the patient from going to such places and take measures if the patients is already living in such conditions.

Atrial Fibrillation - Atrial fibrillation is an irregular heart rate beating that can increase your complications related to the heart like heart failure or a risk of stroke. During atrial fibrillation, the two upper chambers of the heart (atria) are out of coordination with the two lower chambers of the heart (ventricular) - irregular and irregularly throbbing. Atrial fibrillation often involves heartbeat, shortness of breath and weakness. Atrial fibrillation can be formed in blood clots inside the atria. This is because blood tendency to make blood clots happens when it is not moving. The quivering atria does not transfer to all the ventricles of blood. Some blood only pools inside the Atria, and still the pool of blood remains to make clot. They can travel outside the heart and be trapped in the pulmonary artery (due to pulmonary embolism), an artery (the cause of the stroke) for the brain or arteries anywhere in the body. Although atrial fibrillation is not life-threatening itself, it is a problem which require serious attention as it can lead to life-threatening problems in the future. Atrial fibrillation can occur in an unsystematically way, it can come and go without much knowledge of monitoring it. A person can develop an atrial fibrillation which sticks and does not go away and person may require a treatment in such cases.

There are lot of people who are suffering from atrial fibrillation and have no symptoms in general about their condition. They are very much unaware of their condition unless until it is revealed during a physical examination. People with atrial fibrillation symptoms may experience signs and symptoms such as:

- Less ability to exercise
- Fatigue
- Dizziness
- Confusion
- Shortness of breath
- Pain in chest

LITERATURE REVIEW

After considering different research paper, it has been noticed that, it is very hard to find the abnormalities in the heartbeat count of a patient. The average heart rate count for people 18 to 60 years old ranges from 60 to 100 beats/minute Patients are not satisfied with the treatment that doctors usually use to calculate heartbeat. Therefore, there should be a device to track internal changes in the human body.

This treatment can also be very expensive if done in private hospitals and research facilities. But using IoT devices we can come up with a way to make it less expensive and more efficient.

Hossain and Muhammad, 2016, explained in her research that all the promising potential of the emerging Internet of Things (IoT) technologies for interconnected medical devices and sensors have played an important role in the future of health care industry for quality patient care and management tool. With an ever-increasing number of elderly and disabled people, in order to avoid preventable deaths, there is an urgent need for real-time health monitoring infrastructure to analyze patients' health care data. Wearables are being used to monitor patient and gather data for clinical research trials and academic research studies (Patel et al., 2012). But these wearables can be very expensive costing from Rs.1 lakh to Rs.10 lakhs. In this chapter studied how the author has used apple watch and dismantled it to create a health monitoring system using heart beat sensor and accelerometer. Research shows that the rapid spread of wearable devices and smart phones, the Internet of Things-Enabled Technology is developing health care over a traditional hub-based system to a more personal health care system (PHS). PHS will enable faster and safer preventive care, less overall cost, better patient-centric exercises and increased stability. IoT enabled PHS will be implemented by providing highly customized access to rich medical information and skilled medical judgment to each individual by storing the information and using it later for analysis and review. However, empowering the utility of IoT enabled technology in PHS is still very effective in that area, considering the lack of cost effective and accurate smart medical sensors used in the IoT system. Suhas discusses in his paper discuss about the physical parameters like temperature, pulse rate and ECG and how they are achieved and processed using ARM7 LPC 2138 processor and later displayed by using graphical user interface(GUI) (Kale and Khandelwal, 2013). If an important parameter goes out of the normal range, an alert will be sent to the doctor's mobile.

In this paper, they have proposed a for the management of personal welfare information in the form of PWR which provides the basis for integrating the information monitored from various devices and integrating a mobile health platform that ensures preventive and active service (Na and Choi, 2013). They expect that the integrated model of personal welfare management will be a foundation structure for the mobile based health monitoring system, which provides a person with confidence and a better-quality life. This paper describes E-Health Monitoring (EHM) ecosystem and current EHM market areas (Jia, Chen, and Qi, 2012). The paper used a reference model which uses three EHM based technical models combining with various technologies to provide an improved EHM. The Model 1 uses a communication model between device to device communication only, Model 2 used a method in which networking is used to provide the connection between the devices and Model 3 used a platform-based topology combines with network. Model 3 technology is also equipped with an improved support platform providing different services which is a new Model in itself taking inspiration from Model2. They have also proposed some key technologies which can be used in combination with Model 3 providing an improved service support platform.

This paper presents the design and implementation of patient health monitoring architecture using GSM (Baswa et al., 2017). This is based up on the communication devices like mobile phones and wireless sensor networks for the real time analysis of health status. The main focus in this paper is on developing a model that can facilitate the doctors through tele-monitoring. This architecture or device will be useful for individuals who will be at home or at hospital. The device developed will be useful for medical applications.

Figure 1. Health monitoring system

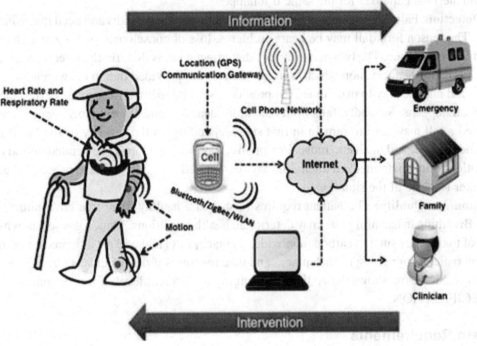

PROPOSED SYSTEM

Remote health care of patients at home is increasing with the popularity of various types of mobile devices, which are able to take care remotely. Along with the cloud, IoT and mobile technologies make it easier for health care teams like doctors, nurses and experts to monitor health conditions of patients by sharing health information. By ensuring guidance awareness about patients, this can bring more responsibility for hospital management. Also, demonstrated the health care system for hospital management so that doctors and parents are allowed to monitor patients' health conditions far away through the Internet. Remote monitoring and guidance awareness are the main focus by sharing information in an authentic way. We are using various kind of IoT sensors for generating different kind of Healthcare information about the individual using the device.

We are using a system of IoT technologies using sensors like heartbeat sensor, temperature sensor, MEMS sensor and gas sensor to keep a track of patient's health. We are also using gas sensor to collect the information about the quality of air surrounding the user and alert the user if the level of air quality is bad. Sensors are connected to a microcontroller which is further connected to an LCD display and GSM Module (used for sending alerts to the caretaker) which is in turn interfaced with Wi-Fi connection in order to store the data on the cloud. If the system detects any abrupt change of values not specified in the normal ranges of temperature, heartbeat, gas (surrounding the user), and MEMS (fall detection), then a message will be sent to the patient's caretaker alerting them to take actions.

Atrial fibrillation can be formed in blood clots inside the atria. This is because blood tendency to make blood clots happens when it is not moving. The quivering atria does not transfer to all the ventricles of blood. Some blood only pools inside the Atria, and still the pool of blood goes to make clot. Thus, we are using a heartbeat sensor or Photo Plethysmography (PPG) sensor to check for the abnormal heartbeat pattern and alert the caretaker for the same if it happens.

Fall Detection: Falls are responsible for 40% of all injury related deaths and need immediate medical attention. The reason for a fall may be heart problems, loss of consciousness, fatigue, exhaustion, diseases and loss of balance. The two major factors that affect a fall is that, firstly, it requires an immediate attention by medical supervision which is in lot of cases not provided due to unawareness of the situation of the fall and the way to overcome is to provide a sensing method to send an alert to the caretaker when the fall happens. Secondly, falls limits the individual movement or independence. A person who experienced a fall may have to remain in that state depending on the severity of the fall if the person become unconscious and unable to move. Person may have to stay alone for extended period of time. At such situation, immediate medical attention may be required which won't have proceeded until unless the caretaker is aware of the situation.

Pollution/Air Quality: The patient requires to stay in a healthy toxic free environment for better recovery. Breathing in harmful gases may deteriorate health conditions. Thus, a gas sensor which detects presence of toxic gases such as carbon monoxide, methane, LPG and will act as a precaution measure to prevent the patient from going to such places and take measures if the patients is already living in such conditions. Table below shows the AQI values ranging to different level of health concerns TECHNICAL SPECIFICATION

Hardware Requirements

Embware emb0005 heartbeat sensor - The heartbeat can be measured on the basis of optical power variation, because during the heartbeat, the light is dispersed or absorbed during its path through the blood. Heart rate is directly related to the sound of the human heart system.

Heartbeat sensor contains a light detector which detects the maximum amount of light passing through the finger. This Bright LED directly corresponds to the number of heart beats. The LED shows bright red color when collecting the amount of light which is later gets detected by the light detector. The color of LED is changing depending on the amount of blood passing through the finger, LED is bright when maximum amount of blood is passing and it will be opaque in color when less light is passing though the finger and the finger detector. The low volume of lights reaches because of this minimum blood flow and the difference can be observed from LED to the detector. The detector signal becomes more diverse with every heart pulse arrival.

Signals collected from the detector are converted into electrical pulse which are amplified by an amplifier. Later these electrical signals are triggered which gives an output of +5V logical level signal.

MQ-9 Gas sensor - MQ-9 gas sensor can detect or measure harmful gases like LPG gas as well as carbon monoxide and methane. The MQ-9 gas sensor can even operate without a microcontroller. It comes with a set of Digital Pin which allows it to be used without a microcontroller. It can measure the gas values in ppm by using the analog pin. It used +5V and thus can be used with most microcontrollers.

Temperature sensor - LM35 is a temperature sensor which measures the temperature in Degree Centigrade. It uses integrated analog signals to provide the electrical output. It is very easy to use the LM35 sensor because of its built-in calibration interfacing and low output impedance. No external calibration or trimming is needed to provide specific accuracy to the LM35 sensor.

Wifi module (ESP8266)– It is a low-cost microchip which uses a System on Chip (SoC) module. It is a Wi-Fi enabled microchip. It has all the microcontroller capabilities with full usage over TCP/

Figure 2. Heartbeat sensor

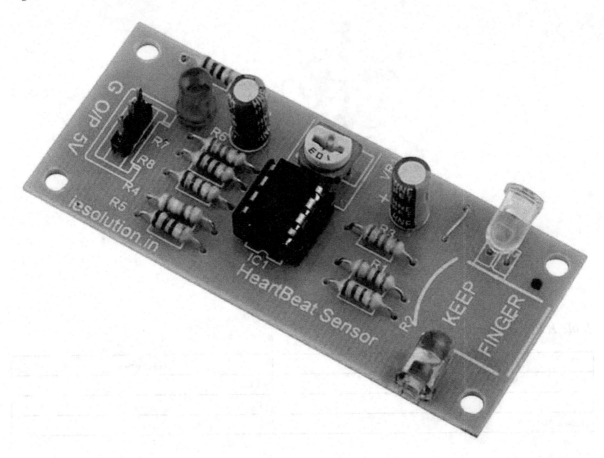

Figure 3. Heartbeat sensor principle

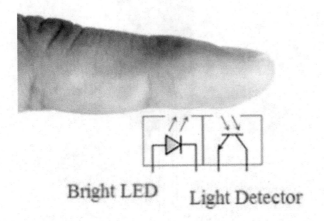

Bright LED   Light Detector

Sensor Principle

Figure 4. Top view

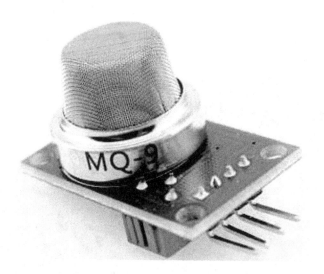

Table 1. Pin description MQ9

Arduino UNO	Gas Sensor
5V	VCC
GND	GND
Analog A0	A0

Figure 5. Temperature sensor

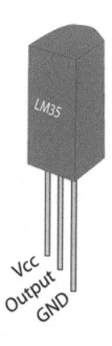

Table 2. Pin description LM35

Pin No	Function	Name
1	Supply voltage; 5V (+35V to -2V)	Vcc
2	Output voltage (+6V to -1V)	Output
3	Ground (0V)	Ground

Figure 6. Wi-Fi module

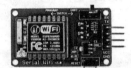

IP commands and protocols. Each of the ESP8266 are preprogrammed with a set of commands called AT-Command set, which enables it to be used with any Arduino device and gives access to all Wi-Fi networking tasks like any Wi-Fi. It provides almost same capabilities as Wi-Fi shield offers. It is capable of offloading networking functions or either hosting an application from another processor.

GSM module -The SIM card mounted GSM modem after getting digit direction by SMS from any mobile phone send that information to the MC through sequential correspondence. While the program is executed, the GSM modem gets direction 'STOP' to build up a yield at the MC, the contact purpose of which are utilized to cripple/turn off the start switch.

Transformer - In transformer the step-down converters are used for converting high voltage into low voltage. In transformer the converter when output voltage is less than the input voltage it is called as a step-down converter, and the converter when output voltage is greater than the input voltage is called as step-up converter. There are two types of transformers, step-up and step-down transformers which are

Figure 7. GSM module

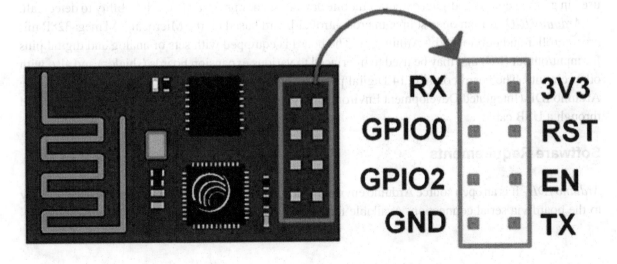

Figure 8. Architecture of GSM

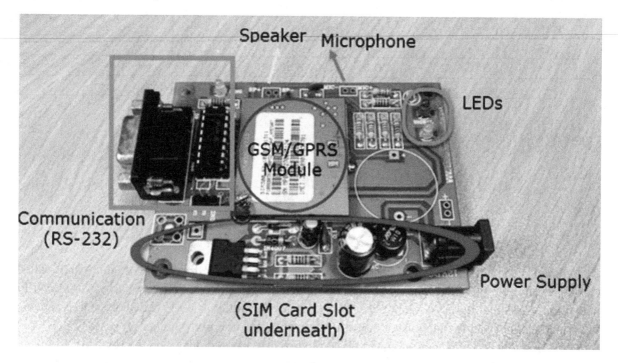

used when we require to step up or step down the voltage levels. In our application 230V AC is converted into 12V AC using a step-down transformer.

MEMS - Micro-electromechanical systems (MEMS)is an innovation that consolidates PCs with modest mechanical gadgets, for example, sensors, valves, riggings, mirrors, and actuators installed in semiconductor chips. In order to sense the acceleration and angular position we use the sensor ADXL 335 MEMS based accelerometer. It is a 3-axis system, which provides analog output corresponding to the 3 axis X, Y and Z axes of the orthogonal coordinate system. Some commercial applications of MEMS include Inkjet printers which often use thermal bubble ejection to deposit ink on the paper. This sensor finds its use in modern car in detecting/measuring the acceleration of the car. This application is widely used in gaming consoles, digital cameras, mobile devices. In our project we use this ability to detect fall.

ArduinoUNO -It is an open source microcontroller board based on the Microchip ATmega328P microcontroller and developed by Arduino.cc. The board is equipped with sets of analog and digital pins for input/output (I/O) that may be used to interfaced to various expansion boards (shields) and also with other circuits. The board contains 14 Digital pins, 6 Analog pins and they are programmable with the Arduino IDE (Integrated Development Environment) via a type-B USB cable. Arduino can be powered through a USB cable.

Software Requirements

Arduino IDE - It is an open source Arduino environment and it enables us to type and upload code directly to the board via serial connection. Available for Mac OS X, Windows and Linux, this environment is

Figure 9. Transformer

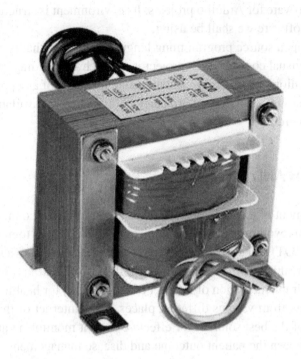

Figure 10. Arduino UNO

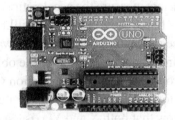

Figure 11. Architecture of Arduino Uno

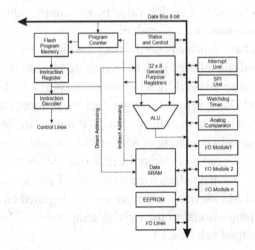

the omnipresent go to software for Arduino projects. Its environment is structured using Java and based off Processing, another software we shall be using.

Processing - It is an open source programming language and IDE that is aimed at supporting computer programming in a visual context. Each project is a sketch – providing various computational and graphics functions. This allows us to acquire instant visual feedback of any process. A major advantage of this processing possesses is wide-array of 3rd party libraries that are available for use. It is built upon the Java model similar to arduino.

DESIGN APPROACH AND DETAILS

In the advanced development of technology, IoT makes all objects interconnected and it is been recognized as the next technical revolution. One such application in healthcare to monitor the patients" health status. Internet of things(IOT) makes medical pieces of equipment more efficient by allowing real time monitoring of patient's health in which sensor acquire data of patient and reduces human error. The significant challenges in implementation of internet of things(IOT) for health applications are monitoring the data of all patients from various different places. Thus internet of things(IOT) in the medical field brings out the one of the best solution for effective patient monitoring at reduced cost and it also reduces the trade -off between the patient outcome and disease management.

Sensors

MEMS - Accelerometer - Accelerometers measure the acceleration, most likely due to motion of a body. However, when the accelerometer is fixed, only the gravity pulling down on it is sensed. The device detects linear acceleration along three perpendicular axes. If one was to sample the x, y and z axes data, they would get an accurate idea regarding the orientation of the object.

The analog values the microcontroller gets are the acceleration values along each axis. However, one firstly should calibrate their device to ensure accuracy of the values keeping the device in a position shown in the figure above. As we know that both X and Y-axis readings must be 0 when it is parallel to the ground while the reading of Z-axis must be the maximum. Adjust correcting factor to obtain this. In the above given orientation, the values in g's must be this – (0g, 0g, 1g). Here simple mathematical manipulation tells us to divide corrected analog value by maximum value. Thus, we now we have successfully converted the voltage values into g's value.

Heartbeat sensor - The pulse oximeter is used detect the pulse rate is based on the phenomenon of absorption characteristics of red and infrared light of oxygenated and deoxygenated hemoglobin i.e. Oxygenated hemoglobin absorbs more infrared light (wavelength approx 850 nm – 1 mm) and allows more red light to pass through it and Deoxygenated (oxygen lacking/reduced) hemoglobin absorbs more red light and it allows more infrared light to pass through it. Red light is in the range of 600 - 750 nm wavelength light band. Infrared light is in the range of 850 - 1000 nm wavelength light band. Pulse oximeter therefore uses a light emitter with red and infrared LEDs that shines through a reasonably translucent site with good blood flow. The normal values used as threshold are 60 - 100.

Temperature Sensor - The LM35 series are the precision integrated circuit temperature sensors, and its output voltage is linearly proportional to the Celsius temperature. The LM35 is operates at -55° to +120°C. We have set the threshold value as 40.

Table 3. Air quality conditions

Air Quality Index (AQI) Values range:	Levels of Health Concern/air quality conditions are:
0 to 50	Good
51 to 100	Moderate
101 to 150	Unhealthy for Sensitive Groups
151 to 200	Unhealthy
201 to 300	Very Unhealthy
301 to 500	Hazardous

Gas sensor - The MQ series of gas sensors generally use a small heater inside along with an electrochemical sensor. They are sensitive for various range of gases. As the output of the gas sensors is resistive, we use a resistor to that is connected between the output pin and ground. No other component is required. Moreover, there is no specific value for the load resistor that is present . Its value could range from 2kΩ to 47kΩ. Lowering the value reduces the sensitivity . More higher the value the less accurate it will be for higher concentrations of gas. This output voltage can therefore be directed to any given ADC or any other comparator circuit and accordingly the gas value would be calculated using the lookup table. These sensors can be easily be directly connected to micro controllers with internal ADC or with Arduino.

GSM Module- The role of GSM module is to send message whenever there is any value which is a cause of concern i.e any abnormal reading that states that the person well being is at risk like when temperature is higher than 40' C or if a person is fallen or abnormal pulse rate.

A GSM/GPRS modem is a class of wireless modem, designed for communication over the GSM and GPRS network. It requires a SIM (Subscriber Identity Module) card just like mobile phones to activate communication with the network. Also, they have IMEI (International Mobile Equipment Identity) number similar to mobile phones for their identification.

1. The MODEM needs AT commands also known as attention commands. These commands are communicated through serial communication for interacting with processor or controller.
2. The controller/processor sends these commands.
3. After the MODEM receives a command it sends back a result.
4. The MODEM supports different AT commands, which can be sent to interact with the GSM and GPRS cellular network by the processor/controller/computer.

In our project we have given the number of the caretaker, to send messages in case of emergencies.

Data Storage and Monitoring

All the data gathered from the sensors is stored at real time basis in the cloud. This is done by interfacing the Wi-Fi module with the microcontroller. The patient is provided with an account which is password protected. The doctor can use this data for further analysis.

Figure 12. Block diagram

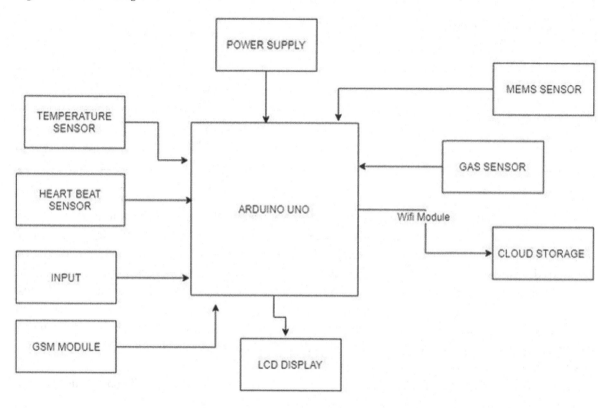

Figure 13. Steps for data analysis

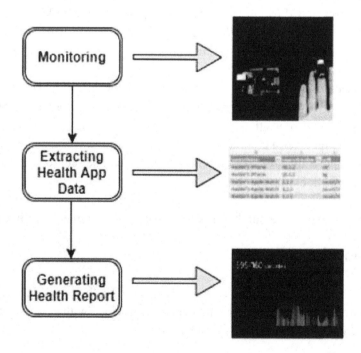

Figure 14. Implementation

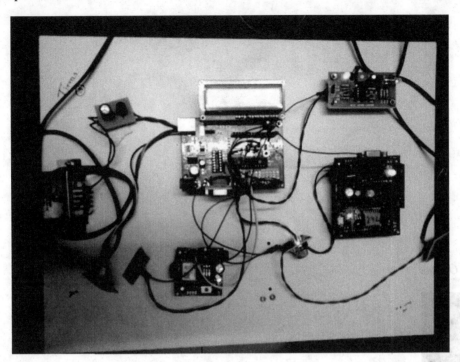

Figure 15. Messages received

Yesterday • 12:13 PM

Fall_Detect_Temp=032_HB=067
_Gs=019_MEMS=015

Fall_Detect_Temp=032_HB=000
_Gs=016_MEMS=067

Fall_Detect_Temp=029_HB=000
_Gs=016_MEMS=056

Wed 12:15 PM • **via Jio 4G**

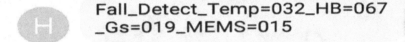

Proposed Architecture

The heartbeat sensor, gas sensor, mems, temperature sensor is interfaced with the microcontroller Arduino uno.

A LCD is attached which displays the values of the sensors.

A gsm module is attached which helps to send the message to the number fed, here the hospital/caretaker.

Figure 16. Login form

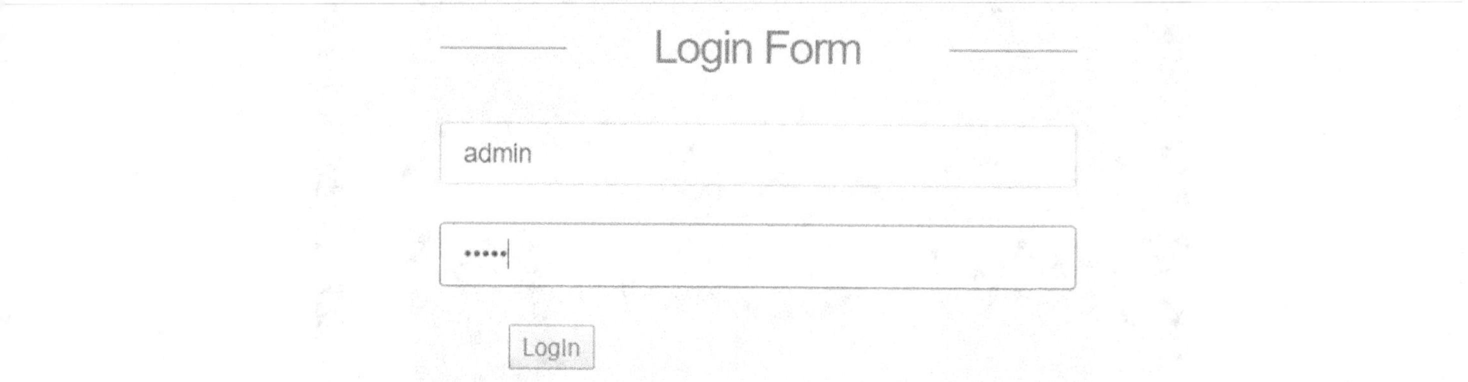

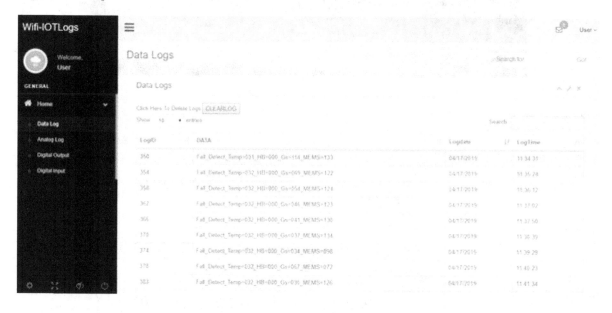

Figure 17. Output

A cloud storage is created. The user can set the password and share data with the doctor. Further, this data can be used for analysis and research purposes. All the data obtained from sensors are stored in the cloud storage. The patient can access the data by logging into this form. The form is password protected. This feature allows patient to share the data only with the doctor and the caretaker he wishes to share it with.

The Log table shows the date and time changes were detected.

Figure 18. Messages received

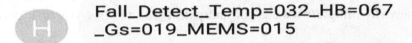

Yesterday • 12:13 PM

Fall_Detect_Temp=032_HB=067 _Gs=019_MEMS=015

Fall_Detect_Temp=032_HB=000 _Gs=016_MEMS=067

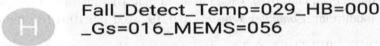

Fall_Detect_Temp=029_HB=000 _Gs=016_MEMS=056

Wed 12:15 PM • **via Jio 4G**

RESULTS AND DISCUSSION

We have created a project which allows remote healthcare monitoring. This is specifically designed for patients suffering by chronic illness or heart disease such as atrial fibrillation. The system is composed of various sensors to provide information on different physiological aspects of the body. Currently we have only considered factors such as heartbeat rate, temperature, body fall and presence of toxic gas in the surrounding. We have successfully implemented the design and obtained reading of each sensor value respectively. Vast amount of data that a healthcare device sends in a very short time owing to their real- time application is hard to store and manage if the access to cloud is unavailable. It is tough for healthcare providers such as doctors and hospitals to acquire data from various sources and then individually analyze it manually. System that work on the concept of Internet of things can collect and analyze the data in real-time. This reduces the need to store the raw data. This all can happen overcloud with the providers only getting access to final reports with graphs. The Wi-Fi module efficiently stores all the data in the cloud, which can be accessed from anywhere at any period of time.

In case of life-threatening circumstances, on time alert is important. IoT allows devices to gather vital data and transfer that data to doctors for real-time tracking, while dropping notifications to people about critical parts.

The GSM module is effective in sending messages to the caretaker along with all the information related to the patient. The technology driven setup cuts down the expense, by chopping down pointless visits, using better quality assets, and improving the allotment and planning. These features make our project suitable for patients who require immediate attention in case of emergencies.

REFERENCES

Abawajy, J. H., & Hassan, M. M. (2017). Federated internet of things and cloud computing pervasive patient health monitoring system. *IEEE Communications Magazine, 55*(1), 48–53. doi:10.1109/MCOM.2017.1600374CM

Baswa, M., Karthik, R., Natarajan, P. B., Jyothi, K., & Annapurna, B. (2017, December). Patient health management system using e-health monitoring architecture. In *2017 International Conference on Intelligent Sustainable Systems (ICISS)* (pp. 1120-1124). Piscataway, NJ: IEEE. 10.1109/ISS1.2017.8389356

CDC. (n.d.). Retrieved from https://www.cdc.gov/dhdsp/data_statistics/fact_sheets/fs_atrial_fibrillation.html

Gelogo, Y. E., Oh, J. W., Park, J. W., & Kim, H. K. (2015, November). Internet of things (IoT) driven U-Healthcare system architecture. In *2015 8th International Conference on Bio-Science and Bio-Technology (BSBT)* (pp. 24-26). Piscataway, NJ: IEEE.

Hossain, M. S., & Muhammad, G. (2016). Cloud-assisted industrial internet of things (IIoT)–enabled framework for health monitoring. *Computer Networks*, *101*, 192–202. doi:10.1016/j.comnet.2016.01.009

Jia, X., Chen, H., & Qi, F. (2012, October). Technical models and key technologies of e-health monitoring. In *2012 IEEE 14th International Conference on e-Health Networking, Applications and Services (Healthcom)* (pp. 23-26). Piscataway, NJ: IEEE.

Kale, S., & Khandelwal, C. S. (2013, March). Design and implementation of real time embedded tele-health monitoring system. In *2013 International Conference on Circuits, Power and Computing Technologies (ICCPCT)* (pp. 771-774). Piscataway, NJ: IEEE. 10.1109/ICCPCT.2013.6528842

Manoj, A. S., Hussain, M. A., & Teja, P. S. (2019). Patient Health Monitoring Using IoT. Mobile Health Applications for Quality Healthcare Delivery, 30.

Na, H., & Choi, Y. (2013, October). Conceptual design of personal wellness record for mobile health monitoring. In *2013 IEEE 2nd Global Conference on Consumer Electronics (GCCE)* (pp. 410-411). Piscataway, NJ: IEEE. 10.1109/GCCE.2013.6664873

Patel, S., Park, H., Bonato, P., Chan, L., & Rodgers, M. (2012). A review of wearable sensors and systems with application in rehabilitation. *Journal of Neuroengineering and Rehabilitation*, *9*(1), 21. doi:10.1186/1743-0003-9-21 PMID:22520559

Proceedings of the International Conference on Intelligent Sustainable Systems (ICISS 2017) IEEE Xplore Compliant - Part Number:CFP17M19-ART, ISBN:978-1-5386-1959-9.

Raja, S. (2018). Chronic Health Patient Monitoring System Using IOT. International Journal on Recent and Innovation Trends in computing and communication, 6(3), 114-119.

Riazul Islam, S. M., & Kwak, DKabir, M. H., Hossain, M., & Kwak, K.-S. (2015). The internet of things for health care: A comprehensive survey. *IEEE Access: Practical Innovations, Open Solutions*, *3*, 678–708. doi:10.1109/ACCESS.2015.2437951

Sekhar, Y. R. Android based health care monitoring system. Department Of ECE, Vignan's University, Vadlamudi, India.

Shanin, F., Das, H. A., Krishnan, G. A., Neha, L. S., Thaha, N., Aneesh, R. P., ... Jayakrishan, S. (2018, July). Portable and Centralised E-Health Record System for Patient Monitoring Using Internet of Things (IoT). In *2018 International CET Conference on Control, Communication, and Computing (IC4)* (pp. 165-170). Piscataway, NJ: IEEE. 10.1109/CETIC4.2018.8530891

Sharma, A., Choudhury, T., & Kumar, P. (2018, June). Health monitoring & management using IoT devices in a Cloud Based Framework. In *2018 International Conference on Advances in Computing and Communication Engineering (ICACCE)* (pp. 219-224). Piscataway, NJ: IEEE. 10.1109/ICACCE.2018.8441752

Zhang, Y. & Sun, S. (2013, April). Real-time data driven monitoring and optimization method for IoT-based sensible production process. In 2013 10th IEEE international conference on networking, sensing and control (ICNSC) (pp. 486-490). Piscataway, NJ: IEEE.

Chapter 11
IoT–Based Health Services Framework for Endless Ailment Administration at Remote Areas

Rajkumar Rajaseskaran

https://orcid.org/0000-0002-0983-7259
Vellore Institute of Technology, India

Mridual Bhasin
Vellore Institute of Technology, India

K. Govinda
Vellore Institute of Technology, India

Jolly Masih
Erasmus University, The Netherlands

Sruthi M.
Vellore Institute of Technology, India

ABSTRACT

The objective is to build an IoT-based patient monitoring smart device. The device would monitor real-time data of patients and send it to the Cloud. It has become imperative to attend to minute internal changes in the body that affect overall health. The system would remotely take care of an individual's changes in health and notify the relatives or doctors of any abnormal changes. Cloud storages provide easy availability and monitoring of real-time data. The system uses microcontroller Arduino Nano and sensors – GY80, Heartbeat sensor, Flex sensor, and Galvanic Skin (GSR) sensor with a Wi-Fi Module.

INTRODUCTION

Continuous measurement of patient parameters such as heart rate and rhythm, respiratory rate, blood

DOI: 10.4018/978-1-7998-1090-2.ch011

pressure, blood-oxygen saturation, and many other parameters have become a common feature of the care of critically ill patients. When accurate and immediate decision-making is crucial for effective patient care, electronic monitors frequently are used to collect and display physiological data. Increasingly, such data are collected using non-invasive sensors from less seriously ill patients in a hospital's medical-surgical units, labor and delivery suites, nursing homes, or patients' own homes to detect unexpected life-threatening conditions or to record routine but required data efficiently. usually think of a patient monitor as something that watches for—and warns against—serious or life-threatening events in patients, critically ill or otherwise. Patient monitoring can be rigorously defined as "repeated or continuous observations or measurements of the patient, his or her physiological function, and the function of life support equipment, for the purpose of guiding management decisions, including when to make therapeutic interventions, and assessment of those interventions"

A patient monitor may not only alert caregivers to potentially life-threatening events; many also provide physiologic input data used to control directly connected life support devices.

Motivation

Incorporating the patient monitoring system in chronic disease management can significantly improve an individual's quality of life. It allows patients to maintain independence, prevent complications, and minimize personal costs. This system facilitates these goals by delivering care right to the home. In addition, patients and their family members feel comfort knowing that they are being monitored and will be supported if a problem arises. Key features of this system like remote monitoring and trend analysis of physiological parameters, enable early detection of deterioration; thereby, reducing number of emergency department visits, hospitalizations, and duration of hospital stays. The need for wireless mobility in healthcare facilitates the adoption of this system both in community and institutional settings. The time saved as a result of the patient monitoring system implementation increases efficiency, and allows healthcare providers to allocate more time to remotely educate and communicate with patients.

The objective of the proposed system is to design a system that will be portable and easily wearable like a watch, and in any critical condition, an alert or a message will be sent to the doctor or any family member. So, with that can easily save many lives with just a small tap of a finger.

With the advancements in technology all over the world, health monitoring systems are used in every field such as hospitals, home care units, sports and many more. This health monitoring system is used for chronicle disease patients who have daily check-up. Normally it is difficult to keep track on abnormalities in heartbeat count for patient itself manually. Patients are not well versed with manual treatment that doctors normally use for tracking the count of heartbeat, skin response, body temperature, etc. There are various instruments available in market to keep track on internal body changes. But there are many limitations in maintenance part due to their heavy cost, size of instruments and mobility of patients. Researchers have designed different health monitoring systems based on different requirements. So, I will look to design a system as that will be portable and easily wearable like a watch, and in any critical condition, an alert or a message will be sent to the doctor or any family member. So, with that can easily save many lives with just a small tap of a finger.

The GY80 sensor includes gyroscope, temperature sensor, pressure sensor, accelerometer, and magnetometer reducing the cost of the system altogether. The sensors in GY80 increase the accuracy of Fall Detection in individuals to 100% (with a consistency of 99.38%). Fall Detection and Gait movements from the sensors are recorded and anomalies can be detected by comparison with the data from patients of Parkinson's disease, for whom the locomotory system functions anomalously. The heartbeat sensor is responsible for gathering the pulse rates and its abnormal behavior for different age groups while GSR sensor monitors the sweat gland activities through the conductance properties of skin, which is the indicative of Sympathetic Nervous System responses and as such emotional behavioral of the individual.

Consistent assessment of patient parameters, for example, heart rate and beat, blood pressure, blood-sugar levels, ECG and numerous different parameters have turned into a typical component for the care of fundamentally sick patients. Whenever exact and prompt management is significant for successful patient care, electronic screens and monitors are utilized to gather and show physiological information. Progressively, such information is gathered utilizing non-obtrusive sensors from less sick patients in a healing facility's medicinal surgical units, work and conveyance suites, nursing homes, or patients' own particular homes to recognize unforeseen dangerous conditions or to record routine however required information proficiently. typically think about a vital sign monitoring device as something that looks for and alerts us against serious or perilous occurrences in patients, fundamentally sick or not. Patient monitoring can be rigorously defined as "repeated or continuous observations or measurements of the patient, his or her physiological function, and the function of life support equipment, for the purpose of guiding management decisions, including when to make therapeutic interventions, and assessment of those interventions".

A patient monitoring device may not just alert specialists to possibly dangerous occurrences; a lot of them likewise give physiologic information used to control specifically associated life bolster gadgets. Incorporating the patient monitoring system in chronic disease management can significantly improve an individual's quality of life. It allows patients to maintain independence, prevent complications, and minimize personal costs. This system facilitates these goals by delivering care right to the home. In addition, patients and their family members feel comfort knowing that they are being monitored and will be supported if a problem arises. Key features of this system like remote monitoring and trend analysis of physiological parameters, enable early detection of deterioration; thereby, reducing number of emergency department visits, hospitalizations, and duration of hospital stays. The need for wireless mobility in healthcare facilitates the adoption of this system both in community and institutional settings. The time saved as a result of the patient monitoring system implementation increases efficiency and allows healthcare providers to allocate more time to remotely educate and communicate with patients.

Literature Survey

Internet of things plays essential role in many applications like health monitoring system, remote sensing, and disease. It is to build and design a sensing and also data conditioning system to get the accurate heart rate, ECG, body temperature, body positioning, skin-response etc. To-day several devices are commercially available for personal health care, fitness, and activity awareness.

The patient monitoring system based on Internet of things project and the real-time parameters of patient's health are sent to cloud using the internet connection. The user can get these details anywhere in the world because the parameters are sent to remote Internet location so that user can get the information.Such a disruptive technology could have a transformative impact on global healthcare systems and drastically reduce healthcare costs and improve speed and accuracy for diagnoses.

Luigi Atzori et al., 2010 in his paper addresses the Internet of Things. The main advantage of this enabling factor is promising paradigm is the combination of some technologies and communications solution. Tracking technologies and identification, wireless and wired sensor as well as actuator networks, well developed communication protocols also distributed intelligence for smart objects are just most important. The results of Internet of things are synergetic activities gathered in various fields of knowledge, like telecommunications, informatics, social science and electronics. This survey is pointed to those who want to approach this complicated discipline and contribute to its development. Eleonara Borgia et al., 2014 in this paper the Internet of Things (IoT) means that a new paradigm that makes a combination of aspects and technologies which are coming from various approaches. To form system some devices are combined together such devices are Internet Protocol, sensing technologies, communication technologies, and embedded device etc. The system where the real and digital worlds meet and are continuously in symbiotic interaction. The building block of the IoT vision is a smart object. The smart objects mean they are not only able to collect the information from the environment and interact/ control the physical world, but also to be interconnected with each other through Internet to exchange data as well as information. In this paper they present some key words and features as well as the driver technologies of IoT. Gennaro Tartarisco et al., 2012 in this paper includes the information about how to build or develop a new computational technology based on clinical decision support systems, information processing, wireless communication and also data mining kept new premises in the field of Personal Healthcare systems. This architecture is developed to gather and manage a huge amount of data which supporting the physicians in their process of decision through a continuous similar remote monitoring model. This architecture is useful to evaluating stress state of individual subject perfect for stress monitoring during the period of normal activities described. Some novel integrated processing approach are based on the factors are autoregressive model; artificial neural networks are helpful for identifying stress conditions. The architecture is designed to get the classification terms of stress conditions. Franca Delmastro et al., 2012 in this paper the estimation of wireless communication technologies and providing a continuous remote support to patients and new instruments to develop the workflow of the hospital personnel.

This paper mainly represents the survey of wireless communication technologies which are presently applied in eHealth system. The eHealth system main aim is providing a continuous and remote support to patients and well instruments to improve the workflow of hospital personnel. The inquiry of advantages and drawbacks of present technologies also shows the definition of new research issues and possible result and solutions for future eHealth systems.

Long Hu et al., 2015 designed a centralized controller to manage physical devices and provide an interface which is helpful for collecting data. This physical device also provides the facilities like transmission and processing to develop a more flexible health surveillance application. Recently the humans are facing dangerous problems like unexpected death the reason is heart attack. So, to avoid this kind of problems the internet of things such as HealthIoT is required. The required information of patients is conducted by using the wearable technology and robotics. The basic infrastructure of health surveillance is realized with the help of HealthIoT system. This HealthIoT system also provides the facility of the management infrastructure. It opens a new research direction of HealthIoT and smart homes.

Figure 1. Voltage regulator IC

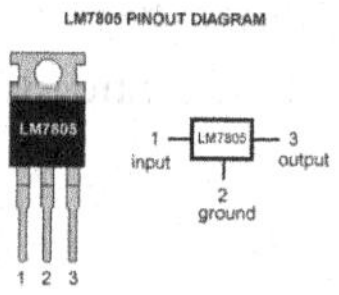

COMPONENTS OF THE PROPOSED FRAMEWORK

5V Power Supply

In this device, a power supply for converting mains AC voltage to a regulated DC voltage was made. For making a power supply designing of each and every component is essential. So, the components that are needed for making this regulator are:

- Voltage regulator
- Capacitors
- 1k Resistor
- Led diode

Requires a 5V, LM7805 Voltage Regulator IC was used 7805 IC Rating:

- Input voltage range 7V- 35V
- Current rating $I_{c=}$ 1A
- Output voltage range $V_{Max=5.2V,}$ $V_{Min=4.8V}$

To build this power supply, with a 1000 uF capacitor was needed on the input side, and a 100 uF capacitor on the output side. The capacitors help filter the input and output from noise created by the power supply, and/or the load. Larger capacitors on both sides were added to help keep the power supply clean, and noise free. Secondly, there is no way of knowing if our power supply is working, a little LED was also added as a power indicator.

Arduino Nano Microcontroller

The Arduino Nano is a small, complete, and breadboard-friendly board based on the ATmega328 (Arduino Nano 3.x) or ATmega168 (Arduino Nano 2.x). It has more or less the same functionality of the Arduino Duemilanove, but in a different package. It lacks only a DC power jack, and works with a Mini-B USB cable instead of a standard one.

Temperature Sensor

For detecting the temperature, LM35 sensor was used. The LM35 is an integrated circuit sensor that can be used to measure temperature with an electrical output proportional to the temperature (in Celsius).

Figure 2. 9V to 5V convertor circuit diagram

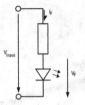

Figure 3. Arduino nano

You can measure temperature more accurately than a using a thermistor. The sensor circuitry is sealed and not subject to oxidation, etc. The LM35 generates a higher output voltage than thermocouples and may not require that the output voltage be amplified.

- Operates from 4 V to 30 V
- Less than 60-μA Current Drain
- Linear + 10-mV/°C Scale Factor
- 0.5°C Ensured Accuracy (at 25°C)
- Rated for Full −55°C to 150°C Range

Heartrate Sensor

The heartbeat sensor is based on the principle of photo plethysmography. It measures the change in volume of blood through any organ of the body which causes a change in the light intensity through that organ (a vascular region). In case of applications where heart pulse rate to be monitored, the timing of the pulses is more important. The flow of blood volume is decided by the rate of heart pulses and since light is absorbed by blood, the signal pulses are equivalent to the heartbeat pulses.

The basic heartbeat sensor consists of a light emitting diode and a detector like a light detecting resistor or a photodiode. The heartbeat pulses cause a variation in the flow of blood to different regions of the body. When a tissue is illuminated with the light source, i.e. light emitted by the led, it either

Figure 4. Temperature sensor

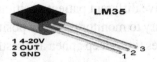

Figure 5. Heart rate sensor

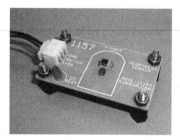

reflects (a finger tissue) or transmits the light (earlobe). Some of the light is absorbed by the blood and the transmitted or the reflected light is received by the light detector. The amount of light absorbed depends on the blood volume in that tissue. The detector output is in form of electrical signal and is proportional to the heartbeat rate.

This signal is actually a DC signal relating to the tissues and the blood volume and the AC component synchronous with the heartbeat and caused by pulsatile changes in arterial blood volume is superimposed on the DC signal. Thus, the major requirement is to isolate that AC component as it is of prime importance.

The digital pulses are given to a microcontroller for calculating the heartbeat rate, given by the formula-

BPM = 60*f

where f is the pulse frequency

GSR Sensor

One of the most sensitive markers for emotional arousal is galvanic skin response (GSR), also referred to as skin conductance (SC) or electro-dermal activity (EDA). EDA modulates the amount of sweat secretion from sweat glands. The amount of sweat glands varies across the human body, being highest in hand and foot regions (200–600 sweat glands per cm2). While sweat secretion plays a major role for thermoregulation and sensory discrimination, changes in skin conductance in hand and foot regions are also triggered quite impressively by emotional stimulation: the higher the arousal, the higher the skin conductance.

Skin conductance is not under conscious control. Instead, it is modulated autonomously by sympathetic activity which drives human behavior, cognitive and emotional states on a subconscious level. Skin conductance therefore offers direct insights into autonomous emotional regulation. It can be used as alternative to self-reflective test procedures, or – even better – as additional source of insight to validate verbal self-reports or interviews of a respondent.

Body Positioning Sensor

The Body Position Sensor monitors five different patient positions (standing/sitting, supine, prone, left and right.) In many cases, it is necessary to monitor the body positions and movements made because of their relationships to particular diseases (i.e., sleep apnea and restless legs syndrome). Analyzing move-

Figure 6. GSR sensor

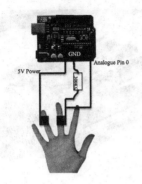

ments during sleep also helps in determining sleep quality and irregular sleeping patterns. The body position sensor could also help to detect fainting or falling of elderly people or persons with disabilities.

Flex Sensor

A flex sensor or bend sensor is a sensor that measures the amount of deflection or bending. Usually, the sensor is stuck to the surface, and resistance of sensor element is varied by bending the surface. Since the resistance is directly proportional to the amount of bend it is used as goniometer, and often called flexible potentiometer.

Wi-Fi-Module

The WiFi module used is ESP8266, which is an impressive, low cost WiFi module suitable for adding WiFi functionality to an existing microcontroller project via a UART serial connection. The module can even be reprogrammed to act as a standalone WiFi connected device by just adding power.

The feature list is impressive and includes:

- 802.11 b/g/n protocol
- Wi-Fi Direct (P2P), soft-AP
- Integrated TCP/IP protocol stack

Figure 7. Positioning sensor

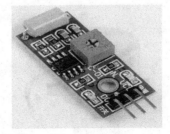

Figure 8. Flex sensor

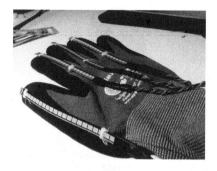

Figure 9. WiFi module

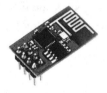

Buzzer

A buzzer is a mechanical, electromechanical, magnetic, electromagnetic, electro-acoustic or piezoelectric audio signaling device. A piezo electric buzzer can be driven by an oscillating electronic circuit or other audio signal source. A click, beep or ring can indicate that a button has been pressed.

16x2 LCD Display

A liquid-crystal display (LCD) is a flat panel display, electronic visual display, or video display that uses the light modulating properties of liquid crystals. Liquid crystals do not emit light directly. 16x2 LCD has 2 horizontal line which comprising a space of 16 displaying character.

It has two types of register inbuilt that is

- Command Register
- Data Register

Figure 10. Buzzer

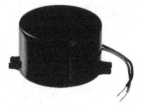

Figure 11. 16x2 LCD

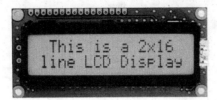

Command register is used to insert a special command into the LCD. While Data register is used to insert a data into the LCD. Command is a special set of data which is used to give the internal command to LCD like Clear screen, move to line 1 character 1, setting up the cursor etc.

- **Arduino IDE:**

Arduino is an open source computer hardware and software company, project, and user community that designs and manufactures single-board microcontrollers and microcontroller kits for building digital devices and interactive objects that can sense and control objects in the physical and digital world.

- **ThingSpeak Server:**

ThingSpeak is an open source Internet of Things (IoT) application and API to store and retrieve data from things using the HTTP protocol over the Internet or via a Local Area Network. ThingSpeak enables the creation of sensor logging applications, location tracking applications, and a social network of things with status updates.

PROPOSED SYSTEM

The proposed Architecture of the Remote Patient Monitoring System warrants the use of various sensors for monitoring patient's health parameters like temperature, heart rate, body positioning, skin response and flex. Also, a buzzer is set up on the device which will be activated if any health parameter goes against the normal values. Various sensors are available in the market and many more are being developed and researched. Here we have used some of the sensors in this project and store the real time sensor data obtained from an Arduino Nano microcontroller chip which is a programmable device having its own IDE. The sensor data is manipulated using a program. Also, a Wi-Fi module is incorporated in the system which has an internet protocol which provides the Arduino board access to the Wi-Fi. This module has a sufficiently effective on-load up handling ability that enables it to be incorporated with the sensors and other application specific gadgets through its GPIOs with insignificant advancement and negligible stacking amid runtime.

The sensor data is sent through the module to a hosted server environment, where the data can be viewed in a presentable format by a healthcare practitioner using a computer or a mobile device.

The Internet of Things idea can empower us to devise a harvest domain information framework with the purpose to assemble the whole healthcare predictive framework. The motivation behind this

Figure 12. System diagram

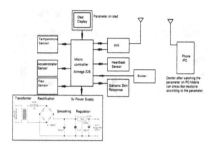

framework is to design a system that will be portable and easily wearable like a watch, and in any critical condition, an alert or a message will be sent to the doctor or any family member. So, with that, can easily save many lives with just a small tap of a finger.

IMPLEMENTATION

The approach to designing the system was very direct and simplistic. The system has four sensors that are gathering real time values provided by the inputs. The buzzer is an additional functionality that is used to detect when any vital signs go awry. The health specialist or doctor can use the remote viewing functionality of the system to give the required suggestions and medication to the patient. And also, the patient itself can know when his/her vital signs are not in the right place and they need to take care of them with the appropriate medication.

IoT based Health Services Framework for Endless Ailment Administration at Remote Areas

RESULTS AND DISCUSSION

First the Arduino Nano Microcontroller was hardwired with a temperature sensor, power supply and an OLED display board. The microcontroller was then programmed to input temperature sensor readings and display it in real time on the OLED display.

Thereafter procured more sensors for heart rate(pulse), body positioning, skin response and flex sensor for signaling and was able to display the readings on the OLED display. also introduced a buzzer to alert an attendant in case the patient reading touched a threshold level. Thereafter I procured a wi-fi module compatible with Arduino Nano and after wiring it with the microcontroller and writing appropriate

Figure 13. Implemented system

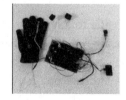

Figure 14. Temperature sensor reading at idle state

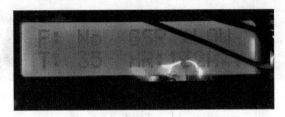

Figure 15. Temperature sensor reading when in contact with patient

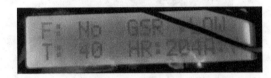

code were able to connect the module to the internet using Wi-Fi internet. Next, we looked for a cloud server where I could send the data procured from the sensors and display the readings. we found a free experimental service compatible with Arduino which could directly display results in a graphical format.

Then, the readings of the idle state and the state where a patient or a person interacts with the sensor were taken in order to test the working of each and every sensor. After that, the graphs of all the sensors over multiple days were taken.

The reading of the LM35 temperature sensor was first taken at the idle state, i.e., the state in which the sensor is in no contact with a person or a patient and the temperature came out to be 35 degrees Celsius as can be seen from the below figure:

Then, the temperature reading was taken when the sensor was in contact with a person or a patient and the reading came out to be 40 degrees Celsius as can be seen from the below figure:

After the temperature sensor, the readings of the heart rate sensor were taken when the sensor was in idle state. As the sensor is light sensitive, the readings come out due to exposure to light. From the figure, it can be seen that the reading came out to be 72 pulses per minute:

Then, the readings were taken when the heart sensor was in contact with a person's or a patient's finger for a required amount of time. It can thus be seen from the below figure that the reading goes up to 96 pulses per minute:

After that the testing of the body positioning sensor was done. At first, the reading was taken when the sensor is held in its upright position. As can be seen from the figure the LCD reads Y, which means that the body is in a normal position:

Figure 16. Heart rate reading when in contact with patient

Figure 17. Heart rate reading when in contact with patient

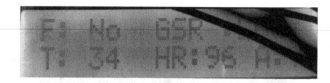

Figure 18. Body positioning sensor reading when in idle state

Figure 19. Body positioning sensor reading when in contact with patient

Then, the sensor was bend in a position and by doing that the reading was changed from Y to N which shows that the body is now in a different position that can lead to various positioning defects in the body:

Then, the Galvanic Skin Response (GSR) sensor was tested in the idle state, where the reading shows LOW as there is no contact with the skin, so there is no conductance:

After that, some water was added to the fingers in order to simulate some sweating in the hands and as can be seen from the figure, the GSR now reads as high as the skin conductance has increased due to simulated sweating:

And finally, the Flex or Bend sensor was tested in the idle state, which is used for gesture by just moving the finger when wearing the glove.

Figure 20. GSR sensor reading when in idle state

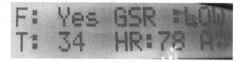

Figure 21. GSR sensor reading when sweating happens

Then, the movement of the finger was made by moving the glove and reading changes from No to Yes, showing that there is some sort of movement of the finger, signaling a gesture.

CONCLUSION AND FUTURE WORK

This chapter for remote patient monitoring works for several sensors like temperature, heart rate, skin response, body positioning. I was able to procure these sensors at inexpensive pricing, was able to generate data from these sensors and display the readings online using a free cloud service. A Wi-Fi module is used to connect to Wi-Fi internet to enable remote monitoring. I was able to see results in graphical format. So, the goals set forth for this project were successfully accomplished.

However, devices for other health parameters were either expensive or not available. So, for a real device which would provide accurate and reliable readings, one would require better sensors which are either slightly expensive or unavailable. A lot of work still needs to be done in the development of such sensors so that such devices could become popular in the medical profession. Till such time, doctors and hospitals would continue to use the traditional medical equipment for health monitoring of a patient. However, I believe that there is scope of remote patient monitoring by doctors by integrating the existing equipment to Internet by developing H/w and S/w interfaces. In fact, there are already some products in the markets with traditional healthcare equipment connected remotely.

For adoption of real medical diagnostic devices which are inexpensive the mindset of the medical fraternity needs to shift from mere profit making to patient care. Researchers in universities need to do more work in developing such devices and bring them to market which at present is the monopoly of a few companies. There is a lot of scope for future work in developing such sensors and devices.

REFERENCES

Atzori, L., Iera, A., & Morabito, G. (2010). The internet of things: A survey. *Computer Networks*, *54*(15), 2787–2805. doi:10.1016/j.comnet.2010.05.010

Barjis, J., Kolfschoten, G., & Maritz, J. (2013). A sustainable and affordable support system for rural healthcare delivery. *Decision Support Systems*, *56*, 223–233. doi:10.1016/j.dss.2013.06.005

BeginnerTopro. (2017, June 30). How to make a 12V to 5V Converter using 7805 IC. Retrieved from https://www.youtube.com/watch?v=8jzOirylcKgza

Borgia, E. (2014). The Internet of Things vision: Key features, applications and open issues. *Computer Communications*, *54*, 1–31. doi:10.1016/j.comcom.2014.09.008

Delmastro, F. (2012). Pervasive communications in healthcare. *Computer Communications*, *35*(11), 1284–1295. doi:10.1016/j.comcom.2012.04.018

Foundations. (2019). Retrieved from https://www.arduino.cc/en/Tutorial/Foundations

Gardner, R. M., & Shabot, M. M. (2006). Patient-Monitoring Systems. In E. H. Shortliffe & J. J. Cimino (Eds.), *Biomedical Informatics. Health Informatics*. New York, NY: Springer.

Heartbeat Sensor - How to Measure Heartbeat. Working and Application. (2019, June 24). Retrieved from https://www.elprocus.com/heartbeat-sensor-working-application/

Hu, L., Qiu, M., Song, J., Hossain, M. S., & Ghoneim, A. (2015). Software defined healthcare networks. *IEEE Wireless Communications*, *22*(6), 67–75. doi:10.1109/MWC.2015.7368826

LM35 Temperature Sensor. (n.d.). Retrieved from http://www.dnatechindia.com/LM35-Temperature-Sensor-Basics.html

Malasinghe, L. P., Ramzan, N. & Dahal, K. J. (2017). Ambient Intell Human Comput. doi:10.100712652-017-0598-x

Mohammadzadeh, N., & Safdari, R. (2014). Patient monitoring in mobile health: Opportunities and challenges. *Medicinski Arhiv*, *68*(1), 57. doi:10.5455/medarh.2014.68.57-60 PMID:24783916

5V. Power Supply using 7805 Voltage Regulator with Design. (2013, May 16). Retrieved from https://electrosome.com/power-supply-design-5v-7805-voltage-regulator/

Tartarisco, G., Baldus, G., Corda, D., Raso, R., Arnao, A., Ferro, M., ... Pioggia, G. (2012). Personal Health System architecture for stress monitoring and support to clinical decisions. *Computer Communications*, *35*(11), 1296–1305. doi:10.1016/j.comcom.2011.11.015

What is GSR (galvanic skin response) and how does it work? (n.d.). Retrieved from https://imotions.com/blog/gsr/

Chapter 12
Opinions on Cyber Security, Electronic Health Records, and Medical Confidentiality:
Emerging Issues on Internet of Medical Things From Nigeria

Ibrahim Taiwo Adeleke
Federal Medical Centre, Bida, Nigeria

Qudrotullaah Bolanle Suleiman Abdul
University of Ilorin Teaching Hospital, Nigeria

ABSTRACT

IoMT has helped to improve health safety and care of billions of people and at least, health-related parameters can now be monitored from home in real time. This chapter deployed a cross-sectional design to determine perceptions of Nigerian healthcare providers toward medical confidentiality and cyber security in the wake of electronic health records and IoMT. Participants' opinions on the workings of EHRs in Nigeria include: security of health records (79.4%); aiding effective healthcare data backup (88.2%); enhancement of medical confidentiality (89.2%); speeding up documentation process (93.1%); and that EHRs will generally bring about positive changes in the country healthcare system. Nearly a third (31.4%) of participants have heard about audit trail, which they admitted (43.1%) have the capabilities to facilitate effective medical confidentiality. Healthcare providers in Nigeria have some concerns over security of patient health information on the Cloud, but are hopeful of the workability of IoMT for its promises to improve healthcare quality.

INTRODUCTION

Internet of things (IoT) is a combination of various technologies that empower a diverse range of ap-

DOI: 10.4018/978-1-7998-1090-2.ch012

pliances, devices and objects to interact and communicate with each other using different networking technologies (Kodali, Swamy & Lakshmi, 2015). In the healthcare context, internet of things (IoT) or internet of medical things (IoMT) extends the Web through the deployment of ubiquitous devices with capabilities for embedded identification, sensing, and data exchange features (Miorandi et al., 2012). In IoT-based healthcare, diverse distributed devices aggregate, analyze and communicate real time medical information to the cloud, thus making it possible to collect, store and analyze the large amount of data in several new forms and activate context based alarms (Kodali, Swamy & Lakshmi, 2015). IoMT plays a key role in the growth of medical information systems. IoT has potentials to collect and integrate possibly more precise, relevant, and high-quality data in real time to monitor processes and outcomes (Gupta, Maharaj & Malekian, 2016). With IoMT, patient's health records and related data can be accessed from anywhere in the world using any Internet-enabled device like PC, tablet or smart phone (Kodali, Swamy & Lakshmi, 2015). A healthcare provider can automatically collect information about the patient, applies decision support rules and as such, speed up treatment process (Chacko & Hayajneh, 2018).

The need to cut cost, improve medical care and adopt electronic health record (EHR) is driving hospitals to implement IT solutions that streamlines procedures such as billing, medical imaging and electronic medical record (EMR) processing. EHR is being defined (NAHIT, 2011) as an electronic record of health-related information on an individual that conforms to nationally recognized interoperability standards and that can be created, managed, and consulted by authorized clinicians and staff across more than one healthcare organization. In other words, EHR is a repository of patient data in digital form, stored and exchanged securely, and accessible by multiple authorized users. It contains retrospective, concurrent, and prospective information and its primary purpose is to support continuing, efficient and quality integrated health (Hayrinen, Saranto & Nykanen, 2008). Electronic health record has evolved to play a major role in healthcare in modern society.

IoMT allows billions of smart devices to communicate and share data, and millions of new devices are connected to the Internet every day (Gartner, 2015). It enables healthcare providers to automatically collect information and apply decision support rules to allow for earlier intervention in the treatment process (Chacko & Hayajneh, 2018). Securing healthcare data requires enforceable security policies and implementing solutions that focus on vulnerabilities, configuration assessments, malware defenses, as well as activity and event monitoring (Chacko & Hayajneh, 2018). There are three main components of information security, which are captured in the CIA Triad of TechTarget (TechTarget, 2015); confidentiality, which limits access to the information in IoT devices; integrity, which ensures that information in IoT devices is trustworthy and accurate and lastly, availability, which guarantees reliable access to the information in IoT devices by authorized people. Traditionally, healthcare organizations have proven to be eminently capable of ensuring the integrity and availability of information within their connected devices.

Yet as cyber security threats intensify, ensuring confidentiality has become increasingly difficult. Storing sensitive information such as EHRs in the Cloud means that precautions must be taken to ensure the safety and confidentiality of the data. Medical confidentiality on the other hand, is the limiting of health information to only those for whom they are appropriate (Adeleke et al., 2011). With the emergence of IoT and Cloud computing, EHR management systems are facing an important platform shift, but such important changes must be approached carefully (Rodrigues, 2013). The adoption of EHRs with information exchange among patients, providers and payers, increased regulation and provider consolidation indicate the need for better information security (Appari, 2010). Although EHRs provide considerable benefits to patients and healthcare providers, there have been concerns (Adeleke et al., 2015; Hoffman, 2007; Taitsman, Grimm & Agrawal, 2013) over confidentiality, integrity, and availability of the data.

Similarly, the rate at which encrypted messages are being sent over the internet makes them susceptible to the dangers of hacking and other cyber threats (Alhassan et al., 2016). Evidence (Hoffman, 2007) has shown that confidentiality of patient's health records is being threatened and that such violations tend to increase in the wake of computerization, IoMT and centralization of health records. These necessitate the need for an efficient, secure, accurate, reliable way of securing user information such as data encryption as recommended in a recent study (Waziri et al., 2016).

In Nigeria, healthcare providers have shown a lack of adequate understanding of their respective responsibilities toward medical confidentiality (Adeleke, 2011; Adeleke et al., 2015b; Aliyu et al., 2015) and were reported to lack the right computing knowledge and skills (Bello et al., 2004; Adeleke et al., 2014; Adeleke et al., 2014b; Adeleke et al., 2015c; Adeleke et al., 2015d; Abodunrin & Akande, 2009). As such, it can be said that they may be short of major prerequisites to the successful adoption and implementations of EHRs and IoMT in the country. Likewise, providers of healthcare services in Nigeria though have the right skills for appropriate documentation (Adeleke et al., 2012), they lack the will to ensure quality healthcare documentation (Adeleke et al., 2012; Abdulkadir et al., 2011). In terms of policy making, the World Health Report in year 2000 ranked Nigeria 187 out of 191 countries in healthcare infrastructure and health services provision (Idowu, Adagunodo, & Adedoyin, 2016) and Nigerian healthcare policy makers as well, lack a clear understanding of the usefulness of hospital information systems (Idowu, Adagunodo, & Adedoyin, 2016).

The aim of this chapter is to present knowledge, attitude and opinion of Nigerian healthcare providers toward medical confidentiality and cyber security in the wake of electronic health records and Internet of medical things.

This chapter is structured as follow. In the first section, the authors introduce our work. The second section describes the background in Internet of medical things., electronic health records, cyber security and medical confidentiality. In the third section, the authors describe the methods and materials deployed in the course of the study. This includes the setting, design, population, sampling techniques, sample size and ethics. In the fourth section, findings from the study are narrated. The fifth section discusses the study's findings in relation to previous studies and prevailing realities. Finally, the authors offer our conclusion and look to the future as it relates to the work.

BACKGROUND

Since its emergence, internet of medical things has helped to improve health safety, and care of billions of people (Sun et al., 2018). Nowadays, health-related parameters can be monitored from home in real time and outcome transferred to cloud storage after processing (Sun et al., 2018). The most promising benefits of IoMT might be in increasing workforce productivity, cost savings, operation efficiencies, improved patient experience and care, and reduction in human error (Riggings & Wamba, 2015; Alsmirat et al., 2016 and Joyia et al., 2017). Studies in the last decade have tuned their focus on security, data privacy, and concerns on trust associated with IoMT (Gubbi et al., 2013, Atzori, Iera, & Morabito, 2010 and Perera, 2014). A more recent study reveals that 78% of the IoMT users were apprehensive of the technology owing to personal data hacking distress (Irdeto, 2017).

Solangi et al., (2018) alerted "Although currently data security and privacy may be insignificant, they could be amplified fully in future so policymakers should proactively address the issues and carefully weigh the cost associated with IoT against the enormous projected benefits. IoT privacy and security issues are much in excess of a thought of individualistic or individual damages. It is a fundamental component of a strong and independent society. Protecting it as innovation advances is both an individual and social concern". In spite of these, Chen et al., opined "future healthcare systems specifically ehealth, would be embedded with IoMT to provide advanced medical services with more secure and efficient authentication for users". Likewise, Kulkar & Sathe (2014) reasoned "The Internet of things will change our society, and will bring seamless 'anytime, anywhere' personalized healthcare and monitoring over fast reliable and secure networks. This implies that we are approaching the end of the divide present between digital, virtual and physical worlds".

MATERIALS AND METHODS

This study was carried out at the venue of the 19th Annual National Conference/Annual General Meeting of the Islamic Medical Association of Nigeria (IMAN) held between 2nd and 8th July 2018 in Birni Kebbi, Nigeria. The study design was cross-sectional survey of major key contributors and users of patients' health records, which include medical practitioners, health records professionals, nurses, medical laboratory scientists and pharmacists. The study participants were recruited from among the healthcare providers in attendance at the venue of the above mentioned conference with an average annual attendance of 500. A total sample size of 217 using the online sample size calculator, Survey System sample size calculator, was recruited. A 25-item questionnaire that elicit data on participants' socio-demographic characteristics, computer and internet use, knowledge on medical confidentiality, awareness on cyber threats, workability of electronic health records in the wake of IoMT was deployed. The statistical software SPSS version 16 was used to compute the data. Analysis carried out on the data include descriptive and the use of chi square to elicit relationships. Tables and charts were also deployed for illustrations. The ethics approval to conduct this study was obtained from the Health Research Ethics Committee of Federal Medical Centre, Bida. Informed consent was explicitly worded on the first page of the instrument. This was done in order to solicit participants' permission before the administration of questionnaire.

PERCEPTIONS OF NIGERIAN HEALTHCARE PROVIDERS ON THE SUBJECT

One hundred and two (45.3%) of the 225 questionnaires distributed were returned and analyzed. Most participants were males (81.4%), nearly a third (32.4%) were nurses and more than one-third were below ten years in professional practice. Two-third of participants possess personal laptop and more than half (54.9%) surf the internet daily. The majority of participants (91.2%) enjoy working with computer while a two-third of them preferred working with computer to manual. Overwhelmingly, the majority of participants acknowledged inherent benefits of information and communication technologies especially in healthcare delivery system.

Participants' opinions on the workings of EHRs in Nigeria include security of health records (79.4%); aiding effective healthcare data backup (88.2%); enhancement of medical confidentiality (89.2%); speeding up documentation process (93.1%) and that EHRs will generally bring about positive changes in the country healthcare system. Nonetheless, a notable portion of participants (59.8%) opined that technology freely opens health information to cyber threats, that patient health records can be hacked like Facebook account (50.0%), all which may negatively affect (20.6%) medical confidentiality.

Many (60.8%) participants have heard about cyber security mostly (41.2%) through social media and nearly a third (31.4%) has heard about audit trail, which they admitted (43.1%) have the capabilities to facilitate effective medical confidentiality. Overall, participants envisioned holistic paperless (54.9), feasibility (95.1%) and workability (62.7%) of full EHRs implementation in the country.

PERCEPTIONS OF NIGERIAN HEALTHCARE PROVIDERS ON THE SUBJECT IN THE LIGHT OF PREVIOUS STUDIES

Although the Nigerian healthcare system has not fully embraced ICT owing to some reported human and political challenges (Adeleke et al., 2014), most participants in this current study appreciate the gains of ICT and they prefer working with ICT than the proliferated paper-based system. Most of these participants have heard about cyber security in their course of accessing the social media platforms and nearly a third have heard about audit trial, for its capability to ensure confidentiality in an electronic environment. However, a recent study from Nigeria reveals that most of those who are supposed to promote the tenets of medical confidentiality in the country are mixed with unqualified personnel mostly at private medical offices in the country (Adeleke et al., 2018). Traditionally, it is upon the healthcare practitioners to promote the tenets of medical confidentiality. As the country's healthcare system is said to be flooded with unqualified practitioners, this may pose danger to medical confidentiality.

Although more than half of participants opined that emerging technologies open health information freely to cyber threats, the study shows healthcare providers who believe in the workings of electronic health records especially for its enhancement of medical confidentiality, assurances of data security and potentialities of stimulating positive changes in the country's healthcare delivery systems. The apprehensions held by participants in this study as regard concerns over security in the use of IoMT is in tandem with that of Solangi et al., (2018), who opined that security threats with IoMT could be amplified in future. Nevertheless, opinions on positive workability of IoMT agree with reports from Kulkar & Sathe (2014) and Solangi et al., (2018) futuristic opinion. Findings from this study show a group of healthcare providers with an improved attitude toward patient's health records and clinical documentation. It could be recalled that earlier studies found them to lack adequate understanding of their respective responsibilities toward medical confidentiality (Adeleke, 2011; Adeleke et al., 2015b; Aliyu et al., 2015); lack the right computing knowledge and skills (Bello et al., 2004; Adeleke et al., 2014; Adeleke et al., 2014b; Adeleke et al., 2015c; Adeleke et al., 2015d; Abodunrin & Akande, 2009); though have the right skills for appropriate documentation (Adeleke et al, 2012), but, lack the will to ensure quality healthcare documentation (Adeleke et al., 2012; Abdulkadir et al., 2011).

SOLUTION AND RECOMMENDATIONS

Healthcare providers require continuing professional education especially on Internet of things. Authorities and stakeholders in the Nigerian healthcare system should rise up to adopt and implement electronic health records to move the system forward for improved healthcare quality.

FUTURE RESEARCH DIRECTIONS

Studies in future should focus advancement of IoMT such that current concerns are addressed.

CONCLUSION

Healthcare providers in Nigeria though hold some concerns over security of patient's health information on the cloud, are hopeful of the workability of IoMT, for its promises to improve healthcare quality.

ACKNOWLEDGMENT

The thank Mr. A. A. Adebisi for his assistance during data collection; Mr. Usman Isah for his assistance during electricity power fluctuation; Drs. Yaqub Ibn Muhammad and Tajudeen Abiola both officials of IMAN, for the enabling environment during data collection.

The authors specially appreciate the 102 participants in this study.

REFERENCES

Abodunrin, A. L., & Akande, T. M. (2009). Knowledge and perception of e-health and telemedicine among health professionals in LAUTECH Teaching Hospital, Osogbo, Nigeria. *Int J Health Res.*, *2*(1), 51–58.

Adeleke, I. T., Adekanye, A. O., Jibril, A. D., Danmallam, F. F., Inyinbor, H. E., & Omokanye, S. A. (2014). Research knowledge and behaviour of health workers at Federal Medical Centre, Bida: A task before learned mentors. *El Med J.*, *2*(2), 105–109. doi:10.18035/emj.v2i2.71

Adeleke, I. T., Adekanye, A. O., Onawola, K. A., Okuku, A. G., Adefemi, S. A., Erinle, S. A., & ... & AbdulGhaney, O. O. (2012). Data quality assessment in healthcare: A 365-day chart review of inpatients' health records at a Nigerian tertiary hospital. *Journal of the American Medical Informatics Association*, *19*, 1039–1042. doi:10.1136/amiajnl-2012-000823

Adeleke, I. T., Asiru, M. A., Oweghoro, B. M., Jimoh, A. B., & Ndana, A. M. (2015). Computer and internet use among tertiary healthcare providers and trainees in a Nigerian public hospital. *American Journal of Health Research*, *3*(1), 1–10. doi:10.11648/j.ajhr.s.2015030101.11

Adeleke, I. T., Erinle, S. A., Ndana, A. M., Anaman, T. C., Ogundele, O. A., & Aliyu, D. (2015). Health information technology in Nigeria: Stakeholders' perspectives of nationwide implementations and meaningful use of the emerging technology in the most populous black nation. *American Journal of Health Research*, *3*(1), 17–24. doi:10.11648/j.ajhr.s.2015030101.13

Adeleke, I. T., Ezike, S. O., Ogundele, O. A., & Ibraheem, S. O. (2015). Freedom of information act and concerns over medical confidentiality among healthcare providers in Nigeria. *IMAN Medical Journal*, *1*(1), 21–28.

Adeleke, I. T., Lawal, A. H., Adio, R. A., & Adebisi, A. A. (2014). Information technology skills and training needs of health information management professionals in Nigeria: A nationwide study. *The HIM Journal, 44*(1), 1–9. doi:10.12826/18333575 PMID:27092467

Adeleke, I. T., Salami, A. A., Achinbee, M., Anama, T. C., Zakari, I. B., & Wasagi, M. H. (2015). ICT knowledge, utilization and perception among healthcare providers at National Hospital Abuja, Nigeria. *American Journal of Health Research., 3*(1), 1–10. doi:10.11648/j.ajhr.s.2015030101.17

Adeleke, I. T., Suleiman-Abdul, Q. B., Aliyu, A., Ishaq, I. A., & Adio, R. A. (2018, Sept. 20). Deploying unqualified personnel in health records practice – role substitution or quackery? Implications for health services delivery in Nigeria. [Epub ahead of print]. *Health Information Management*. doi:10.1177/1833358318800459 PMID:30235948

Aliyu, D., Adeleke, I. T., Omoniyi, S. O., Samaila, B. A., Adamu, A., & Abubakar, A. Y. (2015). Knowledge, attitude and practice of nursing ethics and law among nurses at Federal Medical Centre, Bida. *American Journal of Health Research, 3*(1), 32–37. doi:10.11648/j.ajhr.s.2015030101.15

Alsmirat, M. A., Jararweh, Y., Obaidat, I., & Gupta, B. B. (2016). Internet of surveillance: A cloud supported large-scale wireless surveillance system. J Supercomput. 1;73(3):973-992. doi:10.100711227-016-1857-x

Appari, A., & Johnson, M. E. (2010). Information security and privacy in healthcare: Current state of research. *Int. J. Internet and Enterprise Management, 6*(4), 279–314. doi:10.1504/IJIEM.2010.035624

Atzori, L., Iera, A., & Morabito, G. (2010). The internet of things: A survey. *Computer Networks, 54*(15), 2787–2805. doi:10.1016/j.comnet.2010.05.010

Bello, I. S., Arogundade, F. A., Sanusi, A. A., Ezeoma, I. T., Abioye-Kuteyi, E. A., & Akinsola, A. (2004). Knowledge and utilization of information technology among health care professionals and students in Ile-Ife, Nigeria: A Case Study of a University Teaching Hospital. *Journal of Medical Internet Research, 6*(4), e45. doi:10.2196/jmir.6.4.e45 PMID:15631969

Chacko, A., & Hayajneh, T. (2018). Security and privacy issues with IoT in healthcare. *EAI Endorsed Transactions on Pervasive Health and Technology., 4*(14), e2.

Chen, M., Gonzalez, S., Vasilakos, A., Cao, H., & Leung, V. C. M. (2011). Body area networks: A survey. *Mobile Networks and Applications, 16*(2), 171–193. doi:10.100711036-010-0260-8

Gartner Says 6.4 Billion Connected "Things" Will Be in Use in 2016, Up 30 Percent From 2015. Available at www.gartner.com/newsroom/id/3165317

Gubbi, J., Buyya, R., Marusic, S., & Palaniswami, M. (2013). Internet of things (IoT): A vision, architectural elements, and future directions. *Future Generation Computer Systems, 29*(7), 1645–1660. doi:10.1016/j.future.2013.01.010

Hayrinen, K., Saranto, K., & Nykanen, P. (2008). Definition, structure, content, use and impacts of electronic health records: A review of the research literature. *International Journal of Medical Informatics, 77*(5), 291–304. doi:10.1016/j.ijmedinf.2007.09.001 PMID:17951106

Hoffman, S. (2007). In Sickness, Health, and Cyberspace: Protecting the security of electronic private health information. *Boston College Law Review. Boston College. Law School*, 48(2), 331–386.

Idowu, B., Adagunodo, R., & Adedoyin, R. (2006). Information technology infusion model for health sector in developing country: Nigeria as a case. *Technology and Health Care*, 14(2), 69–77. PMID:16720950

Irdeto organization. (2017). Irdeto Global Consumer Piracy Survey.

Joyia, G. J., Liaqat, R. M., Farooq, A., & Rehman, S. (2017). Internet of medical things (IoMT): Applications, benefits and future challenges in healthcare domain. *Journal of Communication*. doi:10.12720/jcm.12.4.240-247

Adeleke, I. T., Adekanye, A. O., Adefemi, S. A., Onawola, K. A., Okuku, A. G., Sheshi, E. U., ... & Tume, A. A. (2011). Knowledge, attitude and practice of confidentiality of patients' health records among healthcare professionals at Federal Medical Centre, Bida. *Nigerian Journal of Medicine*, 20(2), 228–235. PMID:21970234

Kodali, R. K., Swamy, G., & Lakshmi, B. (2015). An implementation of IoT for healthcare. *IEEE Conference Paper*. 10.1109/RAICS.2015.7488451

Kulkar, A., & Sathe, S. (2014). Healthcare applications of the Internet of things: A review. *International Journal of Computer Science and Information Technologies*, 5(5), 6229–6232.

Abdulkadir, A., Yunusa, G., Tabari, A., Anas, I., Ojo, J., Akinlade, B., ... & Uyobong, I. (2011). Medical record system in Nigeria: Observations from multicentre auditing of radiographic requests and patients' information documentation practices. *J. Med. Med. Sci.*, 2(5), 854–858.

Miorandi, D., Sicari, S., De Pellegrini, F., & Chlamtac, I. (2012, September). Internet of things: Vision, applications and research challenges. *Ad Hoc Networks*, 10(7), 1497–1516. doi:10.1016/j.adhoc.2012.02.016

National Alliance for Health Information Technology. NAHIT releases HIT definitions. Electronic health records. Available at https://www.healthcare-informatics.com/news-item/nahit-releases-hit-definitions

Perera, C., Zaslavsky, A., Christen, P., & Georgakopoulos, D. (2014). Context aware computing for the internet of things: A survey. *IEEE Communications Surveys and Tutorials*, 16(1), 414–454. doi:10.1109/SURV.2013.042313.00197

Riggins, F. J. & Wamba, S. F. (2015, January). Research Directions on the Adoption, Usage, and Impact of the Internet of things through the Use of Big Data Analytics. (2015). Presented at *2015 48th Hawaii International Conference on System Sciences*, Kauai, HI, p. 40. doi:10.1109/HICSS.2015.186

Rodrigues, J. P. C., de la Torre, I., Fernández, G., & López-Coronado, M. (2013). Analysis of the Security and Privacy Requirements of Cloud-Based Electronic Health Records Systems. *Journal of Medical Internet Research*, 15(8), e186. doi:10.2196/jmir.2494 PMID:23965254

Solangi, Z. A., Solangi, Y. A., Chandio, S., Abd-Aziz, M. S., Hamzah, M. S., & Shah, A. (2018, May). The future of data privacy and security concerns in Internet of things. *2018 IEEE International Conference on Innovative Research and Development (ICIRD)*. 10.1109/ICIRD.2018.8376320

Sun, W., Cai, Z., Li, Y., Liu, F., Fang, S., & Wang, G. (2018). Security and privacy in the Medical Internet of things: A review. *Hindawi Security and Communication Networks*, 1–9. doi:10.1155/2018/5978636

Taitsman, J. K., Grimm, C. M., & Agrawal, S. (2013). Protecting patient privacy and data security. *The New England Journal of Medicine*, *368*(11), 977–979. doi:10.1056/NEJMp1215258 PMID:23444980

TechTarget. Confidentiality, integrity, and availability (CIA triad). Available at https://whatis.techtarget.com/definition/Confidentiality-integrity-and-availability-CIA

Waziri, V. O., Alhassan, J. K., Ismaila, I., & Egigogo, R. A. (2016). Securing file on cloud computing system using encryption software: a comparative analysis. *International Conference on Information and Communication Technology and Its Applications (ICTA 2016)*. 97-104.

APPENDIX

Table 1. Percentage of those who prefer computer to manual documentation

		Frequency	Percent	Valid Percent	Cumulative Percent
Prefer computer to manual					
Valid	Yes	69	67.6	67.6	67.6
	No	21	20.6	20.6	88.2
	I don't know	5	4.9	4.9	93.1
	NR	7	6.9	6.9	100.0
	Total	102	100.0	100.0	

Table 2. Feasibility of EHRs in Nigeria

		Frequency	Percent	Valid Percent	Cumulative Percent
EHR implementation in Nigeria is feasible					
Valid	Yes	97	95.1	95.1	95.1
	No	3	2.9	2.9	98.0
	NR	2	2.0	2.0	100.0
	Total	102	100.0	100.0	

Table 3. Hospitals with full implementation of EHRs in Nigeria

		Frequency	Percent	Valid Percent	Cumulative Percent
Hospitals with full EHRs operation in Nigeria					
Valid	Yes	23	22.5	22.5	22.5
	No	44	43.1	43.1	65.7
	I don't know	31	30.4	30.4	96.1
	NR	4	3.9	3.9	100.0
	Total	102	100.0	100.0	

Table 4. Functionality of EHRs to enhance medical confidentiality

		Frequency	Percent	Valid Percent	Cumulative Percent
EHR will enhance confidentiality					
Valid	Yes	91	89.2	89.2	89.2
	No	5	4.9	4.9	94.1
	I don't know	4	3.9	3.9	98.0
	NR	2	2.0	2.0	100.0
	Total	102	100.0	100.0	

Figure 1. Electronic health records will bring about positive changes to Nigerian healthcare systems

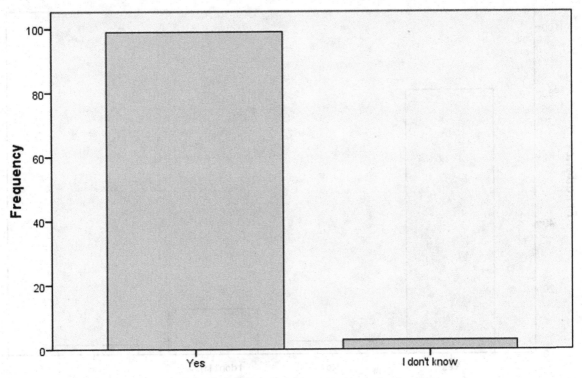

Figure 2. Electronic health records secure patients' health records

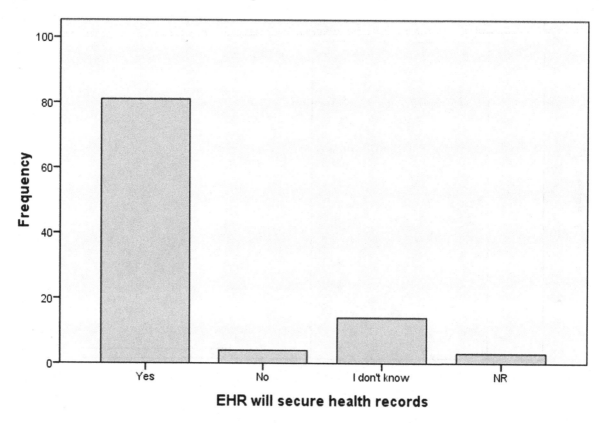

Figure 3. Sources of awareness on cyber security among participants

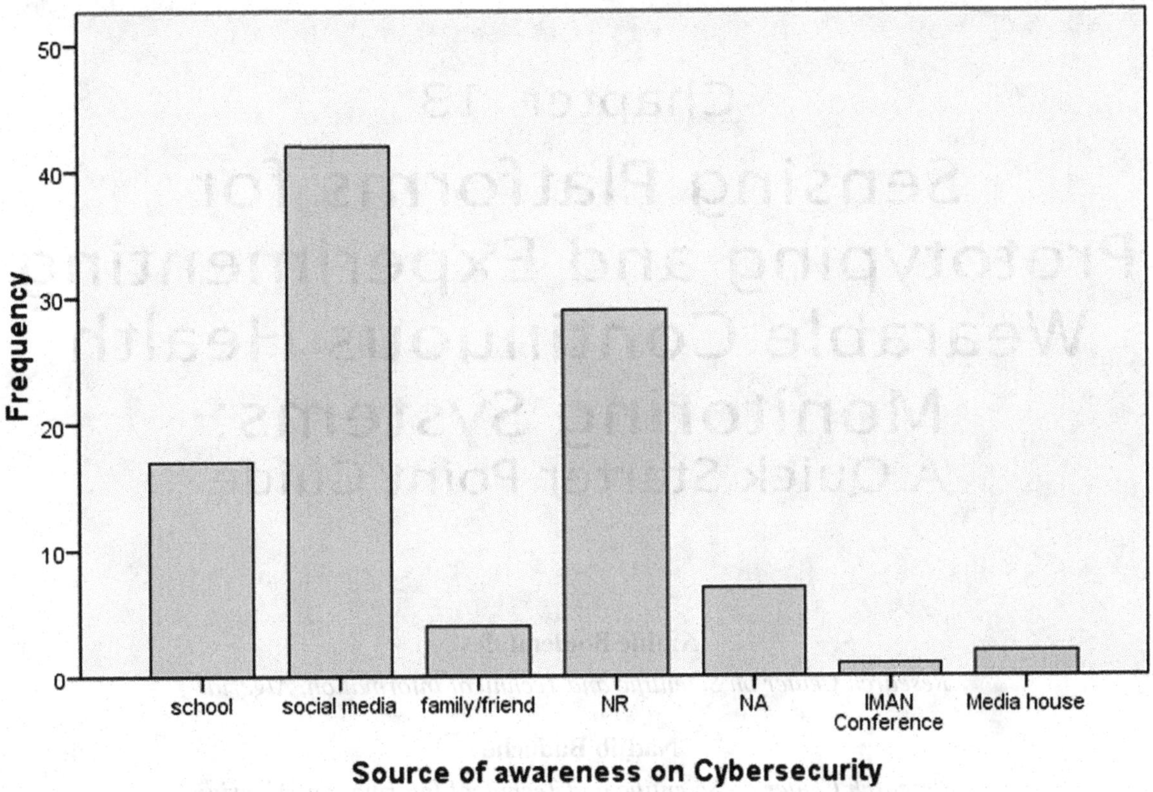

Chapter 13

Sensing Platforms for Prototyping and Experimenting Wearable Continuous Health Monitoring Systems:
A Quick Starter Point Guide

Amine Boulemtafes

Research Center on Scientific and Technical Information, Algeria

Nadjib Badache

Research Center on Scientific and Technical Information, Algeria

ABSTRACT

Continuous monitoring generally imposes a set of constraints including form factor, energy consumption, and mobility support in order to enable anywhere and anytime monitoring. Sensors, within this context, play an important role as the first building block of such systems and the main entry point for the monitoring process. Therefore, to experiment continuous health-monitoring systems in real-like conditions, sensing platforms need to meet a number of related requirements and constraints, especially for mobility factor. This chapter aims to present an overview of popular sensing platforms meeting appropriate constraints, allowing experimenters and researchers to start prototyping and experimentation projects for continuous health monitoring. For that, a number of requirements and constraints for continuous monitoring prototyping are firstly identified, then sensing platforms are classified into three proposed and compared categories, namely, ready-to-use, ready-to-compose kits, and do-it-yourself platforms. On that basis, a set of interesting platforms are reviewed and compared under each category.

DOI: 10.4018/978-1-7998-1090-2.ch013

INTRODUCTION

Wearable health monitoring systems' (WHMS) goal of enhancing life's quality of persons without disturbing their daily activities requires a number of features to be satisfied. In fact, form factor, energy consumption as well as mobility support enabling an anywhere and anytime monitoring, are major concerns to consider in order to allow a continuous monitoring. In this context, sensors play an important role as they represent the first building block and the main entry point for the monitoring process (Boulemtafes, Rachedi, & Badache, 2015; Boulemtafes & Badache, 2016).

Besides, prototyping and experimenting systems through test beds are important steps before attaining the final realization stage and achieving pretending goals. Within this perspective, and in order to experiment continuous health monitoring in real-like conditions, sensing platforms meeting appropriate factor and constraints should be used.

This work aims to present a quick overview of popular sensing platforms for prototyping and experimenting health monitoring systems, particularly heart and motion-based monitoring applications, such as cardiovascular risk factors prediction, Myocardial Infarction detection, gait analysis, sleep efficiency prediction, or fall detection and risk assessment.

Starting from identifying constraints' requirements to be fulfilled, the goal of this work is not to review all available sensing platforms but rather, to present a set of interesting models of platforms along with their main features, allowing experimenters and researchers to start prototyping and experimentation projects. The presented sensing platforms are reviewed and compared according to a proposed classification comprising three categories namely ready-to-use, ready-to-compose kits and do-it-yourself platforms.

CONTINUOUS MONITORING AND PROTOTYPING CONSTRAINTS' REQUIREMENTS

Ensuring continuous health monitoring implies inevitably dealing with a set of related constraints, particularly, keeping connectivity and coping with its intermittence, which is considered as one of the main concerns regarding mobile users (Boulemtafes et al., 2015). However, from sensing devices point of view, a number of criteria should be also taken into consideration in order to enable continuous and convenient monitoring. Two major constraints are: (1) The probability of relying on devices' batteries for long periods. In fact, recharging devices might be disturbing, or even impossible if there's no access to a power supply, like in case of mobility; and (2) Relying on wearables, which need not to disturb the monitored user and his daily activities (Maciuca, Popescu, Strutu, & Stamatescu, 2013; Boulemtafes & Badache, 2016).

Consequently, sensing platforms should ideally follow a number of recommendations in order to cope with continuous monitoring (Boulemtafes et al., 2015; Boulemtafes & Badache, 2016), principally:

- Sensing platforms should be as much as possible lightweight and unobtrusive in order to minimize disruption of the user and his daily activities.
- Sensing platforms should communicate through wireless networks in order to offer freedom of movement.
- Sensing platforms should be energy-efficient in terms of operation and processing, as well as in terms of communication. This aims to keep continuous monitoring as long as possible, like by

using low energy short range communication standards, especially when adopting a mobile base station between sensing platforms and the remote side.

However, in a prototyping configuration and for experimentation purposes, some of these requirements could be somehow overridden in some cases such as for the unobtrusiveness constraint.

Besides, since prototyping implies customization and development of actions and scenarios, platforms should moreover allow open access to sensing parameters, operations and collected data.

SENSING PLATFORMS

Various sensing devices and platforms for health monitoring are available. They are made either to be used directly with predefined sensors, or to allow adding custom ones. Some platforms allow even composing personalized wearables. Besides, a set of components from boards to sensors are available in order to mount customized platforms.

The authors propose to classify sensing platforms into three main categories, namely, ready-to-use, ready-to-compose kits and do-it-yourself platforms (see Table 3 for summary and comparison). The proposed categories are described below, along with review and comparison of a set of interesting platforms.

1. Ready-to-Use

Ready-to-use (R2U) sensing platforms means no assembling required, so that you can start playing directly. Although such platforms are typically not expandable and thus limited in terms of sensing and communication choices, they are however generally easy to use, lightweight and designed so as to meet energy efficiency needs, while they offer interesting set of sensors.

R2U platforms are either provided with a special application to deal with sensed data, or offer an API (Application Programming Interface) for developers, sometimes in addition to the special application, in order to communicate with the platform and have more access to sensors and data collected ("MetaWear Android API," 2017). Provided API might be however restricted by some providers (Irfan Husain, 2014). Platforms without API are of course not what best suit research prototyping. However, they can be managed to be used in some cases, as in (Benharref & Serhani, 2014) where blood sugar readings retrieved from the provided application are entered into the prototype's application.

A set of interesting R2U sensing platforms (see Figure 1) for prototyping WHMS are presented below (see Table 1 for comparison), along with their main continuous-monitoring-friendly advantages.

a. ECG Necklace, is a biomedical sensor used to measure body parameters related to ECG (Electrocardiogram) and activity signals. This patient-friendly designed platform seems to be suited for prototyping continuous monitoring, especially as it offers a long battery lifetime, allows in-device data storage, communicates through efficient Bluetooth Smart data connection (i.e. Bluetooth Low Energy, BLE), and provides an open technology for researchers ("Maastricht Instruments - ECG Necklace," n.d.).

b. Polar H10, is a heart rate monitor strap designed at the base for fitness. However, with an open access to sensed data, a tested accuracy, a long battery lifetime and a Bluetooth Smart communication, Polar H10 seems to be suitable for continuous monitoring prototyping ("Polar Electro - H10 heart rate sensor", n.d.; Wang et al., 2017).

Figure 1. Figure 1. (a) ECG Necklace, (c) MetaHealth, (d) Shimmer unit, (e) MetaMotion C and round clip support, and (f) MySignals SDP main box

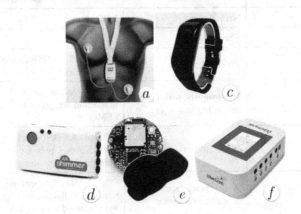

c. MetaHealth, is a development board for biometric monitoring, relying on BLE communication, and offering optical heart rate (OHR), galvanic skin response (GSR), thermistor, and 6-axis of motion (accelerometer + gyroscope) sensors. The overall is packed into one small board bundled into a wrist water-resistant band. Moreover, MetaHealth provides an API for interacting with the board and its sensors ("MbientLab - MetaHealth," n.d.).

d. Shimmer, are a set of wearable sensor platforms enabling simple and effective biophysical and kinematic data capture in real-time. Shimmer platforms integrates a Bluetooth 2.1 RN42 radio and have very low power consumption. Available sensors include 10-axis IMU (included on most of units featuring a motion processor for on-board 3D orientation estimation), ECG, EMG, GSR and PPG (Photoplethysmography, from earlobe and finger). Moreover, the platform offers an API for development ("Shimmersensing - Wearable body sensors | Wearable technology," n.d.).

e. MetaMotion *C,* is another board made by the developers of MetaHealth. The platform is interesting for motion-based applications such as fall detection. It features 10-axis of motion sensing (accelerometer, gyroscope and barometer) with built-in advanced 9-axis sensor fusion algorithms, luminosity/ambient light and temperature sensing, BLE communication, small round form factor and API for interaction. Moreover, the board offers different wearable options like wrist band or belt clip-on ("MbientLab - MetamotionC," n.d.).

f. MySignals SDP, is a ready to use development platform for medical devices and eHealth applications allowing to measure more than 10 biometric parameters, including ECG, temperature, blood sugar and pressure, EMG, GSR, and SpO2. Sensors are plugged via wires into a small box integrating BLE and WiFi interfaces for external communications. Moreover, the platform provides an API for interaction and development ("MySignals - eHealth and Medical IoT Development Platform," n.d.).

Different other R2U sensing platforms used for research experimentation can be found in the literature, such as Alivetec Bluetooth ECG/Accelerometer sensor (Gay & Leijdekkers, 2007), Zephyr BioHarness (Triantafyllidis, Koutkias, Chouvarda, & Maglaveras, 2013), or iBGStar (Benharref & Serhani, 2014).

It should be lastly noted that some R2U platforms can also be considered as boards (i.e., The third category "do-it-yourself platforms" described below), and thus be expanded in terms of sensing capabilities. Genuine 101 platform ("Genuino 101," n.d.) for example, by integrating built-in 6-axis accelerometer

Table 1. Presented R2U platforms comparison

Platform	Position	Sensors	Comm.
ECG Necklace	Neck & chest	ECG	BLE
Polar H10	Chest	Heart rate	BLE
MetaHealth	Wrist	OHR via PPG / GSR / (6-axis) Accelerometer, gyroscope / Thermistor	BLE
Shimmer	Wrist/fingers, waist/ chest depending on sensor	(10-axis) Accelerometer, gyroscope, magnetometer, pressure / GSR / PPG / ECG / EMG	BT 2.1 (RN 42)
MeatMotion C	Wrist, clothes	(10-axis) Accelerometer, gyroscope, magnetometer, pressure (barometer) / Temperature/ Ambient light	BLE
MySignals SDP	Wrist, chest, ...etc. depending on sensor	ECG / EMG / Temperature / Body position / Snoring / Glucometer / Spirometer / GSR / SpO2 / Blood pressure / Air flow	BLE, WiFi

/ gyroscope and Bluetooth LE capabilities, enables to work directly on motion sensing applications such as fall detection. Besides, by supporting custom sensors, the platform also allows to further expand its scope of applications ("Arduino - Genuino 101 CurieBLE Heart Rate Monitor," n.d.).

2. Ready-to-Compose Kits

Ready-to-compose (R2C) kits are generally made for learning and prototyping, and allow composing custom sensing platforms. Unlike R2U platforms, R2C kits typically support various biosensors, and may propose different communication interfaces. However, R2C kits may not be always as unobtrusive as R2U platforms, although such a constraint is not necessarily considered as a drawback in case of experimentation settings.

Three interesting R2C kits (see Figure 2) made for e-Health and bio-measurement, particularly heart-based monitoring, are described below (see Table 2 for comparison):

a. BITalino is a low-cost toolkit, intended for learning and prototyping body-signals based applications. It requires no electrical skill, and comes in three kit versions: (a) board kit, an all-in-one board with pre-connected sensors ready to use; (b) freestyle kit, comprising broken blocks used to create custom

Figure 2. Figure 2. (b) MySignals HDP and (c) MtM Sensors kit (Health kit)

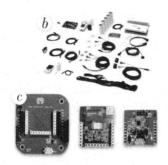

Table 2. Presented R2C kits comparison

	Bitalino kit	MySignals HDP	MtM Health / Motion SK
Assembly	Depending on kit version: Ready to use, easy custom wearables design, or plug-and-play	Easy assembly through boards plugging and wires	Easy assembly through boards plugging
Convenience	Seems to be unobtrusive	Might be obtrusive due to possible wired communication between sensors and main board	• Small factor • Seems to be unobtrusive
Sensing	• EMG, ECG, EDA, EEG and accelerometer • Third party sensors support	• ECG, EMG, Temperature, Body position, Snoring, Glucometer, Spirometer, GSR, SpO2, Blood pressure, Air flow • Custom sensors support	• (Health) Pulse and SpO2 • (Motion) Accelerome-ter and gyroscope
Communication	BLE	• On-board radios: BLE, WiFi • Extra radios: 4G/3G/GPRS, Bluetooth, ZigBee	BLE

wearables with standard or third-party sensors; and (c) plugged kit, a plug-and-play platform to use sensors interchangeably. BITalino kits rely on the BLE interface for energy-efficient communications and provide a set of sensors, including EMG (Electromyogram), ECG, EDA (Electrodermal activity), EEG (Electroencephalogram) and accelerometer. Third-party sensors can also be used ("BITalino – Biomedical Equipment," n.d.).

b. MySignals Hardware Development Platform (HDP), is a more hardware-focused model of MySignals SDP. It is designed to work on top of an Arduino and to be controlled using its SDK. In addition to the sensors and radios (ie. BLE and WiFi) available for MySignals SDP, the HDP version also supports custom sensors and extra radios including 4G/3G/GPRS, Bluetooth and ZigBee ("MySignals - eHealth and Medical IoT Development Platform," n.d.).

c. MtM+'s development Sensor Kits (SK), are small factor IoT (Internet of Things) development kits offering turnkey solutions for rapid Internet of Things product development. Two main kits are especially interesting, namely, Health and Motion Sensors kits. The Health kit comprises essentially a multi-function board for communication (BLE) and processing, an extension board for adding third-party boards and serving as a bridge for programming, and a sensing board for pulse and SpO2 monitoring. A battery board can also be added in order to obtain a standalone device.

Besides, with the same boards structure as Health kit, Motion Sensors Kit works on the basis of accelerometer and gyroscope sensors, allowing to target motion-based applications such as fall detection ("MtM+ Technology Corporation - IoT Development Kit," n.d.; "RF Design - Nordic-powered Bluetooth low energy development kit offers complete turnkey solution for rapid Internet of Things product development," 2016).

3. Do-it-Yourself

Do-It-Yourself (DIY) alternative is another interesting option for sensing platforms in prototyping and experimentation settings. In fact, available sensors, boards, and even sewable electronic pieces used in interactive textiles ("Arduino - ArduinoBoardLilyPad," n.d.; "MCHobby - LilyPad Temperature Sensor," n.d.; "LilyPad Accelerometer," n.d.) enable to create different kind of custom sensing platforms (see Figure 3). DIY are particularity interesting as they allow composing custom sensing platforms with a reduced cost. However, they typically require assembly, which might be complicated. Communication, such as for programming, with DIY platforms is generally made via serial communication protocols such as I2C (Inter-Integrated Circuit) or SPI (Serial Peripheral Protocol). However, API interface might be available in some components (Zhang, Passow, Jovanov, Stoll, & Thurow, 2013).

Developers and retails like Pololu, Sparkfun, Cooking-hacks, or Adafruit propose a set of electronics, from boards to sensors, enabling to compose custom platforms for health monitoring. Interesting sensors include:

- IMUs for motion sensing applications, comprising accelerometer, gyroscope, barometer, altimeter and magnetometer ("Pololu - AltIMU-10 v5 Gyro, Accelerometer, Compass, and Altimeter," n.d.; "Adafruit 10-DOF IMU Breakout," n.d.; "LilyPad Accelerometer," n.d.).
- Temperature, both skin and ambient ("SparkFun Digital Temperature Sensor Breakout," n.d.; "Omega technologies - Precision Thermistor Sensors for Surface Temperature Measurements," n.d.; "Overview | TMP36 Temperature Sensor | Adafruit Learning System," n.d.; "MCHobby - LilyPad Temperature Sensor," n.d.).
- Pulse or heart beat ("SparkFun Electronics - Pulse Sensor," n.d.; "World Famous Electronics llc. - Heartbeats in your projects," n.d.).
- ECG ("MCHobby - ECG-EKG/EMG shield pour Arduino," n.d.; "MCHobby - Câble pro ECG-EKG/EMG pour électrode gel," n.d.; "Electrode ECG à gel," n.d.).

Regarding the available boards for hosting sensors, interesting ones include:

- Arduino ("Arduino," n.d.).
- Raspberry Pi ("Raspberry Pi - Teach, Learn, and Make with Raspberry Pi," n.d.).
- Genuino (Arduino) 101 ("Arduino - Genuino 101," n.d.).
- BLEduino, a BLE integrated Arduino ("ElecFreaks - BLEDuino," 2016).
- (Discontinued) C.H.I.P. platform, with built-in BLE/WiFi modules ("Chip Community - Next Thing Co. has ceased operations," 2019).
- Lilypad Arduino ("Arduino - ArduinoBoardLilyPad," n.d.) for sewable electronics.

Other parts might also be needed depending on the selected boards and sensors, such as ECG or BLE shields for Arduino ("MCHobby - ECG-EKG/EMG shield pour Arduino," n.d.; RedBear - BLE Shield – Retired," n.d.).

Through reviewing the literature, it turns out that various research works rely on the DIY concept for experimentation and prototyping. Zhang et al. (2013) described a low-power monitoring prototype, made using a micro-controller with an energy-efficient processor, an ANT transceiver, and a temperature sensor. Kunnath et al. (2013) presented a low-power and lightweight wearable hardware comprising an ECG front-end and a low-power accelerometer. Jalaliniya and Pederson (2012), willing to recognize kids' sickness, built a wearable device using a digital temperature sensor, a pulse sensor, a Mini Pro Arduino microcontroller, and a Bluetooth Mate Gold communication module to communicate with mobile application. Many other DIY prototypes can be mentioned such as an activity monitor presented

Figure 3. ECG/EMG shield (a) for Arduino or BLEduino. Electrodes can be connected using Cable pro (b) - Images copyright : Olimex Ltd

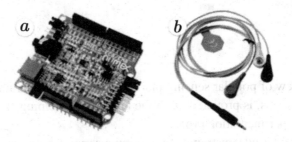

in (Wang, Liu, & Wang, 2013), a sensor node for skin temperature as described in (Dementyev, Behnaz, & Gorbach, 2013), or even a Smartshoe designed by the authors of (Majumder et al., 2013).

DISCUSSION

Sensing platforms for prototyping and experimenting WHMS can be classified into three main categories, namely: ready-to-use, ready-to-compose kits and do-it-yourself platforms (see Table 3 for comparison).

R2U platforms are interesting in terms of convenience, quick deployment and ease of programming and interaction through APIs. However, such platforms are generally not expandable and thus might be limited in terms of sensors and communication interfaces, although some might offer quite interesting set of sensors such as MySignals SDP.

Besides, R2C kits are generally more flexible in terms of sensing and communication capabilities. However, they require assembly and might lack of unobtrusiveness and readiness to use.

Table 3. Sensing platforms categories

	R2U platforms	R2C kits	DIY kits
Readiness to use	Ready	Assembly needed (generally easy)	Assembly needed (possibly more complicated than R2C kits)
Convenience	Generally unobtrusive and convenient	Some might be obtrusive	Depend on electronics used (hosting board, sensors, ...)
Programming	Generally easy through open or restricted API	Depending on kit, via provided API, SDK (Software Development Kit), ...	Generally through serial protocols like I2C and SPI, or possibly via API for some components
Expandability	Generally not expandable and limited in terms of sensing and communication	• Sometimes expandable in terms of sensing through third party sensors • Some might allow different communication interfaces	Depend on electronics used (hosting board, sensors, communication interfaces, ...)

Lastly, DIY platforms are an interesting option for reducing costs while allowing better prototyping customization. However, DIY platforms may require more complicated assembly and programming than R2C kits and R2U platforms.

CONCLUSION

In this chapter, an overview of popular sensing platforms, meeting constraints of prototyping continuous health monitoring systems, is provided, with the aim to be a helping starting point for researchers willing to start WHMS experimentation projects.

A number of requirements and constraints for continuous monitoring prototyping were firstly identified, then sensing platforms were classified into three proposed and compared categories, namely, ready-to-use, ready-to-compose kits, and do-it-yourself platforms. On that basis, a set of interesting platforms were reviewed and compared under each category.

Selecting sensing platforms for prototyping WHMS depends on target application requirements and constraints, especially regarding sensing and communication. For continuous monitoring, energy-efficiency and wireless communication are likely to be the most important criteria to observe in an experimentation configuration. Other constraints might be also relevant depending on target purposes, such as sensors position which may impact accuracy ("MIT Technology Review - The Struggle for Accurate Measurements on Your Wrist," 2015), or sensing method to adopt like using ECG or PPG for heart activity measurements (Gonçalves, Pinto, Silva, Ayres-de-Campos, & Bernardes, 2016).

DISCLAIMER

- None of the presented sensing platforms were actually tested or evaluated within this work. Information provided in this document, were essentially retrieved from official hardware developers' websites and online retails.
- It should be noted that sensing platforms described in this work, are presented only as potential platforms for health monitoring experimentation purposes. This document doesn't guarantee that such platforms could be effectively used as medical devices or substitute medical professionals. Similar disclaimers are stated by some hardware developers such as in ("MySignals - eHealth and Medical IoT Development Platform," n.d.) and ("BITalino – Biomedical Equipment," n.d.).

REFERENCES

Adafruit. (2012, July 29). *Overview | TMP36 Temperature Sensor | Adafruit Learning System*. Retrieved from https://learn.adafruit.com/tmp36-temperature-sensor

Adafruit. (n.d.). *Adafruit 10-DOF IMU Breakout - L3GD20H + LSM303 + BMP180*. Retrieved from https://www.adafruit.com/products/1604

Arduino. (n.d.). *Arduino - Genuino 101 CurieBLE Heart Rate Monitor*. Retrieved from https://www. arduino.cc/en/Tutorial/Genuino101CurieBLEHeartRateMonitor

Arduino. (n.d.). *Arduino*. Retrieved from https://www.arduino.cc/

Arduino. (n.d.). *ArduinoBoardLilyPad*. Retrieved from https://www.arduino.cc/en/Main/ArduinoBoard-LilyPad/

Arduino. (n.d.). *Genuino 101*. Retrieved from https://store.arduino.cc/product/GBX00005

Benharref, A., & Serhani, M. A. (2014). Novel cloud and SOA-based framework for E-Health monitoring using wireless biosensors. *IEEE Journal of Biomedical and Health Informatics*, 18(1), 46–55. doi:10.1109/JBHI.2013.2262659 PMID:24403403

BITalino. (n.d.). *BITalino – Biomedical Equipment*. Retrieved from http://www.bitalino.com

Boulemtafes, A. & Badache, N. (2016). Wearable Health Monitoring Systems: An Overview of Design Research Areas. In mHealth Ecosystems and Social Networks in Healthcare (pp. 17-27). Cham, Switzerland: Springer.

Boulemtafes, A., Rachedi, A., & Badache, N. (2015, November). A study of mobility support in wearable health monitoring systems: Design framework. In *2015 IEEE/ACS 12th International Conference of Computer Systems and Applications (AICCSA)* (pp. 1-8). Piscataway, NJ: IEEE.

Chip Community. (2019, Feb. 2). *Next Thing Co. has ceased operations*. Retrieved from http://www. chip-community.org/index.php/Main_Page

Dementyev, A., Behnaz, A., & Gorbach, A. M. (2013, January). 135-hour-battery-life skin temperature monitoring system using a Bluetooth cellular phone. In *2013 IEEE Topical Conference on Biomedical Wireless Technologies, Networks, and Sensing Systems* (pp. 25-27). Piscataway, NJ: IEEE. 10.1109/ BioWireleSS.2013.6613663

ElecFreaks. (2016, Jan. 15). *BLEDuino*. Retrieved from https://www.elecfreaks.com/wiki/index. php?title=BLEDUINO

Gay, V., & Leijdekkers, P. (2007). A health monitoring system using smart phones and wearable sensors. *International Journal of ARM*, 8(2), 29–35.

Gonçalves, H., Pinto, P., Silva, M., Ayres-de-Campos, D., & Bernardes, J. (2016). Electrocardiography versus photoplethysmography in assessment of maternal heart rate variability during labor. *SpringerPlus*, 5(1), 1079. doi:10.118640064-016-2787-z PMID:27462527

Irfan Husain, M. D. (2014, Feb. 14). *New Healthpatch biosensor captures a wide range of information with just an adhesive, disposable patch*. Retrieved from https://www.imedicalapps.com/2014/02/vital-connect-wearable-biosensor-healthpatch/

Jalaliniya, S. & Pederson, T. (2012, October). A wearable kids' health monitoring system on smartphone. In *Proceedings of the 7th Nordic Conference on Human-Computer Interaction: Making Sense Through Design* (pp. 791-792). New York, NY: ACM. 10.1145/2399016.2399150

Kunnath, A. T., Nadarajan, D., Mohan, M., & Ramesh, M. V. (2013, August). Wicard: A context aware wearable wireless sensor for cardiac monitoring. In *2013 International Conference on Advances in Computing, Communications and Informatics (ICACCI)* (pp. 1097-1102). Piscataway, NJ: IEEE. 10.1109/ICACCI.2013.6637330

Maastricht Instruments. (n.d.). *ECG Necklace*. Retrieved from http://www.maastrichtinstruments.nl/portfolio/ecg-necklace-body-area-network/

Maciuca, A., Popescu, D., Strutu, M., & Stamatescu, G. (2013, September). Wireless sensor network based on multilevel femtocells for home monitoring. In *2013 IEEE 7th International Conference on Intelligent Data Acquisition and Advanced Computing Systems (IDAACS)* (Vol. 1, pp. 499-503). Piscataway, NJ: IEEE. 10.1109/IDAACS.2013.6662735

Majumder, A. J. A., Zerin, I., Uddin, M., Ahamed, S. I., & Smith, R. O. (2013, October). SmartPrediction: A real-time smartphone-based fall risk prediction and prevention system. In *Proceedings of the 2013 Research in Adaptive and Convergent Systems* (pp. 434-439). New York, NY: ACM. 10.1145/2513228.2513267

MbientLab. (2017). *MetaWear Android API*. Retrieved from https://mbientlab.com/androiddocs/latest/

MbientLab. (n.d.). *MetaHealth*. Retrieved from https://mbientlab.com/product/metahealth-bundle/

MbientLab. (n.d.). *MetamotionC*. Retrieved from https://mbientlab.com/product/metamotionc/

MCHobby. (n.d.). *Câble pro ECG-EKG/EMG pour électrode gel*. Retrieved from https://shop.mchobby.be/shields/695-cable-pro-ecg-ekgemg-pour-electrode-gel-3232100006959-olimex.html

MCHobby. (n.d.). *ECG-EKG/EMG shield pour Arduino*. Retrieved from https://shop.mchobby.be/shields/693-ekg-emg-shield-pour-arduino-3232100006935-olimex.html

MCHobby. (n.d.). *Electrode ECG à gel*. Retrieved from http://shop.mchobby.be/shields/696-electrode-ecg-a-gel-3232100006966.html

MIT Technology Review. (2015, June 22). *The Struggle for Accurate Measurements on Your Wrist*. Retrieved from https://www.technologyreview.com/s/538416/the-struggle-for-accurate-measurements-on-your-wrist/

MtM+ Technology Corporation (n.d.). *IoT Development Kit*. Retrieved from https://www.mtmtech.com.tw/kit.html

MySignals. (n.d.). *eHealth and Medical IoT Development Platform*. Retrieved from http://www.mysignals.com/

Omega Engineering. (n.d.). *Precision Thermistor Sensors for Surface Temperature Measurements*. Retrieved from http://www.omega.com/pptst/ON-409_ON-909.html

Polar Electro. (n.d.). *H10 heart rate sensor*. Retrieved from https://www.polar.com/us-en/products/accessories/h10_heart_rate_sensor#features

Pololu (n.d.). *AltIMU-10 v5 Gyro, Accelerometer, Compass, and Altimeter (LSM6DS33, LIS3MDL, and LPS25H Carrier)*. Retrieved from https://www.pololu.com/product/2739

Raspberry Pi Foundation. (n.d.). *Raspberry Pi — Teach, Learn, and Make with Raspberry Pi*. Retrieved from https://www.raspberrypi.org/

RedBear. (n.d.). *BLE Shield - Retired*. Retrieved from https://redbear.cc/product/retired/ble-shield.html

RF Design. (2016, Sept. 1). *Nordic-powered Bluetooth low energy development kit offers complete turnkey solution for rapid Internet of Things product development*. Retrieved from http://rf-design.co.za/nordic-powered-bluetooth-low-energy-development-kit-offers-complete-turnkey-solution-rapid-internet-things-product-development/

Shimmersensing. (n.d.). *Wearable body sensors | Wearable technology*. Retrieved from http://shimmersensing.com/products/

SparkFun Electronics. (n.d.). *LilyPad Accelerometer – ADXL335 - DEV-09267*. Retrieved from https://www.sparkfun.com/products/9267

SparkFun Electronics. (n.d.). *LilyPad Temperature Sensor - DEV-08777*. Retrieved from https://www.sparkfun.com/products/8777

SparkFun Electronics. (n.d.). *Pulse Sensor - SEN-11574*. Retrieved from https://www.sparkfun.com/products/11574

SparkFun Electronics. (n.d.). *SparkFun Digital Temperature Sensor Breakout – TMP102*. Retrieved from https://www.sparkfun.com/products/11931

Triantafyllidis, A. K., Koutkias, V. G., Chouvarda, I., & Maglaveras, N. (2013). A pervasive health system integrating patient monitoring, status logging, and social sharing. *IEEE Journal of Biomedical and Health Informatics*, 17(1), 30–37. doi:10.1109/TITB.2012.2227269 PMID:23193318

Wang, C., Liu, C., & Wang, T. (2013). A remote health care system combining a fall down alarm and biomedical signal monitor system in an android smart-phone. Int. J. Adv. Comput. Sci. Appl, 4.

Wang, R., Blackburn, G., Desai, M., Phelan, D., Gillinov, L., Houghtaling, P., & Gillinov, M. (2017). Accuracy of wrist-worn heart rate monitors. *JAMA Cardiology*, 2(1), 104–106. doi:10.1001/jamacardio.2016.3340 PMID:27732703

World Famous Electronics. (n.d.). *Heartbeats in your projects*. Retrieved from http://pulsesensor.com/

Zhang, W., Passow, P., Jovanov, E., Stoll, R., & Thurow, K. (2013, August). A secure and scalable telemonitoring system using ultra-low-energy wireless sensor interface for long-term monitoring in life science applications. In *2013 IEEE International Conference on Automation Science and Engineering (CASE)* (pp. 617-622). Piscataway, NJ: IEEE. 10.1109/CoASE.2013.6653979

Chapter 14

Big Data, Data Mining, and Data Analytics in IoT-Based Healthcare Applications

Isakki Alias Devi P

Ayya Nadar Janaki Ammal College, India

ABSTRACT

IoT seriously impacts every industry. The healthcare industry has experienced progression in digitizing medical records. Healthcare services are costlier than ever. Data mining is one of the largest challenges to face IoT. Big Data is an accumulation of data. IoT devices receive lots of data. Big data systems can do a lot of data analytics. The tools can also be used to perform these operations. The big health application system can be built by integrating medical health resources using intelligent terminals, internet of things (IoT), big data, and cloud computing. People suffer from many diseases. A big health system can be applied to scientific health management by detecting risk factors for the occurrence of diseases. Patients can have special attention to their health requirements and their devices can be tuned to remind them of their appointments, calorie count, exercise check, blood pressure variations, symptoms of any diseases, and so much more.

INTRODUCTION

The global population is aging and the chronic diseases are growing day by day. While technology can't stop the population from ageing, it can make healthcare easier in terms of ease of use. The combination of latest information technology with healthcare system will diminish the problems. A new paradigm, known as the Internet of Things (IoT), is an extensive applicability in healthcare industry also. Big data and data analytics are the in-demand. IoT devices collect lots of data. It is not possible for queries. If IoT devices collect data, Big data will analyze data. The information can be measured faster.

According to S. Haller et al. "A world where physical objects are seamlessly integrated into the information network, and where the physical objects can become active participants in business pro-

DOI: 10.4018/978-1-7998-1090-2.ch014

cesses. Services are accessible to interact with these 'smart object' over the Internet, query their state and information associated with them, account security and privacy issues."

IoT is the next generation of Internet which will contain trillions of nodes representing various objects from many ubiquitous sensor devices to large web servers (Dey et al., 2018). IoT incorporates the classical networks with the emerging technologies such as ubiquitous computing, cloud computing, data mining, sensor networks, RFID technology, etc. From the perspective of technology, IoT is an integration of sensor networks, which include RFID, and ubiquitous network (Lee & Yoon, 2017). From the perspective of economical view, IoT integrates new related technologies and applications, productions and services, R. & D., industry and market. Convenience, efficiency and automation are the goals of IoT.

Needs of IoT

- Quantified health will be the future of healthcare. The data affect the performance, and so that IoT is needed for better outcomes with respect to health tracking.
- IoT ensures that all information is considered to make better decisions for patients. It is possible by updating the health information of patients on the cloud.
- The primary area of focus is prevention because health care expenses are very high.
- Patient satisfaction is possible by IoT. Through internet-connected devices, valuable patient's data will be gathered.
- IoT allows care teams to collect various data points on personal fitness like heart-rate, temperature, sleep routine etc.,

Challenges to Adopt IoT in Healthcare

The challenges are storage, security and data management (Pang, 2013). There are reliability and security issues with data along with the lack of infrastructure and training among providers. Another problem is the poor internet access. The medical resources are limited. The development of medical resources is not balanced. 80% people are living in areas with limited medical resources but 80% medical resources are provided to the big cities only. One third of diseases could be completely prevented, one third could be detected early and one third could be done with regular treatment to save people. In general, the status of health is from health to low-high risk status. The application of this paradigm in healthcare industry is a mutual hope because it allows medical centers to function proficiently and patients to obtain better treatment. With the help of this technology-based healthcare method, there are unique benefits which improve the quality and efficiency of healing and accordingly the patient's health will be improved.

Internet-connected devices have been used for patients in various forms. Data comes from fetal monitors, electrocardiograms, temperature monitors or blood glucose levels, health information is essential for patients. These measures are needed follow-up interaction with a healthcare professional. The smart technology quickly became an asset in healthcare is when linked with home medication dispensers. These dispensers routinely upload data to the cloud when medication is not taken.

Internet-of-things technology implementations have issues about personal data privacy and security. IoT devices can be used to save the patient's life. IoT in healthcare may be life threatening if not secured. In 2012, an episode of *Homeland* demonstrated a hacked pacemaker inducing a heart attack. Former Vice President Dick Cheney subsequently asked that the wireless capabilities of his pacemaker be disabled.

In 2016, Johnson & Johnson notified one of its connected insulin pumps was susceptible to attack. "In 2017, St. Jude released patches for weak remote monitoring system of implantable pacemakers".

U.S. Food and Drug Administration (FDA) have published lots of guidelines for establishing end-to-end security for the connected medical devices. "In late 2018, the FDA signed a memorandum of agreement with the Department of Homeland Security to implement a new medical device cyber security framework to be established by both agencies".

- Uses of IoT for Business
  - 53% of IoT projects are used for optimizing current businesses and 47% is used for business investment.
  - Target audiences are consumers (42%), business (54%) and internal use by employees (5%) .
- Challenges in IoT Projects
  - 96% of developers faced challenges with their IoT projects
  - IoT does not deliver full potential due to data challenges.
  - Only 8% are able to analyze IoT data in a timely manner.
  - 86% of stakeholders in business roles say that data is important to their IoT projects.
  - 94% face challenges to collect IoT data.
- Better IoT data collection and analysis
  - 70% developers make better, meaningful decisions with improved data
  - 86% can report faster and flexible analytics and increase the ROI of their IoT investments.

BIG DATA

Big data is defined as huge sets of data that can only be analyzed by computers to reveal patterns (Doukas & Maglogiannis, 2012), trends and associations, mainly with regards to human behavior. The term "big data", with regards to healthcare, is the intersection of mathematics, statistics, computer science and healthcare. The adoption of this expertise is not only about quality care for patients, but the sustainability of healthcare systems on the whole. It also raises the issues such as data privacy, data discrimination and data security (Ali & Ebu-Elkheir, 2012).

Big health is an industry which characterized by people-center, managing a person's health from birth to death. The domain of big health covers health products, health service, health finance field.

Big Data is defined in terms of 3V's:

1. Volume (how much data)
2. Velocity (how fast the data is processed)
3. Variety (different formats of data).

A small volume of complex data, a huge volume of simple data, or sophisticated analytics and predictions from any of the data benefits from the Big Data technology modernization. Big Data is classified into three main types:

Structured Data

Structured Data refers to the data which is already stored in databases. It reports about 20% of total existing data. It is used in computer-related activities. There are two sources of structured data which are machines and humans (Raghupathi & Raghupathi, 2014). All the data received from sensors, web logs and financial systems can be classified under machine-generated data. Human-generated structured data includes all the data as human input into a computer, such as his demographic details. When the user surfs on the internet, or even makes a game movement, data is created. This can be used by companies to predict their customer behavior and take the necessary decisions.

Unstructured Data

The structured data exists in the traditional row-column databases. But the unstructured data is opposite to structured data. These do not have any clear format in storage. The remaining data are created, about 80% of the total account for unstructured big data. Most of the data belongs to this category.

Unstructured data are also categorized based on its source into machine generated and human generated. Machine generated data contains all the satellite images, the scientific data from various experiments captured by different technology. Human generated unstructured data is resided enormously on the internet, since it contains social media data, mobile data and lot of website content.

Semi-Structured Data

Information that is not in the traditional database format as structured data, but contain some organizational properties which make it easier to process, are included in semi-structured data. NoSQL documents are semi structured, since they contain keywords that can be used to process the document effectively.

VARIETIES OF BIG DATA

Big Data is focused on three main varieties:

1. Transactional data—these include data from invoices, payment orders, delivery records, claim activities and cost data. These are useful for payers and providers in healthcare.
2. Machine or clinical data—this can be data gathered from industrial equipments, real-time data from sensors and wearable techs as well as web logs that track user behaviors online.
3. Social data—this can be coming from social media services, such as Facebook Likes, Tweets and YouTube views which gives insights on patients behavior.

Original business value comes from combining these big data with traditional data such as patient records, medical history, location details, and medication management to generate new decisions. In the healthcare arena, the amount of patient and consumer health data has grown largely because of computer-based information systems. In recent years, the adoption of wearable technology, biosensors and mHealth increase the amount of biological data being captured. In a clinical setting, these data include details which come from electronic patient records outcomes (ePRO), electronic health records

Figure 1. Big data value chain

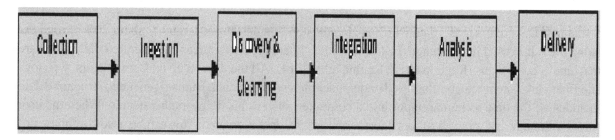

(EHR) and other software sources. It is calculated that there are over 10.7 billion objects and devices connected to the internet today. It is expected to cultivate to 50 billion by 2020 according to a recent report by Cisco and DHL.

Big Data Value Chain

Big data value chain contains 6 phases such as:

1. Collection
2. Ingestion
3. Discovery & Cleansing
4. Integration
5. Analysis
6. Delivery

Figure 1 shows big data value chain with 6 phases.

1. **Collection**: Structured, unstructured and semi-structured data from multiple sources.
2. **Ingestion**: Loading vast amounts of data onto a single data store.
3. **Discovery & Cleansing:** Understanding format and content; clean up and formatting.
4. **Integration**: Linking, entity extraction, entity resolution, indexing and data fusion.
5. **Analysis**: Intelligence, statistics, predictive and text analytics, machine learning.
6. **Delivery**: Querying, visualization, real time delivery in enterprise-class availability.

BIG DATA AND INTERNET OF "MEDICAL" THINGS

Big data become valuables to healthcare industry in what's known as the internet of things (IoT). Data scientist uses big data to reorganize healthcare of patients. The diseases can be detected and treated by algorithms. Devices are helpful for human health. This data will be checked against genetic profile. Death rates will be reduced. Any device which generates data about a person's health and sends that data into the cloud, will be part of IoT. This data also has lot of variations and in terms of huge amount of medical data from different age groups, or high variability of veracity in terms of incomplete patient records and so on (Dey et al., 2018).

Medical big data has different features compared to big data from other fields. It is hard to frequently access. It is structured in comparison and has legal complications associated with its use (Doukas & Maglogiannis, 2012).In order to get value from the connected digital health environments, it is important to have a platform on which to create and manage applications, to run analytics, to receive, store and secure data. The term "connected health" is described that how healthcare is connecting in the digital health industry. Health information systems confirm great potential in improving the efficiency in the delivery of care, a reduction in overall costs to the health care system. It is necessary to organize and process the ever-increasing quantity of data which is digitally collected and stored within the health care organizations.

Many patients are using mobile applications (apps) to manage their health needs. The devices and mobile apps are now progressively used and integrated with telemedicine via the medical Internet of Things (mIoT). mIoT is a very tedious way of the digital transformation in healthcare industry. It allows new business paradigms to emerge changes. Wearables and mobile apps support fitness, health education, tracking of symptom, etc. All those platform analytics can raise the relevancy of data interpretations together data outputs.

Applications of Big Data in Healthcare

Big data is the collection of data sets. It is very tedious to process using hand database management tools or traditional data processing applications. Companies utilize big data to ensure higher profitablility.

Early Disease Detection

Big data analytics can guess the start of epidemics. It goes one step ahead and predicts the location of carriers. This was happened in the issue of Ebola to negate its spread. The body composition data can predict the side effects of certain medicine as well as the spread of diseases. This is important information for doctors.

Personalized Medicine

Big data makes a real personalized healthcare industry. This involves creating genetic profile for the patients based on which perfect healthcare plan is created. The plan is also collaborated with social and lifestyle habits. This helps to predict the issues of diseases as well as provides recommendations for better treatment.

Clinical Trials

Big data can be used for on-scale clinical trials. This can be started with the selection of a sample set, The doctors can scan through medical profiles which meet their requirements. Then, Big data can enable to track which was not happened earlier. The trial success rate has increased.

Increased Profits Via High Cost Patients

A minority group of patients report for major healthcare spending. The high cost patients never bother about money and they used to do master check up twice in a year.

Loss of Privacy Because of Big Data

Healthcare transformation comes with many challenges.

1. Access to healthcare
2. Consumer Engagement
3. Cost efficiency
4. Levels and quality of care

Fortunately, companies taking advantage of big data are gaining deeper insights into patient health and creating exceptional customer experiences. Suppose, for example, Linda is seeing her physician for her annual physical checkup. She has the problems such as diabetic, stress, irritable, low blood pressure. In a big data world, Linda's physician has a 360 degree view of her healthcare history. Her appointments, diets, exercise, labs, vitals, prescriptions, treatments, allergies, etc., will be recorded.

Big Data Standardization Challenges

- Big Data use cases, definitions, vocabulary and reference architectures (e.g. system, data, platforms, online/offline)
- Specifications and standardization of metadata including data provenance
- Application models (e.g. batch, streaming)
- Query languages including non-relational queries to support diverse data types (XML, RDF, JSON, multimedia) and Big Data operations
- Domain-specific languages
- Semantics of eventual consistency
- Advanced network protocols for efficient data transfer
- General and domain specific ontology and taxonomies for describing data semantics including interoperation between ontology
- Big Data security and privacy access controls
- Remote, distributed, and federated analytics (taking the analytics to the data) including data and processing resource discovery and data mining
- Data sharing and exchange
- Data storage, e.g. memory storage system, distributed file system, data warehouse, etc.
- Human consumption of the results of big data analysis (e.g. visualization)
- Interface between relational (SQL) and non-relational (NoSQL)
- Big Data Quality and Veracity description and management

DATA MINING AND DATA ANALYTICS IN IoT

Many data mining tools are useful to face those challenges effectively. So the propagation of the IoT would be the next stage of the big data concept. Big data analysis can drive the digital interruption of the healthcare industry, business processes and decision making. Data mining is used to extract targeted data from a very large dataset. The technique involves traversing through the huge volume of data using data mining methods of association, classification, compilation and so on (Imadali, 2012).

Association is used to create interrelationships between two or more data sets to identify a pattern. It enables the deduction of general tendencies among data sets. Other significant part of data mining techniques is classification and clustering. Classification is used to assign data into particular target classes to precisely predict what will occur within the class (Jara, Zamora-Izquierdo, & Skarmeta, 2012, 2013; Jiawei & Kamber, 2011). Clustering is the process of grouping similar data records.

Role of Data Analytics in Internet of Things (IoT)

IoT and big data are linked together to perform various operations. Data which is consumed and produced in IoT keep growing at an expanding rate. This incursion of data is increasing rapidly. In 200, there will be approximately 30.73 billion IoT connected devices. The data generated from IoT devices will turn as value. If it subjects to analysis, data analytics will bring into the picture. Data analytics can be used to examine big and small data sets with varying data properties to extract meaningful conclusions. These conclusions are in the form of trends, patterns, and statistics. It helps for the organization to make good and effective decisions in business.

Merging Data Analytics and IoT for the Businesses

Data Analytics are useful for the growth of IoT applications. An analytics tools will allow an organization to make use of their variety of dataset. The following lists must be considered:

- **Volume:** There are huge amount of clusters of data sets. IoT applications can make use of those data sets. The organizations are needed to manage these data and analyze the same for extracting required patterns. These datasets along with real time data must be analyzed effectively with the help of data analytics software.
- **Structure:** IoT applications contain data sets that have a structure as unstructured, semi-structured and structured data sets.
- **Driving Revenue:** The data analytics in IoT investments will allow organizations to gain an detailed approach into customer preferences. This leads to the development of offers as per the customer's expectations. It will improve the revenues of the organizations in an effective manner.

Optimize the Processes With Data

There are different types of data analytics that can be applied in the IoT investments. Some of these types have been described below:

- **Streaming Analytics:** This form of data analytics refers as event stream processing and it analyzes huge in-motion data sets. Real-time data streams are analyzed in this process to detect urgent situations and immediate actions. IoT applications based on financial transactions, air fleet tracking, traffic analysis etc. can benefit from this method.
- **Spatial Analytics:** This data analytics method is used to analyze geographic patterns to determine the spatial relationship between the physical objects. Location-based IoT applications, such as smart parking applications can benefit from this form of data analytics.
- **Time Series Analytics:** This form of data analytics is based upon the time-based data which is analyzed to reveal associated patterns and trends. IoT applications, such as weather forecasting applications and health monitoring systems can benefit from this form of data analytics method.
- **Prescriptive Analysis:** This form of data analytics is the combination of descriptive and predictive analysis. It is applied to comprehend the best steps of action which can be taken in a particular situation. Commercial IoT applications can make use of this form of data analytics to gain better conclusions.

Healthcare is one of the leading sectors of every country. The utilization of data analytics in IoT based healthcare applications can provide breach in this area. The reduction of the healthcare costs, enhancement of telehealth monitoring, and remote health services, increased diagnosis and treatment can be achieved using the same. The utilization of data analytics shall be promoted in the area of IoT to gain improved revenues, competitive gain, and customer engagement.

DATA MINING PROCESSES

IoT data mining processes are divided into multiple stages, as follows:

- Data is integrated according to different data sources.
- Data is cleaned, so it can be easily extracted and processed.
- Some parts of data are extracted and prepared for future processing.
- Sophisticated algorithms are used to identify patterns.
- Data is restructured and presented to the users in a articulate way.

The enormous amount of data produced by IoT devices can be converted into knowledge using data mining techniques. Technologies are used to mine certain useful trends and patterns which are unknown, to enhance the performance of the organizations. All the organizations are growing rapidly with the help of data mining functionalities. Data mining helps to find out something in the huge data which is profitable to the organization. The primary aim of knowledge discovery in databases is to discover the novel patterns in the large data sets. It is the blend of artificial intelligence, machine learning and statistics. Data mining transforms a data set into meaningful structure and extracts information which helps to gain deep knowledge into the raw data collected from various IoT applications.

But there also are challenges that need to be overcome such as issues related to data structure, security, standardization, storage and transfer. With the use of technology and potential data mining tools like Hadoop, big data can be investigated more quickly and in a less cumbersome way. With the large quantities of medical data available, we feel confident that we can uncover important and solid information regarding people's health. If this presumption is valid and the analysis outcomes are dependable, this could be the start of a new phase of total illnesses prevention or even eradication.

Therefore, IoT forms a network of physical objects or things which might be embedded with electronics, sensor and network connectivity by which the devices can collect and exchange data (Höller et al., 2014). The perfect association between IoT and Data Mining result into a new emerging technology which benefits to the society. Different applications generate huge amount of heterogeneous data. As the data in IoT application is generated continuously from different sources like wireless sensor networks, RFID etc.

Imadali (2012) differentiated types of data from IoT into "data about things" and "data generated by things". Data about things refers to data that describe things themselves and data generated by things refers to data generated by things. This new type of data (i.e., data captured by sensor or RFID) has been defined as a kind of "big data" (Jara, Zamora-Izquierdo, & Skarmeta, 2012). The huge amount of data generated by IoT applications and potential of KDD motivated us to analyze a data mining framework for IoT applications.

Clustering for IoT

Clustering algorithms (Raghupathi & Raghupathi, 2014) divide data into meaningful groups. The patterns in the same group are similar in some sense and patterns in different group are dissimilar in the same sense. This is an unsupervised learning technique. For example, search engine uses clustering method to group web pages into different groups like news, videos, images, blogs etc.

Clustering is an efficient way to enhance the performance of IoT on the integration of identification, sensing, and actuation. New clustering algorithms are developed for the WSNs that are found on IoT (Uttarkar & Kilkarni, 2014). One of the clustering algorithms which considers the energy conservation of WSN is the low-energy adaptive clustering hierarchy (LEACH) (Zhang & Zhang, 2011).

Classification for IoT

Classification is an important technique in data mining. It predicts the output based on the given training data. This is called supervised learning technique. In this technique, a training data is given by the use of which a classifier model is build and based on this model the future pattern is predicted.

For IoT applications, classification algorithms are divided into 2 types – outdoor and indoor. The example for the outdoor IoT is traffic jam problem. The smart phones and other smart devices are used to predict the traffic situations and communicate them to the users. Some classification algorithms are there to solve the traffic jam problem, where the classifiers predict and suggest the less jammed route to the driver based on the previous traffic conditions.

DATA MINING CHALLENGES WITH THE IoT

In healthcare industry, lots of data mining challenges exist. Enormous numbers of patients, doctors, and other details are to be maintained.

Increasingly Large Volumes of Data

As new applications become progressively more complex, developers are facing pressure to process large data sets. Certain applications require data scientists to extract and analyze plenty of petabytes of data. According to EMC, IT support companies are under pressure to facilitate their customers for better solutions and manage huge data.

Data Sets Aren't Homogenous

Before the IoT comes, most applications received data from a single source. Since data were already structured in the same format, data scientists rarely encountered compatibility issues. The IoT has introduced a new layer of complexity for data analysis. Data is created from many different sources in multiple formats, such as web documents, CSV sheets, and SQL tables. Before big data analytics tools can process it, data must be cleaned and convert it into a single structure.

Integrity of Different Sources

Each system uses its own methodology to develop data, which will always introduce some level of uncertainty. Unfortunately, a feasible solution to this challenge has yet to present itself, but the barriers should be nominal for most real-world applications.

Need for Real-Time Analysis

Some applications need data to be extracted and processed in real time. This can be a challenge when analyzing data sets that are petabytes in size.

Solutions to These Challenges

If data mining problems have surfaced with the IoT, new solutions have been developed to solve them. Hadoop and big data extraction tools are important to make it easier. Many companies are expected to get the advantage of Hadoop as IoT becomes widely implemented.

Big Data Hadoop Architecture

Big Data Hadoop Architecture supports for analytic solution using open source Apache Hadoop framework. In Big Data Hadoop architecture, big volumes, variety, and velocity of data are collected from online and stored in HDFS file system. Hadoop architecture also provides HBase and RDBMS for processing and storing big data in the traditional format and useful for users on Big Data Architectures.

Hadoop acts like an information coordinator. It enables specialists to discover relationships in informational indexes with numerous factors. This is the reason for using Hadoop with healthcare information. The big data landing zone can be set up on Hadoop cluster to collect huge data which are stored in HDFS file system (Jara, Zamora-Izquierdo, & Skarmeta, 2012). Map Reduce programming is for online marketing analysts and various algorithms in Hadoop cluster to perform Big data analysts and core java programming language is implemented for Algorithms. The data regarding the previous medical history of patients provide better service from hospitals.

Big Data Hadoop Challenges

The major Big Data Challenges are associated with as follows:

- Capturing data
- Storage
- Cure
- Sharing
- Searching
- Transfer
- Analysis

To fulfill the all above challenges, organizations get help from enterprise servers.

Health Cloud and Health Big Data

Big health system is required to create health IoT. The quantity of networking devices is more nowadays and the enormous amount of data increases much faster. Traditional computing models and data analysis techniques are far from satisfying the massive concurrent user's demands and wobbly growth of data. Therefore, the combination of cloud computing and big data is used to build a platform for big health services. The health big data based on mobile health cloud must have the following features:

- **Heterogeneity**: This is mainly reflected in two aspects: the different parts of the body, different categories of different organizations and different countries and regions can store health data with different medical standards with different storage format. There is a possibility of structured relational data and semi-structured data. CDA (Clinical Document Architecture) is one of the examples. There are text, images, video, audio, and other unstructured data, such as medical records, X-ray, ultrasound, cardiac EEG. With the development of new technology, same kinds of data can be changed in the structure: for example, with the development of medical technology, complete blood test indicators can be measured. It will predictably lead to inconsistent format of historical data.
- **High Correlation**: Medical health data include the body's vital signs which are closely linked and related each other. Small portions of the data, does not accurately identify the function of the body. For example, human leukocyte data which are high and not able to determine the illness. Its causes are acute infection, tissue injuries, hepatitis, and leukemia. However, if the white blood cells in urine is high, the patients may be affected by renal disease.

In addition to the above two basic features, mobile medical big data has the following three characteristics:

- **Real-Time**: The detected data must be real-time due to the nature of health care. It also requires timely treatment.
- **Time and Space Correlation**: Healthcare has important time and space characteristics which manifested in two aspects: First, the different regions people have certain differences. For example, the range of hemoglobin of the persons at high altitude is usually higher than others. In addition, the same physiological parameters of the human body at different times will have certain variations. For example, the blood pressure is relatively high during day time. It is relatively low at night. The human adrenal cortex hormone is high during the day and low at night. With mobile smart devices and sensing devices, the data with time and space properties can be collected.
- **Low Proportion of Valid Data**: Mobile smart devices and conventional sensing devices cannot provide accurate test results like professional medical devices. For example, in the collection process of heart rate data, only the heart rate beyond the normal range will attract patients and medical personnel's attention.

IoT-BASED APPLICATIONS

As per the reports submitted by the P&S Market Research, there will be a compound annual growth rate (CAGR) of 37.6% in the healthcare Internet of Things industry between the years 2015 and 2020. People can enjoy personalized attention for their health requirements and their devices can be tuned to remind them of their appointments, calorie count, exercise check, blood pressure variations and so much more.

The patient medical record (MR) contains emergency data and medical case profiles. The clinical documentation (CD) is a digital or analog record which tracks all the treatment related activities. MR and CD are important for hospital information system (HIS). The clinical documentation serves as the benchmark medical information document for further clinical activities. It must be accurate. It further can serve to generate complete patient medical records. A hospital information system (HIS) must ensure that the patient's health records, as well as the clinical documentation, are always available. They must be reliable, and ensure data privacy.

Furthermore, remote monitoring of patient's health helps to reduce the length of hospital stay. IoT has applications in healthcare that benefit patients, families, physicians, hospitals, and healthcare related organizations. Devices in the form of wearables like fitness bands, wirelessly connected devices like blood pressure and heart rate monitoring cuffs, glucometer etc. provide patients access to personalized attention. These devices are tuned to remind calorie count, exercise check, appointments, blood pressure variations and much more. If any disturbances produced in the routine activities of a person, alert mechanism will send signals to family members and concerned health providers. IoT devices tagged with sensors are used to track real time location of medical equipment like wheelchairs, defibrillators, nebulizers, oxygen pumps and other monitoring equipment. Deployment of medical staff at different locations can also be analyzed in real time.

There are plenty of opportunities for health insurers with IoT-connected intelligent devices. Insurance companies can leverage data captured through health monitoring devices for their underwriting and claims operations. This data will enable them to detect fraud claims and identify prospects for underwriting. IoT devices bring transparency between insurers and customers in the underwriting, pricing, claims handling, and risk assessment processes. In the light of IoT-captured data-driven decisions

Figure 2. Four step IoT architecture

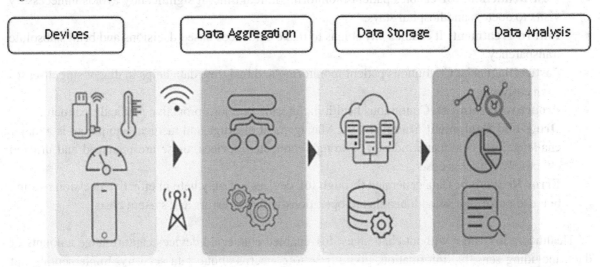

in all operation processes, customers will have adequate visibility into underlying thought behind every decision made and process outcomes.

Insurers can offer incentives to their customers for sharing health data generated by IoT devices. They can reward customers for using IoT devices to keep track of their routine activities and adherence to treatment plans and precautionary health measures. This will help insurers to reduce claims significantly. IoT devices can enable insurance companies to validate claims through the data captured by these devices. The proliferation of healthcare-specific IoT products opens up immense opportunities. And the huge amount of data are generated by these connected devices hold the potential to transform healthcare.

IoT has a four-step architecture which are basically four stages process (See Figure 2). All four stages are connected in a mode that data is processed at one stage and yield the value to the next stage. Integrated values in the process deliver dynamic business prospects.

Step 1: It consists of deployment of interconnected devices such as sensors, actuators, monitors, detectors, camera systems etc. These devices are used to collect the data.

Step 2: Data received from sensors and other devices are in analog form and need to be aggregated and converted to the digital form for further data processing.

Step 3: Once the data is digitized and aggregated, this is pre-processed, standardized and moved to the data center or Cloud (El-Sayed, 2018).

Step 4: Final data is managed and analyzed at the required level. Advanced Analytics can be applied and gives business insights for effective decision-making.

IoT is redefining healthcare by ensuring better care, improved treatment outcomes and reduced costs for patients, and better processes and workflows, improved performance and patient experience for healthcare providers.

The major advantages of IoT in healthcare include:

- **Cost Reduction**: IoT enables patient monitoring in real time. It significantly avoids unnecessary visits to doctors and hospital stays.
- **Future Treatment:** It enables physicians to make evidences based decisions and brings absolute transparency
- **Faster Diagnosis:** Continuous patient monitoring and real time data helps in diagnosing diseases at an early stage.
- **Proactive Treatment**: Continuous health monitoring provides proactive medical treatment.
- **Drugs and Equipment Management:** Management of drugs and medical equipment is a major challenge in a healthcare industry. Through connected devices, these are managed and utilized effectively with less costs
- **Error Reduction:** Data generated through IoT devices not only help in effective decision making but also make sure smooth healthcare operations with less errors and system costs.

Healthcare IoT is not without challenges. IoT-enabled connected devices capture huge amounts of data, including sensitive information, giving rise to concerns about data security. Implementing apt security measures is crucial. IoT explores new dimensions of patient care through real-time health monitoring and access to patients' health data. This data is a goldmine for healthcare stakeholders to improve patient's health and experiences while making revenue opportunities and improving healthcare operations. Being prepared to harness this digital power would prove to be the differentiator in the increasingly connected world.

Wearables and mobile applications support fitness, health education, disease's symptoms tracking, and care coordination (El-Sayed, 2018). All these platform analytics can raise the relevancy of data interpretations, reducing the amount of time that end users spend piecing together data outputs. The details are gained from big data analysis and will drive the digital disruption of the healthcare world and useful to make real time decisions. The applications of IoT in the healthcare industry are numerous:

1. Real Time Location Services

The doctors can use real time location services and track the devices to treat patients and give medications. Medical devices like wheelchairs, scales, defibrillators, nebulizers, pumps or monitoring equipment can be tagged with sensors and located with IoT. Apart from real time location services, there are IoT devices which help in environmental monitoring (Imadali, 2012). The system with IoT sensors are designed to track the moments of caretaking and care giving process. This provides to track locations of patients and medical equipment. It is called as location-as-a-service. The system is designed to improve the satisfaction of staffs and patients. Ex: AwarePoint.

2. Prediction of the Patients in PACU

With the help of Internet of Things, clinicians can predict the arrival of patients who are located in the Post-Anesthesia Care Unit (PACU). Doctors can also monitor the status of patients in real time.

3. Hand Hygiene Compliances

There is a hand hygiene monitoring system that would identify the degree of cleanliness. According to the Center for Disease Control and Prevention in United States, about one patient out of every 20 gets infections due to lack of hand hygiene in hospitals. Many patients lose their lives because of infections.

The communications in the hand hygiene monitoring systems can be done in real time. If a clinician comes closer to a patient's bed without washing his hands, the device will start buzzing. The information about the healthcare worker, his/her ID, time and location will all be fed into a database and this information would be forwarded to the concerned authorities.

4. Tighten Budgets and Improve Patient Journey

The healthcare industry must keep a watchful eye on the budget and at the same time have updated infrastructure to provide better patient experiences. It is now possible for the medical staff to access patient information from the cloud.

The goal is to give quality medical care to patients, and by spending a small amount on IT infrastructure. The hospitals can provide high quality care to patients at affordable rates. IoT aims to give better treatment for patients by:

- Room lighting through personal control
- Communicate with family and friends through email services
- Immediate attention to patient needs

5. Remote Monitoring

Remote health monitoring is significant in the application of Internet Of Things. Through monitoring, adequate healthcare can be given to people who need help. Lots of people die daily, because of not getting timely medical attention. With IoT, devices fit with sensors will notify the healthcare providers about the changes in the functions of body.

These devices are capable of handling complex algorithms and analyzing them. So, the patients can be able to receive proper attention and medical care. The collected patient information would be stored in the cloud. The patients do not need to stay in the hospitals continuously. If there are any variations in the daily activity of a person, alerts will send to the family members and their health providers immediately. These monitoring devices are provided in the form of wearables too.

6. Glucose Level Monitoring Scheme

Glucose Level Sensing Diabetes is a metabolic disease that increases the blood glucose level for a certain amount of time. The monitoring of glucose shows variations in blood patterns, activities and in the formation of meal. A real-time glucose level monitoring scheme was introduced in Istepanian et al. (Uttarkar & Kulkarni, 2014).

7. ECG Monitoring

An electrocardiogram (ECG) monitors the electrical movement of the human heart, determining the heart rate, QT intervals, myocardial ischemia, and diagnosis of arrhythmias (Zhang & Zhang, 2011).

8. Body Temperature Monitoring

Body Temperature Monitoring of human body temperature is an essential measure of medical services since it may be considered a vital indication of preservation of homeostasis (Kamal, Dey, Ashour, 2017). Istepanian et al. (Uttarkar & Kulkarni, 2014) verified the m-IoT strategy using body temperature sensors located in TelosB motes.

9. Medical Alert System

The medical alert system can be worn by a patient as clothing or jewelry. It feeds into a series of connected sensors. Those are useful to measure the health and welfare of the wearer. If a patient falls out of bed, or unconscious for too long period, an alert will be sent to family or friends who can help. Ex: Zanthion.

- **Medication Dispensing Device by Philips**: The patients will not miss a dose anymore. It is suitable for elderly patients.
- **Niox Mino by Aerocrine**: It measures Intric Oxide in a patient's breath.
- **Uro Sense by Future Path Medical**: It is for catheterized patients to check their body temperature and urine results.
- **GPS SmartSole**: This is a shoe-tracking wearable device for dementia patients who used to forget.

Benefits of IoT in Healthcare

a. Research

The resources in the current medical research have lack of real-world information. It uses controlled environments. IoT opens lot of ways to a variety of data and information through analysis and real time data. IoT can deliver data that is far better to standard analytics through making use of instruments. It helps in healthcare by providing more reliable data, which provides better solutions.

b. Devices

The current devices are improving with more power and precision (Jara, Zamora, & Skarmeta, 2012). IoT has the potential to unlock existing technology. It leads us towards better solutions. It fills the gap between the way which deliver healthcare and the equipment. It then detects errors and try to reveal the patterns and missing elements in healthcare.

c. Care

IoT empowers the professionals to use their knowledge and the proper training in a better way to crack the problems. It helps to utilize better data and equipment. Finally, better actions can be happened. IoT allows the professionals to exercise their talents.

d. Medical Information Distribution

This is a most significant innovation of IoT applications in healthcare. The distribution of accurate information to patients remains one of the challenges in medical care. IoT devices can not only improved health in the patient's life but also to facilitate the professional practice.

e. Emergency Care

The emergency services are suffered by the limited resources and sometimes disconnected also. The effective automation and analytics is the best solution in the healthcare industry. An emergency situation can be analyzed from a long distance (Uttarkar & Kulkarni, 2014). The providers can access the profiles of the patients during their arrival at hospitals. It is very essential care to the patients for their life. The losses can be reduced and emergency healthcare is well-improved.

CONCLUSION

With the help of big data, data mining and data analytics, IoT is really helpful for the patients and doctors. IoT will attain the goals of reduced costs and better health once it fully gets adopted the healthcare industry.

A new revolution of personalized preventative health coaches will emerge in this health industry. They are digital health advisors. These workers will possess the skills and the ability to manipulate the medical data. The coaches will help their clients to resolve chronic illness, improve cognitive function and achieve improved mental health.

REFERENCES

Ali, N., & Abu-Elkheir, M. (2012). Data management for the internet of things: Green directions. In *Proc. IEEE Globecom Workshops*, pp. 386–390. 10.1109/GLOCOMW.2012.6477602

Dey, N., Hassanien, A. E., Bhatt, C., Ashour, A., & Satapathy, S. C. (2018). Internet of Things and Big Data Analytics toward Next Generation Intelligence (pp. 3–549). Berlin, Germany: Springer International Publishing. doi:10.1007/978-3-319-60435-0

Doukas, C. & Maglogiannis, I. (2012). Bringing IoT and cloud computing towards pervasive healthcare. *Sixth international conference on innovative mobile and internet services in ubiquitous computing (IMIS)*. Piscataway, NJ: IEEE. 10.1109/IMIS.2012.26

El-Sayed, H., Sankar, S., Prasad, M., Puthal, D., Gupta, A., Mohanty, M., & Lin, C.-T. (2018). Edge of Things: The Big Picture on the Integration of Edge, IoT and the Cloud in a Distributed Computing Environment. *IEEE Access: Practical Innovations, Open Solutions*, *6*, 1706–1717. doi:10.1109/ACCESS.2017.2780087

Höller, J., Tsiatsis, V., Mulligan, C., Karnouskos, S., Avesand, S., & Boyle, D. (2014). *From machine-to-machine to the internet of things: Introduction to a new age of intelligence*. Amsterdam, The Netherlands: Elsevier.

Imadali, S., Karanasiou, A., Petrescu, A., Sifniadis, I., Vèque, V., & Angelidis, P. (2012, October). eHealth service support in IPv6 vehicular networks. In *2012 IEEE 8th International Conference on Wireless and Mobile Computing, Networking and Communications (WiMob)* (pp. 579-585). Piscataway, NJ: IEEE.

Jara, A. J., Zamora, M. A., & Skarmeta, A. F. (2012). Knowledge acquisition and management architecture for mobile and personal health environments based on the internet of things. *IEEE 11th international conference on trust, security and privacy in computing and communications (TrustCom)*. 10.1109/TrustCom.2012.194

Jara, A. J., Zamora-Izquierdo, M. A., & Skarmeta, A. F. (2013). Interconnection framework for mHealth and remote monitoring based on the internet of things. *IEEE Journal on Selected Areas in Communications*, *31*(9), 47–65. doi:10.1109/JSAC.2013.SUP.0513005

Jiawei, H., & Kamber, M. (2017). *Data Mining: Concepts and Techniques*. Morgan Kaufmann.

Kamal, M. S., Dey, N., & Ashour, A. S. (2017). Large scale medical data mining for accurate diagnosis: A blueprint. In S. U. Khan, A. Y. Zomaya, & A. Abbas (Eds.), *Handbook of Large-Scale Distributed Computing in Smart Healthcare* (pp. 157–176). Cham: Springer. doi:10.1007/978-3-319-58280-1_7

Lee, H. C., & Yoon, H.-J. (2017). Medical big data: Promise and challenges. *Kidney Research and Clinical Practice*, *36*(1), 3–11. doi:10.23876/j.krcp.2017.36.1.3 PMID:28392994

Pang, Z. (2013). Ecosystem analysis in the design of open platform-based in-home healthcare terminals towards the internet-of-things. In *15th international conference on advanced communication technology (ICACT)*. IEEE.

Raghupathi, W., & Raghupathi, V. (2014). Big data analytics in healthcare: Promise and potential. *Health Information Science and Systems, Springer*, *2*(3), 2–10. PMID:25825667

Uttarkar, R., & Kulkarni, R. (2014). Internet of Things: Architecture and Security. *International Journal of Computers and Applications*, *3*(4).

Zhang, X. M., & Zhang, N. (2011). An open, secure and flexible platform based on internet of things and cloud computing for ambient aiding living and telemedicine. In *2011 international conference on computer and management (CAMAN)*. IEEE.

Chapter 15
Predictive Modeling for Improving Healthcare Using IoT:
Role of Predictive Models in Healthcare Using IoT

Jayanthi Jagannathan
Sona College of Technology, India

Udaykumar U.
Sona College of Technology, India

ABSTRACT

The chapter covers the challenges faced in real-world healthcare services such as operating room bottlenecks, upcoming newborn medicines, managing datasets, and sources. It includes future directions that address practitioner difficulties. When IoT is merged with predictive techniques, it improves the medical service performance rate tremendously. Finally, the chapter covers the case studies and the tools that are in use to motivate the researchers to contribute to this domain.

INTRODUCTION

The usage of predictive analytics in healthcare can be achieved by merging different data repositories, which has the patient information that includes disease information, food & lifestyle habits. If we collect an information about individual, the task of prediction would be easier. The models can be customized based on the data points, to a specific patient or group of patients that ultimately leads to more precise and effective treatments that are bound to improve the overall efficacy of the healthcare system while at the same time reducing costs (Desikan et al., 2013). Healthcare organizations develop more sophisticated big data analytics capabilities, they are beginning to move from basic descriptive analytics towards the realm of predictive insights (Lindeman, 2018). Predictive analytics may only be the second of three steps along the journey to analytics maturity, but it actually represents a huge leap forward for many organizations. Instead of simply presenting information about past events to a user, predictive analytics

DOI: 10.4018/978-1-7998-1090-2.ch015

estimate the likelihood of a future outcome based on patterns in the historical data. This allows clinicians to receive alerts about potential events before they happen, and therefore make more informed choices about how to proceed with a decision. The importance of being one step ahead of events is most clearly seen in the realms of intensive care, surgery, or emergency care, where a patient's life might depend on a quick reaction time and a finely-tuned sense of when something is going wrong.

How and why are hospitals putting predictive analytics to work? The goal is often to improve operational efficiency or to proactively provide services that prevent greater problems and spending. Many hospitals have started with applications aimed at reducing readmissions and predicting which patients are at risk of developing sepsis. Other common use cases focus on optimizing staffing and resources. These following examples show how predictive analytics helps hospitals leverage their past data to learn what is likely to happen in the future, identify actionable insights, and intervene to reduce costs. These interventions often directly improve patient care and operational efficiencies

LITERATURE REVIEW

Operating Room Bottlenecks

The University of Chicago Medical Center (UCMC) (2017) used predictive analytics to tackle the problem of operating room delays. Such delays are aggravating for clinicians, patients, and families and they are wasteful since ORs are expensive to run. But delays are hard to prevent, with so many individuals and teams working on each surgical case. When one procedure ends, there is a sequence of certain tasks that must be completed before the next surgery can start.

UCMC combined real-time data with a complex-event processing algorithm to improve workflows, create notifications, and streamline the handoffs from one team to the next for each step of the OR process. The effort decreased turnover time 15% to 20% (four minutes per room), which was expected to save the hospital up to $600,000 annually. The new system also increased visibility into what was causing each delay and how to intervene in real time to get things back on track.

Newborn Antibiotics

Kaiser Permanente (2015) led the development of a risk calculator that has reduced the use of antibiotics in newborns. Antibiotics are necessary for a small percentage of newborns who are at risk for early onset neonatal sepsis, an infection that can lead to meningitis or death. Researchers developed a risk prediction model after drawing data from the EHRs of about 600,000 babies and their mothers. The approach better targets newborns who are at the highest risk for sepsis without exposing those at low risk to antibiotics. The effort safely reduced antibiotic use by nearly 50% in newborns delivered at Kaiser's Northern California birthing centers in 2015. It also allowed mothers and babies to stay together in the first few days. Kaiser makes the risk calculator available online.

Care Transitions After Knee and Hip Replacement

Cleveland Clinic (Gartner Research, 2017), feeling the pressures of fixed reimbursements and bundled payments, wanted to find ways to decrease the length of stay for patients receiving total hip and knee replacements. It focused on discharge delays. Often, these were caused by patients' unexpected need for post-acute rehabilitation in a skilled nursing facility. Researchers used analytics to predict which patients would recover successfully at home and which ones required inpatient rehab. The goal was not to prevent a rehab stay, but rather to better prepare for it.

Cleveland Clinic pulled on existing research and a validated prediction model, which drew on variables captured in the physician's office *prior* to surgery. The propensity score was put into the clinical workflow so all providers could use it in their preoperative discussions with patients. The program was successful at taking into account patients' needs, decreasing lengths of stay, driving down costs, and improving the system's patient experience scores in the HCAPHS Care Transition measures.

Patient Data Comes From Two Specific Sources

The data (Bigan, 2019) on which these predictions are built come from two main sources: clinical trials and real-world data gathered as patients receive treatment. Clinical trials are among the most important data sources regarding patient responses to medication, including data on improved outcomes and side-effect risk. These trials typically consist of as many as a thousand patients, and generate data that is very exhaustive, homogeneous (the same measurements are available for all patients), and with clearly defined end points. In point of fact, clinical trial data is the only data source for drugs not yet on the market. (This data is normally the sole property of the pharmaceutical company whose drug is being tested in the trial.)Real-world data is that which has been generated and collected in the field, usually after a drug has been taken off trial and is available to the general public. The data can range from claims or reimbursement data from health insurers to electronic medical records collected by healthcare providers such as private medical doctors or hospitals.

Compared to clinical trial data, data based on real-world evidence is generally available for many more patients, thus providing information on the effectiveness of a drug across the general population. Unlike homogenous clinical trial data, real-world evidence is typically heterogeneous, since not all patients see a doctor at the same time and patient profiles are more diverse than in clinical trial settings. Real-world data also provides more longitudinal information because the patient information can be captured over a longer time span than the typical duration of a clinical trial and does not contain clearly defined end points.

The Power of Combining Data Sources

While relevant analytics (Bigan, 2019) can be implemented using only claims data from payers, more robust data sources that combine claims data with real-world clinical information, such as electronic health records, are richer and may lead to better predictive models. It is possible, for example, to infer a patient's medical status using information based on the drugs they have been prescribed or the physicians who have treated them. A more precise picture, however, can be created when that information is combined with the results of blood tests or other diagnostic tools.

These more precise patient models can then be leveraged to map and predict more general patient journeys. For example, major categories (clusters) of disease-progression trajectories and care pathways can be extracted from the data, and advanced modeling techniques can be devised to predict future patient trajectories as a function of the chosen treatment option. Such models can be used to determine the best therapeutic option at any point in time for a given patient. The challenge is often gaining access to this real-world patient information.

Accessing Real-World Data Can Be a Challenge

Some vendors, especially those serving patients in the United States, sell access to real-world data such as claims, integrated claims or electronic medical records. In some countries and under specific conditions, national payer systems that cover consumption of any medical services, or national registries that cover specific disease areas such as cancer, may make their data available.

Broadly speaking, access to commercial sources tends to be costlier, but usually comes without topical restrictions. While leading commercial sources cover primarily U.S. patients, clinical aspects of a disease derived from these patients can often be transposed to other regions such as Europe, taking into account any differences in clinical practices. Access to European national payer systems may be free or at a minimal cost to reimburse the system for any specific data-preparation expenses, but the institution may limit the ways in which the data can be used for analysis, and it may take longer to access the data. Gaining access to data from the French national payer system, for example, can take as long as six months.

Another limitation (Bigan, 2019) is that, typically, national payer systems cover claims data only. Legislative steps have been taken in some countries to extend coverage to electronic health records, but this process will likely take several years to complete. Fortunately, access to clinical data for very specific disease areas (e.g. cancer) is possible today through dedicated national registries. Real-world evidence can also be accessed by working with a targeted payer or healthcare provider to carry out joint projects.

The Right Fuel for Machine Learning

Clinical trial data lends itself particularly well to artificial intelligence and machine learning because the data usually includes a clear baseline comprised of information collected before treatment initiation, clear outcomes based on measurements during or at the end of the clinical trial and clearly defined end points. To use real-world evidence as a basis for machine learning (Bigan, 2019), however, it is often necessary to reconstruct end points from the longitudinal data. For example, treatment success or failure will not be codified as such in the data: It must be inferred, such as from laboratory data or subsequent treatments or procedures. The advantage of this real-world evidence is that it presents a diversity of patient profiles and prescription patterns that cannot be matched by clinical studies. As such, real-world evidence uniquely enables patient-journey and disease-progression mapping.

Using either clinical trial data or real-world evidence, it is possible to build as many as a hundred or more baseline patient characteristics before the start of treatment, or at a given stage of a disease. These features can include laboratory measurements such as blood and urine tests and genotyping information, concomitant medication, medical history and demographic information. If a given outcome is to be predicted, recursive feature elimination can then be used to determine an optimum feature set, which typically consists of ten or fewer features. Compared to classical statistical analysis, machine learning based on this kind of rich data can make possible highly multi-dimensional multivariate analyses that leverage sophisticated algorithms such as random-forest or gradient-boosted decision trees.

FUTURE DIRECTIONS

Keeping Real-World Practitioners in the Equation

Realizing the full potential of advanced analytics for healthcare applications usually requires going beyond mere predictive models and changing the operating models themselves. To do so, a number of challenges must be addressed. For one, when healthcare practitioners are presented with predictive models, they often display a greater interest in the nature of predictors themselves than in the actual model performance. Before they are willing to adopt a model, practitioners must be convinced that both the predictors—and the way the algorithms use the predictors to arrive at a prediction—make medical sense.

Some medical doctors suggest that algorithms should be so simple that they can be remembered by practitioners. The use of simple decision trees may seem like the best path to communicate the logic behind these models. However, the performance of standard simple decision-tree algorithms, such as CART, is generally insufficient. For this reason, the development of predictive models [12] for healthcare applications usually proceeds into two phases:

Phase One: The best model—the one with the maximum predictive power—is developed.
Phase Two: This optimum model is then translated into simpler, interpretable, actionable tools that comes with a limited number of predictors. An example of such a tool is a fixed-structure decision tree with optimized cutoff values.

Data Alone Not Enough to Inform Medical Decisions

Stakeholders across the healthcare ecosystem are increasing their use of machine learning and artificial intelligence to benefit individual patients and the healthcare ecosystem as a whole. Generalized access to future data sources such as whole-genome sequencing data (Bigan, 2019) and data from personal connected devices such as medical monitoring devices and smartphones will further expand the potential of advanced analytics for healthcare.

At the same time, and no matter what the application, using predictive models to assist in medical decision-making requires the creation of stringent performance requirements. For example, the inclusion of false positives (patients for whom the model falsely predicts disease progression) should be minimized when predicting disease progression, and a specific process must be envisioned to deal with false positives. Such a process might include the addition of medical exams to rule out these false results.

Conversely, when predicting potentially harmful side effects, false negatives (patients for whom the model falsely predicts that they are safe) should be minimized, with attention paid to the background incidence rate of such events in the general population.

The combination of expanding data sources and increasingly sophisticated predictive modeling bodes well for improved patient outcomes and increases in efficiency throughout the healthcare ecosystem. The challenge will come in identifying and accessing the appropriate data sets on which to base these models. Steps must also be taken to make healthcare practitioners both understand the medical sense behind the models and are able to play an ongoing role in providing a real-world check on how the models are applied to actual patients.

Scope of IoT in Health Care

The IoT allows people and things to be connected in terms of time, place, people, network and service (International Telecommunication Union, 2005). The main contributor for the IoT can be attributed to the growth of smart phones and tablets. These mobile devices act as a window to the IoT world. They have the capabilities to perform the wide variety of tasks for the patient & doctors, in addition to providing mobility and connectivity. The mobile revolution is pushing the connectivity of other physical objects seamlessly using the cloud storage. As more and more devices are connecting and communicating with each other, huge volume of data is exchanged. This explosion of data needs to be stored, analyzed with complex data analytic techniques to provide the necessary information for both the patient and doctor. However, in the current trend, only the medical devices within the hospital infrastructure are connected within themselves and this network provides access through medical apps available to the clinicians.

The Internet of Things is a technological platform with widespread mass appeal. It has become popular in all industry segments due to its speed of development, complexity, global reach and novelty. Internet of Things offers a lot of promises in the field of healthcare by increasing efficiency, improving patient care and lowering costs. According to an interesting report from MarketResearch.com, the Healthcare Internet of Things market segment is expected to hit the $117 billion mark by 2020. Some of the methods in which Internet of Things is transforming the healthcare industry are:

- Decreasing Device Downtime through Remote Monitoring & Support – One of the major advantages of this technological innovation is the ability for an IoT device to be tested and diagnosed remotely. For example, a specialist can connect from his own office and run diagnostics on an MRI that has failed. He can identify the root cause and remotely connect to the hospital's technicians to provide hands-on-support. Such interventions in hospitals largely help to lessen medical equipment's idle time and augments systems efficiency.
- Maintaining a Warehouse of Patient Related Data – It is essential for healthcare institutions to maintain and update a database of health-related inferred by or from patients. The Internet of Things enables hospitals to track, monitor and update patient information in a systematic manner. This patient related data could include reported outcomes, medical-device data, and wearables data. Computational methods of analytical support, known as augmented intelligence, are collectively used to analyze information. This type of an enriched database largely assists healthcare professionals in better decision making and providing superior patient care.
- Proactive Replenishment of Supplies– Internet of Things ensures better inventory management in hospitals and healthcare organizations. An IoT-connected medical device can send signals when critical operational components are being depleted. For example, the helium levels in an MRI machine need to be constantly checked to ensure that the equipment operates in a suitable manner. By using IoT-connected devices, field engineers can be sent out to a hospital before an MRI's helium levels dwindle, preventing a total machine stoppage and patient rescheduling. Hence, this technology creates a system of real-time monitoring, tracking and immediate response. Any kind of asset depletion triggers emergency alarms and efforts are made for a rapid replenishment.
- Optimal Utilization of Assets and Operations – Healthcare institutions need to ensure optimum utilization of resources to maximize patient care to the fullest of their abilities. Internet of Things aids in efficient timely scheduling by leveraging utilization to serve a greater number of patients. Cloud based scheduling applications can ensure that machines, hospital staff and infrastructure

is being utilized to its fullest capacity. Microcontrollers that process and wirelessly communicate data can schedule maintenance activities, patient calls and perform inventory management functions. An IoT medical device can provide daily machine utilization statistics that can be employed for well-organized patient scheduling.

ROLE OF IOT IN HEALTHCARE PREDICTIVE MODELING

This is not exactly a secret that healthcare (Xtelligent, n.d.) suffers from a lack of seamless, large-scale health data interoperability. With the ONC(Office of the National Coordinator for Health Information Technology) frowning on vendors that actively block health information exchange, and a concerted industry effort to make data a more accessible asset for a larger number of healthcare organizations, the spirit of interoperability will open up new opportunities for healthcare big data analytics.

The problem is that EHRs contain a relatively limited proportion of the data that could be useful for generating actionable insights. Allergy lists, vital signs, and demographics are all very well, but patients are demanding more nimble reactions and deeper relationships from their providers. Clinical data is where the most successful hospitals start their analytics problems, but to deliver a higher level of consumer satisfaction, providers must know a lot more about their patients and their needs than the EHR (Electronic Health Record) can tell.

The IoT can provide that data, if healthcare organizations build the infrastructure to accept it. Many providers have been able to integrate financial and utilization data to create a portrait of organizational operations, but these sources do not give a clear idea of what patients do on their own time.

The answer is in their devices. Few patients are ever more than arm's length away from their smartphones. They will wear their FitBits or new Apple Watches everywhere; they may have daily interaction with smart pill bottles, food intake apps, sleep monitors, and blood pressure cuffs. These ubiquitous tools are becoming popular with patients who expect simplicity and smarts from their daily interactions with electronic tools, and they are important for tracking how patients behave while healthcare providers aren't looking. Harnessing this data can give savvy organizations an edge when it comes to population health management.

Automated patient-generated data collection systems (Xtelligent, n.d.) will stream data directly into the provider's repository of choice. Once architected, they require little to no action on the part of the patient or the clinician, but simply produce reports that can be analyzed or tracked when necessary. While developing this type of automation can be a difficult task that requires some careful negotiation around physician workflows, researchers and leading organizations have seen success from mining social media data and wearable devices through algorithms that predict behaviors and allow providers a leg up on allocating resources or preempting poor patient choices.

As population health management takes on a greater financial significance and patient-centered care is rewarded with bonuses and incentives, healthcare big data analytics can't afford to ignore these devices as a rich source of pertinent information.

RECENT PREDICTIVE MODELS IN HEALTHCARE

Predictive modeling (Ben, 2018) is at a nascent stage when it comes to healthcare delivery. Although the industry has made enormous strides in the last several years such as better anticipating outcomes among high-risk patient populations healthcare providers' ability to act on the intelligence in a disciplined, rational, risk-adjusted manner still needs to be further developed. That's where applied innovation comes in.

Going forward, advances in healthcare information technology must be designed to help clinically integrated networks manage large, complex patient populations. The goal should be to progress toward a future state where applied machine learning and artificial intelligence will empower physicians, health systems, payers and patients to anticipate challenges, improve outcomes and reduce costs.

Research Becoming Reality

Considerable headway has been made in the last several years, as health systems have begun examining ways to apply predictive modeling techniques to practice.

- For example, some clinically integrated networks are now able to accurately predict potential re-admissions across patient populations of varying risk levels.
- Others are capable of calculating potential savings or losses on overall spend based on historical financial data.

In the age of value-based reimbursement, these are the types of clinical and financial forecasts that organizations must be able to generate and easily interpret on their own.

Much more is on the way, particularly concerning individualized care. Preventive medicine, for instance, could be improved with predictive models that help make diagnoses more accurate and treatment regimens more precise. Genetic predictive modeling research promises to take preventive medicine a step further by helping providers intervene for conditions that have not yet advanced to the point where symptoms have emerged. By tailoring healthcare in this way, providers and payers can help reduce the 20% of care costs wasted every year, (CNBC, 2017) while also improving clinical outcomes and treatment adherence.

NEED FOR IMPROVING HEALTH LITERACY

From a patient-facing perspective (Ben, 2018), the future of analytics may also include leveraging predictive modeling to improve health literacy. A huge number of data sets and analytical models already exist. These instruments could be combined with patient-contributed data to help predict and fill patients' clinical knowledge gaps. That way, patients could more confidently manage their own health and make healthier choices on their own.

Likewise, payers could support this patient engagement by developing algorithms that deliver accurate coverage and cost estimates to patients before they undergo treatments. Comparing affordable, high-quality providers should not only help reduce spending, but also encourage greater efficiency among healthcare organizations that want to stay competitive in their markets.

Vippalapalli and Ananthula (2016) proposed is an economically feasible patient healthcare monitoring system model based on lightweight and affordable wearable sensors in the market. These sensing nodes are established for diagnosis and prevention of diseases using the healthcare data of patients. The devices are designed to be able to collect and share the gathered data among themselves thereby facilitating information analysis and storage. This also eradicates manual inefficiencies in the process. Audrino based wearable device with Body Sensor Networks is proposed for collecting data from the patients. This is combined with "Labview" to offer remote monitoring service.

Mohammad-Parsa Hosseini et al (2017) research work emphases on finding characteristics from a Brain Computer Interface with various sensors like electroencephalography (EEG) and resting state-functional magnetic resonance imaging (rs-fMRI) along with Diffusion Tensor Imaging for data collection from an epileptic brain. The proposed system utilized edge computing methods to provide a context aware real-time solution using invasive as well as noninvasive techniques for monitoring, evaluating and regulating an epileptic brain. This enables detection as well as confirms prompt medical care (surgical or otherwise) in case of incident of an epilepsy seizure. The main goal of this research is to be able to predict an "ictal onset"

Kirtana et al & Lokeswari (2017) proposed a Heart Rate Variability (HRV) measures variation in time interval between consecutive heart beats. HRVanalysis can identify cardiovascular diseases, Diabetic Mellitus, disease states associated with Autonomic Dysrhythmia like Hypertension and different chronic degenerative medical conditions. Observing HRV data will aid detection of such diseases. In this research work, the authors recommended a low-cost and easy to use Remote HRV Monitoring System based on Internet of Things (IoT) technology for Hypertensive patients. In this proposal, HRV parameters are calculated based on the data retrieved using Wireless Zigbee based pulse sensor. This Arduino based systems communicates the data retrieved from monitoring the patient to a backend server using MQTT an IOT protocol. The application server gathers HRV data and visualizes it through various graphs.

Pinto, Cabral, and Gomes (2017) due to a rise in the population of the elderly across the world there needs a growing requirement to provide solutions that provide living assistance to the aged population. In this aspect the Internet of Things is playing vital role in providing a new feature to contemporary healthcare by providing a more personalized, preventive and collaborative form of treatment. This research work presents a living assistance based IoT technology for the elderly that can monitor and register patient's vital requirement as well as provide automatic trigger for alarms in emergency situations. The research work is proposed a solution comprising a wrist band that can connect to the cloud server to monitor and assist elderly people. It claims to be low power/cost solution with Wireless communication capabilities

One Predictive Model Covers All the Bases

While it would be nice if there was "one predictive model to rule them all" (Bradley, 2018) so to speak, that is not the case. Different algorithms will produce different results from the same data, so it's possible that even a well-constructed predictive model will miss certain patterns that become obvious to another. The best approach is to build several predictive models based on different algorithms and run them in parallel to one another. As with any good Venn diagram, the point where all of the models intersect will have the highest probability of being accurate, and thus should be prioritized for attention. Then comes the points where almost all intersect, and so on. This method also help reduce the time spent chasing false positives.

Predictive Modeling Is Only for Large Healthcare Organizations

Predictive modeling is new and requires the construction of complex algorithms (Bradley, 2018), there can be a tendency to think predictive modeling will only work in a large hospital or health system. The reality is that it's just as effective for small-to-mid-size providers. Perhaps more so since they have less margin for error in their financials.

The determinant isn't the size of your organization; it's whether your organization has collected enough historical data to build accurate predictive models and test them to ensure a high degree of reliability. A good rule of thumb is as long as your organization has been collecting data for more than a year, you have the raw materials to look for patterns and trends.

THE TOOLS TO OVERCOME PRACTICAL CHALLENGES

The challenge facing providers today is a practical one: Predictive modeling (Ben, 2018) requires strong data infrastructure, user engagement, staffing and other resources. Yet I believe applied machine learning and artificial intelligence can pave the way for more robust, mainstream predictive models in healthcare.

As algorithms and software tools grow more sophisticated, technology can do the heavy lifting by sorting through vast amounts of data to derive the intelligent insights needed to drive better care decisions and outcomes. Other practical benefits should include:

- Reduction of labor costs and faster data capture for provider organizations
- More effective real-time health monitoring and
- Improved care experience and outcomes for patients. We're not there yet, but we're getting closer to applying predictive modeling principles to everyday care delivery.

When predictive modeling does become more ubiquitous across clinically integrated networks, we are sure to witness clinical and financial performance breakthroughs unlike we have ever seen before.

CONCLUSION

Predictive modeling will really become valuable to healthcare in what's known as the internet of things (IoT) or in this case the IoT of healthcare. For healthcare, any device that generates data about a person's health and sends that data into the cloud (Biotaware, n.d.) will be part of this IoT. Wearables are perhaps the most familiar example of such a device.

In order to get value from the connected digital health environment i.e. IoT, it is important to have a platform on which to create and manage applications, to run analytics, and to receive, store and secure your data. Like an operating system for a laptop, a platform does a lot of things in the background that makes life easier and less expensive for developers, stakeholders, users and you.

The term "connected health" is the term used to described how healthcare is connecting in the digital health industry. A connected health system will maximize healthcare resources and provide increased, flexible opportunities for consumers to engage with clinicians and vice versa to better self-manage their care in the digital health industry. A platform is vital in a connected health system for the digital health industry.

Health information systems (Biotaware, n.d.) show great potential in improving the efficiency in the delivery of care, a reduction in overall costs to the health care system, as well as a marked increase in patient outcomes. With the implementation of this legislation as well as the technologies associated with it, it is imperative to effectively organize and process the ever-increasing quantity of data that is digitally collected and stored within health care organizations.

The paradigm shift of reactive medicine to Proactive and preventive medicine is mainly inspired by economic constraints such as the rising cost of healthcare, as well as continued improvements to the quality of life and long life. Conferring to the Center for Medicare and Medicaid Services(CMS), the cost of medical care in the US in 2016 reached up to 3.6 trillion dollars per year and is expected to increase up to $5.5 trillion by 2025 (Biotaware, n.d.).On the other hand, the global smart healthcare industry is expected to reach $169.30 billion by 2020. It is projected that by 2019, 87% of the healthcare organizations in the US will have adopted IoT technology (Linda, 2017), of which 73% will be used to reduce cost, and 64% will be put to monitor patients.

REFERENCES

Biotaware. (n.d.). *Healthcare Data and Insights Simplified*. Retrieved from https://www.biotaware.com/

Bradley. (2018). Misconceptions about predictive modeling in healthcare. Academic Press.

CNBC. (2017). *Shocking truth: 20% of healthcare expenditures wasted in US and other nations*. CNBC.

Desikan, P., Khare, R., Srivastava, J., Kaplan, R., Ghosh, J., Liu, L., & Gopal, V. (2013). *Predictive Modeling in Healthcare: Challenges and Opportunities. IEEE Life Sciences News Letter*.

ErwanBigan. (2019). *Ground Predictive Healthcare Models in Real-World Medical Dataand in Real World Medical Practice*. Author.

Gartner Research. (2017). *Predictive Algorithms that Healthcare Delivery Organizations Are Using to Improve Outcomes*. Author.

Hosseini, M. P., Tran, T. X., Pompili, D., Elisevich, K., & Soltanian-Zadeh, H. (2017). Deep Learning With Edge Computing for Localization of Epileptogenicity Using Multimodal rs-fMRI and EEG Big Data. *IEEE International Conference on Autonomic Computing*.

International Telecommunication Union. (2005). *The Internet of Things*. Retrieved from http://www.itu.int/osg/spu/publications/internetofthings/InternetofThings_summary.pdf

Kaiser Permanente, Sepsis. (2015). Risk Prediction Model Decreases Use of Antibiotics in Newborns. Author.

Kirtana, R. N., & Lokeswari, Y. V. (2017). An IoT Based Remote HRV Monitoring System for Hypertensive Patients. *IEEE International Conference on Computer, Communication, and Signal Processing*. 10.1109/ICCCSP.2017.7944086

Linda. (2016). *10 Smart Medical Devices That Are Changing HealthCare.* Retrieved from http://www.appcessories.co.uk/connected-smart-medical-devices-that-are-changing-healthcare/

Lindeman, T. (2018). *How hospitals are using predictive analytics.* Academic Press.

Pinto, S., Cabral, J., & Gomes, T. (2017). *We-Care: An IoT-based Health Care System for Elderly People.* IEEE.

Pranam Ben. (2018). Retrieved from www.predictivemodelingnews.com

Vippalapalli, V., & Ananthula, S. (2016). Internet of things (IoT) based smart health care System. *International conference on Signal Processing, Communication, Power and Embedded System (SCOPES),* 1229 – 1233. 10.1109/SCOPES.2016.7955637

Xtelligent. (n.d.). *Healthcare Media Health IT Analytics.* Retrieved from http://www.xtelligentmedia.com/network/HealthITAnalytics

Conclusion

The healthcare domain is still in a state of great distress as the healthcare services are getting costlier than ever. The essential healthcare services would become out of reach to many people and a huge section of society would be prone to chronic diseases. The fact is, technology cannot prevent the population from aging and chronic diseases but it can make the healthcare services more accessible. Disease diagnosis constitutes a great portion of hospital expense whereas a technological revolution can change the medical check-up routine from hospital-centric to patient-centric. Internet of Things (IoT) is a new paradigm which has extensive applicability in vast areas including healthcare. The discharging potentiality of IoT in the healthcare area allows the hospitals to function more effectively and patients get better treatment. This technology could drastically enhance the quality and efficiency of healthcare services. IoT technology has evolved dramatically with the assorted number of wearable's, sensors and handy devices for monitoring the health status. Some of the benefits are:

❖ **Real-time reporting and monitoring**
❖ **End-to-end connectivity and affordability**
❖ **Dynamic data assortment and analysis**
❖ **Patient tracking and alerting**
❖ **Remote medical assistance**

Healthcare IoT is an important area of research because this technology allows us to gather a huge amount of data from patients using non-invasive approaches that would have consumed many years had the data been collected manually. The gathered data can be used for statistical analysis which will support medical research. IoT has an immense impact on medical research and facilitates wide and better treatments.

Incorporating the Internet of Things in Healthcare Applications and Wearable Devices is an essential requirement for building smart healthcare systems. This book addresses how IoT improves the proficiency of healthcare with respect to wireless sensor networks. Delving on topics like sensor integration, and data analytics, this book is ideally designed for computer scientists, bioinformatics analysts, doctors, nurses, hospital executives, medical students, IT specialists, software developers, computer engineers, industry professionals, academicians, researchers, and students seeking current research on how these emerging wireless technologies improve efficiency within the healthcare domain. The book will be relevant to all those involved in the prerequisite and delivery of technology-based healthcare.

P. B. Pankajavalli
Bharathiar University, India

G. S. Karthick
Bharathiar University, India

Compilation of References

5V. Power Supply using 7805 Voltage Regulator with Design. (2013, May 16). Retrieved from https://electrosome.com/power-supply-design-5v-7805-voltage-regulator/

Abawajy, J. H., & Hassan, M. M. (2017). Federated internet of things and cloud computing pervasive patient health monitoring system. *IEEE Communications Magazine*, *55*(1), 48–53. doi:10.1109/MCOM.2017.1600374CM

Abdi, H., & Williams, L. J. (2010). Principal component analysis. *Wiley Interdisciplinary Reviews: Computational Statistics*, *2*(4), 433–459. doi:10.1002/wics.101

Abdulkadir, A., Yunusa, G., Tabari, A., Anas, I., Ojo, J., Akinlade, B., ... & Uyobong, I. (2011). Medical record system in Nigeria: Observations from multicentre auditing of radiographic requests and patients' information documentation practices. *J. Med. Med. Sci.*, *2*(5), 854–858.

Abedalmotaleb, Z., & Thomas, F. (2016). Neighborhood-based interference minimization for stable position-based routing in mobile ad hoc networks. *Future Generation Computer Systems*, *64*, 88–97. doi:10.1016/j.future.2016.03.022

Abodunrin, A. L., & Akande, T. M. (2009). Knowledge and perception of e-health and telemedicine among health professionals in LAUTECH Teaching Hospital, Osogbo, Nigeria. *Int J Health Res.*, *2*(1), 51–58.

Adafruit. (2012, July 29). *Overview | TMP36 Temperature Sensor | Adafruit Learning System*. Retrieved from https://learn.adafruit.com/tmp36-temperature-sensor

Adafruit. (n.d.). *Adafruit 10-DOF IMU Breakout - L3GD20H + LSM303 + BMP180*. Retrieved from https://www.adafruit.com/products/1604

Adeleke, I. T., Adekanye, A. O., Adefemi, S. A., Onawola, K. A., Okuku, A. G., Sheshi, E. U., ... & Tume, A. A. (2011). Knowledge, attitude and practice of confidentiality of patients' health records among healthcare professionals at Federal Medical Centre, Bida. *Nigerian Journal of Medicine*, *20*(2), 228–235. PMID:21970234

Adeleke, I. T., Adekanye, A. O., Jibril, A. D., Danmallam, F. F., Inyinbor, H. E., & Omokanye, S. A. (2014). Research knowledge and behaviour of health workers at Federal Medical Centre, Bida: A task before learned mentors. *El Med J.*, *2*(2), 105–109. doi:10.18035/emj.v2i2.71

Adeleke, I. T., Adekanye, A. O., Onawola, K. A., Okuku, A. G., Adefemi, S. A., Erinle, S. A., & ... & AbdulGhaney, O. O. (2012). Data quality assessment in healthcare: A 365-day chart review of inpatients' health records at a Nigerian tertiary hospital. *Journal of the American Medical Informatics Association*, *19*, 1039–1042. doi:10.1136/amiajnl-2012-000823

Adeleke, I. T., Asiru, M. A., Oweghoro, B. M., Jimoh, A. B., & Ndana, A. M. (2015). Computer and internet use among tertiary healthcare providers and trainees in a Nigerian public hospital. *American Journal of Health Research*, *3*(1), 1–10. doi:10.11648/j.ajhr.s.2015030101.11

Adeleke, I. T., Erinle, S. A., Ndana, A. M., Anaman, T. C., Ogundele, O. A., & Aliyu, D. (2015). Health information technology in Nigeria: Stakeholders' perspectives of nationwide implementations and meaningful use of the emerging technology in the most populous black nation. *American Journal of Health Research, 3*(1), 17–24. doi:10.11648/j.ajhr.s.2015030101.13

Adeleke, I. T., Ezike, S. O., Ogundele, O. A., & Ibraheem, S. O. (2015). Freedom of information act and concerns over medical confidentiality among healthcare providers in Nigeria. *IMAN Medical Journal, 1*(1), 21–28.

Adeleke, I. T., Lawal, A. H., Adio, R. A., & Adebisi, A. A. (2014). Information technology skills and training needs of health information management professionals in Nigeria: A nationwide study. *The HIM Journal, 44*(1), 1–9. doi:10.12826/18333575 PMID:27092467

Adeleke, I. T., Salami, A. A., Achinbee, M., Anama, T. C., Zakari, I. B., & Wasagi, M. H. (2015). ICT knowledge, utilization and perception among healthcare providers at National Hospital Abuja, Nigeria. *American Journal of Health Research., 3*(1), 1–10. doi:10.11648/j.ajhr.s.2015030101.17

Adeleke, I. T., Suleiman-Abdul, Q. B., Aliyu, A., Ishaq, I. A., & Adio, R. A. (2018, Sept. 20). Deploying unqualified personnel in health records practice – role substitution or quackery? Implications for health services delivery in Nigeria. [Epub ahead of print]. *Health Information Management.* doi:10.1177/1833358318800459 PMID:30235948

Adelina, M., Sotiris, N., & Alexandros, A. V. (2019). Adaptive wireless power transfer in mobile ad hoc networks. *Computer Networks, 152*, 87–97. doi:10.1016/j.comnet.2019.02.004

Ahmed, F. (2017). An internet of things (IoT) Application for Predicting the Quantity of Future Heart Attack Patients. *International Journal of Computers and Applications, 164*(6), 36–40. doi:10.5120/ijca2017913773

Ahmed, I. S., Samah, A. G., & Khaled, M. (2017). A Reliable Routing Protocol for Vehicular Ad hoc Networks. *Computers & Electrical Engineering, 64*, 473–495. doi:10.1016/j.compeleceng.2016.11.011

Ahuja, S. P., Mani, S., & Zambrano, J. (2012). A survey of the state of cloud computing in healthcare. *Network and Communication Technologies, 1*(2), 12.

Ajay, K. Y., Santosh, K. D., & Sachin, T. (2017). EFMMRP: Design of efficient fuzzy based multi-constraint multicast routing protocol for wireless ad-hoc network. *Computer Networks, 118*, 15–23. doi:10.1016/j.comnet.2017.03.001

Akyildiz, I. F., Su, W., Sankarasubramaniam, Y., & Cayirci, E. (2002). Wireless sensor networks: A survey. *Computer Networks, 38*(4), 393–422. doi:10.1016/S1389-1286(01)00302-4

Al Ameen, M., Liu, J., & Kwak, K. (2012). Security and privacy issues in wireless sensor networks for healthcare applications. *Journal of Medical Systems, 36*(1), 93–101. doi:10.100710916-010-9449-4 PMID:20703745

AlaaEisa, M., AbdElrazik, S., Hazem El-Bakry, M., Sajjadhasan, M., AsaadHasan, Q., & Samir Zaid, Q. (2016, December). Challenges in Wireless Sensor Networks. In 2016 International Journal of Advanced Research in Computer Science & Technology (IJARCST 2016) (pp. 22-27).

Alemdar, H., & Ersoy, C. (2010). Wireless sensor networks for healthcare: A survey. *Computer Networks, 54*(15), 2688–2710. doi:10.1016/j.comnet.2010.05.003

Al-Fuqaha, A., Guizani, M., Mohammadi, M., Aledhari, M., & Ayyash, M. (2015). Internet of things: A survey on enabling technologies, protocols, and applications. *IEEE Communications Surveys and Tutorials, 17*(4), 2347–2376. doi:10.1109/COMST.2015.2444095

Ali, N., & Abu-Elkheir, M. (2012). Data management for the internet of things: Green directions. In *Proc. IEEE Globecom Workshops*, pp. 386–390. 10.1109/GLOCOMW.2012.6477602

Ali, O., Shrestha, A., Soar, J., & Wamba, S. F. (2018). Cloud computing-enabled healthcare opportunities, issues, and applications: A systematic review. *International Journal of Information Management, 43*, 146–158. doi:10.1016/j.ijinfomgt.2018.07.009

Ali, O., Soar, J., & Shrestha, A. (2018). Perceived potential for value creation from cloud computing: A study of the Australian regional government sector. *Behaviour & Information Technology, 37*(12), 1157–1176. doi:10.1080/0144929X.2018.1488991

Aliyu, D., Adeleke, I. T., Omoniyi, S. O., Samaila, B. A., Adamu, A., & Abubakar, A. Y. (2015). Knowledge, attitude and practice of nursing ethics and law among nurses at Federal Medical Centre, Bida. *American Journal of Health Research, 3*(1), 32–37. doi:10.11648/j.ajhr.s.2015030101.15

Al-Majeed, S. S., Al-Mejibli, I. S., & Karam, J. (2015). Home Telehealth by internet of things (IoT). *Proc. Canadian Conference on Electrical and Computer Engineering.* 10.1109/CCECE.2015.7129344

Almulhim, M. & Zaman, N. (2018). Proposing Secure and Lightweight Authentication Scheme for IoT Based E-Health Applications. In *20th IEEE International Conference on Advance Communication Technology ICACT* 2018.

Alotaibi, M. (2018). *An Enhanced Symmetric Cryptosystem and Biometric-Based Anonymous User Authentication and Session Key Establishment Scheme for WSN.* Piscataway, NJ: IEEE.

Alper, B., Muharrem, T., & Burcu, Y. (2019). P-AUV: Position aware routing and medium access for ad hoc AUV networks. *Journal of Network and Computer Applications, 125*, 146–154. doi:10.1016/j.jnca.2018.10.014

Alsmirat, M. A., Jararweh, Y., Obaidat, I., & Gupta, B. B. (2016). Internet of surveillance: A cloud supported large-scale wireless surveillance system. J Supercomput. 1;73(3):973-992. doi:10.100711227-016-1857-x

Amendola, S., Lodato, R., Manzari, S., Occhiuzzi, C., & Marrocco, G. (2014). RFID technology for IoT-based personal healthcare in smart spaces. IEEE Internet of things Journal, 1(2), 144-152.

Amini, A., Saboohi, H., Ying Wah, T., & Herawan, T. (2014). A fast density-based clustering algorithm for real-time Internet of things stream. *The Scientific World Journal.* doi:10.1155/2014/926020

Aminian, M., & Naji, H. R. (2013). A hospital healthcare monitoring system using wireless sensor networks. *J. Health Med. Inform, 4*(02), 121. doi:10.4172/2157-7420.1000121

Amin, S. U., Hossain, M. S., Muhammad, G., Alhussein, M., & Rahman, M. A. (2019). Cognitive Smart Healthcare for Pathology Detection and Monitoring. *IEEE Access: Practical Innovations, Open Solutions, 7*, 10745–10753. doi:10.1109/ACCESS.2019.2891390

Amna, A. (2015). Real Time Wireless Health Monitoring Application using mobile devices. [IJCNC]. *International Journal of Computer Networks & Communications, 7*(3), 13–30. doi:10.5121/ijcnc.2015.7302

Anwar, M., Abdullah, A. H., Qureshi, K. N., & Majid, A. H. (2017). Wireless body area networks for healthcare applications: An overview. *Telkomnika, 15*(3), 1088–1095. doi:10.12928/telkomnika.v15i3.5793

Appari, A., & Johnson, M. E. (2010). Information security and privacy in healthcare: Current state of research. *Int. J. Internet and Enterprise Management, 6*(4), 279–314. doi:10.1504/IJIEM.2010.035624

Arduino. (n.d.). *Arduino - Genuino 101 CurieBLE Heart Rate Monitor.* Retrieved from https://www.arduino.cc/en/Tutorial/Genuino101CurieBLEHeartRateMonitor

Arduino. (n.d.). *Arduino.* Retrieved from https://www.arduino.cc/

Arduino. (n.d.). *ArduinoBoardLilyPad.* Retrieved from https://www.arduino.cc/en/Main/ArduinoBoardLilyPad/

Arduino. (n.d.). *Genuino 101*. Retrieved from https://store.arduino.cc/product/GBX00005

Atzori, L., Iera, A., & Morabito, G. (2010). The internet of things: A survey. *Computer Networks*, *54*(15), 2787–2805. doi:10.1016/j.comnet.2010.05.010

Azimi, I., Rahmani, A. M., Liljeberg, P., & Tenhunen, H. (2017). Internet of things for remote elderly monitoring: A study from user-centered perspective. *Journal of Ambient Intelligence and Humanized Computing*, *8*(2), 273–289. doi:10.100712652-016-0387-y

Bach, F. R., & Jordan, M. I. (2002). Kernel independent component analysis. *Journal of Machine Learning Research*, *3*(Jul), 1–48.

Barfield, W. (2015). *Fundamentals of wearable computers and augmented reality*. Boca Raton, FL: CRC Press. doi:10.1201/b18703

Barjis, J., Kolfschoten, G., & Maritz, J. (2013). A sustainable and affordable support system for rural healthcare delivery. *Decision Support Systems*, *56*, 223–233. doi:10.1016/j.dss.2013.06.005

Barnaghi, P. M., Bermudez-Edo, M., & Tönjes, R. (2015). Challenges for Quality of Data in Smart Cities. *J. Data and Information Quality*, *6*(2-3), 6–1.

Barson, R. (2016, January). Non-invasive device could end daily finger pricking for people with diabetes.

Barth, A. T., Hanson, M. A., Powell, H. C. Jr, & Lach, J. (2009, June). TEMPO 3.1: A body area sensor network platform for continuous movement assessment. In *2009 Sixth International Workshop on Wearable and Implantable Body Sensor Networks* (pp. 71-76). Piscataway, NJ: IEEE. 10.1109/BSN.2009.39

Baswa, M., Karthik, R., Natarajan, P. B., Jyothi, K., & Annapurna, B. (2017, December). Patient health management system using e-health monitoring architecture. In *2017 International Conference on Intelligent Sustainable Systems (ICISS)* (pp. 1120-1124). Piscataway, NJ: IEEE. 10.1109/ISS1.2017.8389356

Bazzani, M., Conzon, D., Scalera, A., Spirito, M. A., & Trainito, C. I. (2012, June). Enabling the IoT paradigm in e-health solutions through the VIRTUS middleware. In *2012 IEEE 11th International Conference on Trust, Security and Privacy in Computing and Communications (TrustCom)*, (pp. 1954-1959). Piscataway, NJ: IEEE. 10.1109/TrustCom.2012.144

BeginnerTopro. (2017, June 30). How to make a 12V to 5V Converter using 7805 IC. Retrieved from https://www.youtube.com/watch?v=8jzOirylcKgza

Bello, I. S., Arogundade, F. A., Sanusi, A. A., Ezeoma, I. T., Abioye-Kuteyi, E. A., & Akinsola, A. (2004). Knowledge and utilization of information technology among health care professionals and students in Ile-Ife, Nigeria: A Case Study of a University Teaching Hospital. *Journal of Medical Internet Research*, *6*(4), e45. doi:10.2196/jmir.6.4.e45 PMID:15631969

Benharref, A., & Serhani, M. A. (2014). Novel cloud and SOA-based framework for E-Health monitoring using wireless biosensors. *IEEE Journal of Biomedical and Health Informatics*, *18*(1), 46–55. doi:10.1109/JBHI.2013.2262659 PMID:24403403

Berte, D. R. (2018, May). Defining the IoT. In *Proceedings of the International Conference on Business Excellence* (Vol. 12, No. 1, pp. 118-128). Sciendo. 10.2478/picbe-2018-0013

Besant, J. D., Sargent, E. H., & Kelley, S. O. (2015). Rapid electrochemical phenotypic profiling of antibiotic-resistant bacteria. *Lab on a Chip*, *15*(13), 2799–2807.

Bethencourt, J., Sahai, A., & Waters, B. (2007, May). Ciphertext-policy attribute-based encryption. In 2007 IEEE symposium on security and privacy (SP'07) (pp. 321-334). Piscataway, NJ: IEEE.

Bhatia, D., Estevez, L., & Rao, S. (2007, August). Energy efficient contextual sensing for elderly care.In *2007 29th Annual International Conference of the IEEE Engineering in Medicine and Biology Society* (pp. 4052-4055). Piscataway, NJ: IEEE. 10.1109/IEMBS.2007.4353223

Bin, S., Yuan, L., & Xiaoyi, W. (2010, April). Research on data mining models for the internet of things. In 2010 *International Conference on Image Analysis and Signal Processing* (pp. 127-132). Piscataway, NJ: IEEE.

Biotaware. (n.d.). *Healthcare Data and Insights Simplified*. Retrieved from https://www.biotaware.com/

Birkler, J. & Dahl, M. R. (2014). Den digitala patienten. Stockholm, Sweden: Liber.

Bishop, C. M. (2006). Pattern recognition and machine learning. Berlin, Germany: Springer.

BITalino. (n.d.). *BITalino – Biomedical Equipment*. Retrieved from http://www.bitalino.com

Borgia, E. (2014). The Internet of Things vision: Key features, applications and open issues. *Computer Communications*, *54*, 1–31. doi:10.1016/j.comcom.2014.09.008

Boric-Lubecke, O., Gao, X., Yavari, E., Baboli, M., Singh, A., & Lubecke, V. M. (2014, June). E-healthcare: Remote monitoring, privacy, and security. In *2014 IEEE MTT-S International Microwave Symposium (IMS),* (pp. 1-3). Piscataway, NJ: IEEE.

Boulemtafes, A. & Badache, N. (2016). Wearable Health Monitoring Systems: An Overview of Design Research Areas. In mHealth Ecosystems and Social Networks in Healthcare (pp. 17-27). Cham, Switzerland: Springer.

Boulemtafes, A., Rachedi, A., & Badache, N. (2015, November). A study of mobility support in wearable health monitoring systems: Design framework. In *2015 IEEE/ACS 12th International Conference of Computer Systems and Applications (AICCSA)* (pp. 1-8). Piscataway, NJ: IEEE.

Bowman, B. R., & Schuck, E. (1995). *Medical instruments and devices used in the home*. The Biomedical Engineering Handbook.

Bradley. (2018). Misconceptions about predictive modeling in healthcare. Academic Press.

Breiman, L. (2017). Classification and regression trees. Abingdon-on-Thames, UK: Routledge. doi:10.1201/9781315139470

Breiman, L. (1996). Bagging predictors. *Machine Learning*, *24*(2), 123–140. doi:10.1007/BF00058655

Breiman, L. (2001). Random forests. *Machine Learning*, *45*(1), 5–32. doi:10.1023/A:1010933404324

Brickell, E., Camenisch, J., & Chen, L. (2004, October). Direct anonymous attestation. In *Proceedings of the 11th ACM conference on Computer and communications security* (pp. 132-145). ACM.

Bro, R., & Smilde, A. K. (2014). Principal component analysis. *Analytical Methods*, *6*(9), 2812–2831. doi:10.1039/C3AY41907J

Bui, F. M., & Hatzinakos, D. (2008). Biometric methods for secure communications in body sensor networks: Resource-efficient key management and signal-level data scrambling. *EURASIP Journal on Advances in Signal Processing*, 109.

Camenisch, J. (2004, September). Better privacy for trusted computing platforms. In *European Symposium on Research in Computer Security* (pp. 73-88). Springer.

Campello, R. J., Moulavi, D., & Sander, J. (2013, April). Density-based clustering based on hierarchical density estimates. In *Pacific-Asia conference on knowledge discovery and data mining* (pp. 160–172). Berlin, Germany: Springer. doi:10.1007/978-3-642-37456-2_14

Castillejo, P., Martinez, J. F., Rodriguez-Molina, J., & Cuerva, A. (2013). Integration of wearable devices in a wireless sensor network for an E-health application. *IEEE Wireless Communications, 20*(4), 38–49. doi:10.1109/MWC.2013.6590049

Castillo-Effer, M., Quintela, D. H., Moreno, W., Jordan, R., & Westhoff, W. (2004, November). Wireless sensor networks for flash-flood alerting. In *Proceedings of the Fifth IEEE International Caracas Conference on Devices, Circuits and Systems*. (Vol. 1, pp. 142-146). Piscataway, NJ: IEEE. 10.1109/ICCDCS.2004.1393370

CDC. (n.d.). Retrieved from https://www.cdc.gov/dhdsp/data_statistics/fact_sheets/fs_atrial_fibrillation.html

Cecilia, O. (2014). NIGHT-Care: A passive RFID system for remote monitoring and control of overnight living environment. *Procedia Computer Science*, 190–197.

Chacko, A., & Hayajneh, T. (2018). Security and privacy issues with IoT in healthcare. *EAI Endorsed Transactions on Pervasive Health and Technology., 4*(14), e2.

Chase, J. (2013). *The evolution of the internet of things*. Texas Instruments.

Chatman, C. (2010). How cloud computing is changing the face of health care information technology. *Journal of Health Care Compliance, 12*(3), 37–38.

Chavan, More, Thorat, Yewale, & Dhade. (2016). ECG - Remote patient monitoring using cloud computing. Imperial Journal of Interdisciplinary Research, 2(2).

Cheikhrouhou, O., Koubaa, A., Boujelben, M., & Abid, M. (2010). A lightweight user authentication scheme for wireless sensor networks. *IEEE/ACS International Conference on IEEE*. 10.1109/AICCSA.2010.5586995

Chen, F., Deng, P., Wan, J., Zhang, D., Vasilakos, A. V., & Rong, X. (2015). Data mining for the internet of things: Literature review and challenges. *International Journal of Distributed Sensor Networks, 11*(8). doi:10.1155/2015/431047

Chen, M., Gonzalez, S., Vasilakos, A., Cao, H., & Leung, V. C. M. (2011). Body area networks: A survey. *Mobile Networks and Applications, 16*(2), 171–193. doi:10.100711036-010-0260-8

Chen, M., Ma, Y., Li, Y., Wu, D., Zhang, Y., & Youn, C. H. (2017). Wearable 2.0: Enabling human-cloud integration in next generation healthcare systems. *IEEE Communications Magazine, 55*(1), 54–61. doi:10.1109/MCOM.2017.1600410CM

Chiauzzi, E., Rodarte, C., & DasMahapatra, P. (2015). Patient-centered activity monitoring in the self-management of chronic health conditions. *BMC Medicine, 13*(1), 77. doi:10.118612916-015-0319-2 PMID:25889598

Chip Community. (2019, Feb. 2). *Next Thing Co. has ceased operations*. Retrieved from http://www.chip-community.org/index.php/Main_Page

Chiuchisan, I. U. L. I. A. N. A. & Geman, O. A. N. A. (2014). An Approach of a Decision Support and Home Monitoring System for Patients with Neurological Disorders Using Internet of things Concepts. *WSEAS Transaction on Systems, 13*, 460–469.

Chiuchisan, I., Costin, H. N., & Geman, O. (2014, October). Adopting the internet of things technologies in health care systems. In *2014 International Conference and Exposition on Electrical and Power Engineering (EPE)*, (pp. 532-535). Piscataway, NJ: IEEE. 10.1109/ICEPE.2014.6969965

Chiuchisan, I., & Geman, O. (2014). *An approach of a decision support and home monitoring system for patients with neurological disorders using internet of things concepts* (Vol. 13). Wseas Transactions on Systems.

Christin, D., Reinhardt, A., Mogre, P. S., & Steinmetz, R. (2009). Wireless sensor networks and the internet of things: selected challenges. Proceedings of the 8th GI/ITG KuVSFachgesprächDrahtlosesensornetze, 31-34.

Christoph, J., Griebel, L., Leb, I., Engel, I., Köpcke, F., Toddenroth, D., ... Sedlmayr, M. (2015). Secure secondary use of clinical data with cloud-based NLP services. *Methods of Information in Medicine, 54*(03), 276–282. doi:10.3414/ME13-01-0133 PMID:25377309

Clifton, L., Clifton, D. A., Pimentel, M. A. F., Watkinson, P. J., & Tarassenko, L. (2014). Predictive monitoring of mobile patients by combining clinical observations with data from wearable sensors. *IEEE Journal of Biomedical and Health Informatics, 18*(3), 722–730. doi:10.1109/JBHI.2013.2293059 PMID:24808218

CNBC. (2017). *Shocking truth: 20% of healthcare expenditures wasted in US and other nations.* CNBC.

Coates, A., & Ng, A. Y. (2012). Learning feature representations with k-means. In *Neural networks: Tricks of the trade* (pp. 561–580). Berlin, Germany: Springer. doi:10.1007/978-3-642-35289-8_30

Corbett, Ed. (2017, April). *The Real-World Benefits of Machine Learning in Healthcare.* Retrieved from https://www.healthcatalyst.com/clinical-applications-of-machine-learning-in-healthcare

Cortes, C., & Vapnik, V. (1995). Support-vector networks. *Machine Learning, 20*(3), 273–297. doi:10.1007/BF00994018

Costa, C., & Santos, M. Y. (2015). Improving cities sustainability through the use of data mining in the context of big city data. *Lecture Notes in Engineering and Computer Science, 1*, 320–325.

Cover, T. M., & Hart, P. E. (1967). Nearest neighbor pattern classification. *IEEE Transactions on Information Theory, 13*(1), 21–27. doi:10.1109/TIT.1967.1053964

Cristianini, N., & Shawe-Taylor, J. (2000). *An introduction to support vector machines and other kernel-based learning methods.* Cambridge University Press. doi:10.1017/CBO9780511801389

Crossbow Received from Crossbow Technology. Retrieved from http://www.xbow.com

Dargie, W., & Poellabauer, C. (2010). *Fundamentals of wireless sensor networks: theory and practice.* Hoboken, NJ: John Wiley & Sons. doi:10.1002/9780470666388

Dataflair. (n.d.). Received from https://data-flair.training/blogs/iot-applications-in-healthcare

De Meulenaer, G., Gosset, F., Standaert, O.-X., & Pereira, O. (2008). On the energy cost of communication and cryptography in wireless sensor networks. *IEEE International Conference on Wireless and Mobile Computing.* 10.1109/WiMob.2008.16

Delmastro, F. (2012). Pervasive communications in healthcare. *Computer Communications, 35*(11), 1284–1295. doi:10.1016/j.comcom.2012.04.018

Dementyev, A., Behnaz, A., & Gorbach, A. M. (2013, January). 135-hour-battery-life skin temperature monitoring system using a Bluetooth cellular phone. In *2013 IEEE Topical Conference on Biomedical Wireless Technologies, Networks, and Sensing Systems* (pp. 25-27). Piscataway, NJ: IEEE. 10.1109/BioWireleSS.2013.6613663

Derguech, W., Bruke, E., & Curry, E. (2014). An autonomic approach to real-time predictive analytics using open data and internet of things. In *IEEE 11th Intl Conf on Ubiquitous Intelligence and Computing, and IEEE 11th Intl Conf on Autonomic and Trusted Computing, and IEEE 14th Intl Conf on Scalable Computing and Communications and its Associated Workshops (UTC-ATC-ScalCom)* (pp. 204–211). Piscataway, NJ: IEEE. 10.1109/UIC-ATC-ScalCom.2014.137

Desikan, P., Khare, R., Srivastava, J., Kaplan, R., Ghosh, J., Liu, L., & Gopal, V. (2013). *Predictive Modeling in Healthcare: Challenges and Opportunities. IEEE Life Sciences News Letter.*

Devashri, S. (2015). Review on-android based health care monitoring system. International Journal of Innovation Engineering Research and Technology, 1-4.

Dey, N., Hassanien, A. E., Bhatt, C., Ashour, A., & Satapathy, S. C. (2018). Internet of Things and Big Data Analytics toward Next Generation Intelligence (pp. 3–549). Berlin, Germany: Springer International Publishing. doi:10.1007/978-3-319-60435-0

Dohr, A., Modre-Opsrian, R., Drobics, M., Hayn, D., & Schreier, G. (2010). The internet of things for ambient assisted living. In *Seventh International Conference on Information Technology: New Generations (ITNG)*. Piscataway, NJ: IEEE.

Dohr, A., Modre-Opsrian, R., Drobics, M., Hayn, D., & Schreier, G. (2010, April). The internet of things for ambient assisted living. In *2010 Seventh International Conference on Information Technology: New Generations (ITNG)*, (pp. 804-809). Piscataway, NJ: IEEE. 10.1109/ITNG.2010.104

Doukas, C. & Maglogiannis, I. (2012). Bringing IoT and cloud computing towards pervasive healthcare. *Sixth international conference on innovative mobile and internet services in ubiquitous computing (IMIS)*. Piscataway, NJ: IEEE. 10.1109/IMIS.2012.26

Drucker, H., Burges, C. J., Kaufman, L., Smola, A. J., & Vapnik, V. (1997). Support vector regression machines. In Advances in neural information processing systems (pp. 155-161).

Duan, D., Fan, K., Zhang, D., Tan, S., Liang, M., Liu, Y., ... Kobinger, G. P. (2015). Nanozyme-strip for rapid local diagnosis of Ebola. *Biosensors & Bioelectronics*, *74*, 134–141. doi:10.1016/j.bios.2015.05.025 PMID:26134291

Dunsmuir, D., Payne, B. A., Cloete, G., Petersen, C. L., Gorges, M., Lim, J., ... Ansermino, J. M. (2014). Development of mHealth applications for pre-eclampsia triage. *IEEE Journal of Biomedical and Health Informatics*, *18*(6), 1857–1864. doi:10.1109/JBHI.2014.2301156 PMID:25375683

Durairaj, M., & Muthuramalingam, K. (2018). A New Authentication Scheme with Elliptical Curve Cryptography for Internet of Things (IoT) Environments. *Int. J. Eng. Technol.*, *7*(2.26), 119–124. doi:10.14419/ijet.v7i2.26.14364

Dwork, C., & Smith, A. (2009). Differential privacy for statistics: What we know and what we want to learn. *Journal of Privacy and Confidentiality*, *1*(2), 135–154.

Eberhart, R. C. (Ed.). (2014). *Neural network PC tools: a practical guide*. Academic Press.

El Maliki, T. & Seigneur, J.-M. (2007). A survey of user-centric identity management technologies. In *the International Conference on Emerging Security Information, Systems, and Technologies (SECUREWARE 2007)*. Piscataway, NJ: IEEE. 10.1109/SECUREWARE.2007.4385303

ElecFreaks. (2016, Jan. 15). *BLEDuino*. Retrieved from https://www.elecfreaks.com/wiki/index.php?title=BLEDUINO

El-Sayed, H., Sankar, S., Prasad, M., Puthal, D., Gupta, A., Mohanty, M., & Lin, C.-T. (2018). Edge of Things: The Big Picture on the Integration of Edge, IoT and the Cloud in a Distributed Computing Environment. *IEEE Access: Practical Innovations, Open Solutions*, *6*, 1706–1717. doi:10.1109/ACCESS.2017.2780087

ErwanBigan. (2019). *Ground Predictive Healthcare Models in Real-World Medical Dataand in Real World Medical Practice*. Author.

Escobar, L. J. V. & Salinas, S. A. (2016, August). e-Health prototype system for cardiac telemonitoring. In *2016 38th Annual International Conference of the IEEE Engineering in Medicine and Biology Society (EMBC)* (pp. 4399-4402). Piscataway, NJ: IEEE.

Ester, M., Kriegel, H. P., Sander, J., & Xu, X. (1996, August). A density-based algorithm for discovering clusters in large spatial databases with noise. *In Proceedings of International Conference on Knowledge Discovery & Data Mining*, *96*(34), 226–231.

Esteva, A., Robicquet, A., Ramsundar, B., Kuleshov, V., DePristo, M., Chou, K., ... Dean, J. (2019). A guide to deep learning in healthcare. *Nature Medicine, 25*(1), 24–29. doi:10.103841591-018-0316-z PMID:30617335

Evenson, K. R., Goto, M. M., & Furberg, R. D. (2015). Systematic review of the validity and reliability of consumer-wearable activity trackers. *The International Journal of Behavioral Nutrition and Physical Activity, 12*(1), 159. doi:10.118612966-015-0314-1 PMID:26684758

Fadlullah, Z. M., Pathan, A. S. K., & Gacanin, H. (2018, June). On Delay-Sensitive Healthcare Data Analytics at the Network Edge Based on Deep Learning. In 2018 14th International Wireless Communications & Mobile Computing Conference (IWCMC) (pp. 388-393). Piscataway, NJ: IEEE. doi:10.1109/IWCMC.2018.8450475

Fan, Y. J., & Yin, Y. H. (2014, May). IoT-Based smart rehabilitation system. *IEEE Transactions on Industrial Informatics, 10*(2).

Foundations. (2019). Retrieved from https://www.arduino.cc/en/Tutorial/Foundations

Gao, T., Greenspan, D., Welsh, M., Juang, R. R., & Alm, A. (2006, January). Vital signs monitoring and patient tracking over a wireless network. In 2005 IEEE Engineering in Medicine and Biology 27th Annual Conference (pp. 102-105). Piscataway, NJ: IEEE.

Gao, W., Emaminejad, S., Nyein, H. Y. Y., Challa, S., Chen, K., Peck, A., ... Lien, D. H. (2016). Fully integrated wearable sensor arrays for multiplexed in situ perspiration analysis. *Nature, 529*(7587), 509–514. doi:10.1038/nature16521 PMID:26819044

Gardner, R. M., & Shabot, M. M. (2006). Patient-Monitoring Systems. In E. H. Shortliffe & J. J. Cimino (Eds.), *Biomedical Informatics. Health Informatics.* New York, NY: Springer.

Gartner Research. (2017). *Predictive Algorithms that Healthcare Delivery Organizations Are Using to Improve Outcomes.* Author.

Gartner Says 6.4 Billion Connected "Things" Will Be in Use in 2016, Up 30 Percent From 2015. Available at www.gartner.com/newsroom/id/3165317

Gay, V., & Leijdekkers, P. (2007). A health monitoring system using smart phones and wearable sensors. *International Journal of ARM, 8*(2), 29–35.

Geekforgeeks. Retrieved from https://www.geeksforgeeks.org/computer-network-packet-switching-delays/

Gelogo, Y. E., Oh, J. W., Park, J. W., & Kim, H. K. (2015, November). Internet of things (IoT) driven U-Healthcare system architecture. In *2015 8th International Conference on Bio-Science and Bio-Technology (BSBT)* (pp. 24-26). Piscataway, NJ: IEEE.

Glorot, X., & Bengio, Y. (2010, March). Understanding the difficulty of training deep feedforward neural networks. In *Proceedings of the thirteenth international conference on artificial intelligence and statistics* (pp. 249-256).

Gonçalves, H., Pinto, P., Silva, M., Ayres-de-Campos, D., & Bernardes, J. (2016). Electrocardiography versus photoplethysmography in assessment of maternal heart rate variability during labor. *SpringerPlus, 5*(1), 1079. doi:10.118640064-016-2787-z PMID:27462527

Gonzalez, H., Han, J., Li, X., & Klabjan, D. (2006, April). Warehousing and Analyzing Massive RFID Data Sets (Vol. 6, p. 83). Oslo, Norway: ICDE. doi:10.1109/ICDE.2006.171

Goodfellow, I., Bengio, Y., & Courville, A. (2016). *Deep learning.* Cambridge, MA: MIT Press.

Gope, P., & Hwang, T. (2016). BSN-Care:A sensor IoT-based modern healthcare system using body sensor network. *IEEE Sensors, 16*(5), 1368–1376. doi:10.1109/JSEN.2015.2502401

Großsch"adl, J., Szekely, A., & Tillich, S. (2007). The energy cost of cryptographic key establishment in wireless sensor networks. *Proceedings of the 2nd ACM symposium on Information, computer and communications security.* 10.1145/1229285.1229334

Gubbi, J., Buyya, R., Marusic, S., & Palaniswami, M. (2013). Internet of things (IoT): A vision, architectural elements, and future directions. *Future Generation Computer Systems, 29*(7), 1645–1660. doi:10.1016/j.future.2013.01.010

Gupta, V. (2011). Cloud computing in health care. Express Healthcare, Sept.

Gupta, A. K., Sadawarti, H., & Verma, A. K. (2010). Performance analysis of AODV, DSR & TORA routing protocols. *IACSIT International Journal of Engineering and Technology, 2*(2), 226.

Gupta, P., Agrawal, D., Chhabra, J., & Dhir, P. K. (2016, March). IoT based smart healthcare kit. In *2016 International Conference on Computational Techniques in Information and Communication Technologies (ICCTICT)* (pp. 237-242). IEEE. 10.1109/ICCTICT.2016.7514585

Guyon, I., Boser, B., & Vapnik, V. (1993). Automatic capacity tuning of very large VC-dimension classifiers. In Advances in neural information processing systems (pp. 147-155).

Haghi, M., Thurow, K., & Stoll, R. (2017). Wearable devices in medical internet of things: Scientific research and commercially available devices. *Healthcare Informatics Research, 23*(1), 4–15. doi:10.4258/hir.2017.23.1.4 PMID:28261526

Hamidi, H. (2019). An approach to develop the smart health using internet of things and authentication based on biometric technology. Future Gen. Comput. Syst.

Han, W., Gu, Y., Zhang, Y., & Zheng, L. (2014). Data driven quantitative trust model for the Internet of agricultural things. In *International Conference on the internet of things (IoT)* (pp. 31–36). Piscataway, NJ: IEEE. 10.1109/IOT.2014.7030111

Hao, Y., & Foster, R. (2008). Wireless body sensor networks for health-monitoring applications. *Physiological Measurement, 29*(11), R27–R56. doi:10.1088/0967-3334/29/11/R01 PMID:18843167

Hassan Mehmood Khan. (2018). Received from https://iotlearners.com/windows-10-for-the-internet-of-things/

Hassanalieragh, M., Page, A., Soyata, T., Sharma, G., Aktas, M., Mateos, G., . . . Andreescu, S. (2015, June). Health monitoring and management using Internet-of-Things (IoT) sensing with cloud-based processing: Opportunities and challenges. In *2015 IEEE International Conference on Services Computing (SCC),* (pp. 285-292). Piscataway, NJ: IEEE.

Hayrinen, K., Saranto, K., & Nykanen, P. (2008). Definition, structure, content, use and impacts of electronic health records: A review of the research literature. *International Journal of Medical Informatics, 77*(5), 291–304. doi:10.1016/j.ijmedinf.2007.09.001 PMID:17951106

Heartbeat Sensor - How to Measure Heartbeat. Working and Application. (2019, June 24). Retrieved from https://www.elprocus.com/heartbeat-sensor-working-application/

He, K., Zhang, X., Ren, S., & Sun, J. (2016). Deep residual learning for image recognition. In *Proceedings of the IEEE conference on computer vision and pattern recognition* (pp. 770-778).

Hoffman, S. (2007). In Sickness, Health, and Cyberspace: Protecting the security of electronic private health information. *Boston College Law Review. Boston College. Law School, 48*(2), 331–386.

Höller, J., Tsiatsis, V., Mulligan, C., Karnouskos, S., Avesand, S., & Boyle, D. (2014). *From machine-to-machine to the internet of things: Introduction to a new age of intelligence.* Amsterdam, The Netherlands: Elsevier.

Hongsong, C., Zhongchuan, F., & Dongyan, Z. (2011, July). Security and trust research in M2M system. In *Proceedings of 2011 IEEE International Conference on Vehicular Electronics and Safety* (pp. 286-290). IEEE. 10.1109/ICVES.2011.5983830

Hongtao, T., Sanjay, K. B., Choi, L. L., & Wendong, X. (2008). Joint routing and flow rate optimization in multi-rate ad hoc networks. *Computer Networks*, *52*(3), 739–764. doi:10.1016/j.comnet.2007.11.006

Hossain, M. S., & Muhammad, G. (2016). Cloud-assisted industrial internet of things (iiot)–enabled framework for health monitoring. *Computer Networks*, *101*, 192–202. doi:10.1016/j.comnet.2016.01.009

Hosseini, M. P., Tran, T. X., Pompili, D., Elisevich, K., & Soltanian-Zadeh, H. (2017). Deep Learning With Edge Computing for Localization of Epileptogenicity Using Multimodal rs-fMRI and EEG Big Data. *IEEE International Conference on Autonomic Computing.*

Hotelling, H. (1933). Analysis of a complex of statistical variables into principal components. *Journal of Educational Psychology*, *24*(6), 417–441. doi:10.1037/h0071325

Hotelling, H. (1992). Relations between two sets of variates. In *Breakthroughs in statistics* (pp. 162–190). New York, NY: Springer. doi:10.1007/978-1-4612-4380-9_14

Huang, C. H., & Cheng, K. W. (2014, January). RFID technology combined with IoT application in medical nursing system. *Bulletin of Networking, Computing, Systems, and Software*, *3*(1), 20–24.

Huang, P. H., Ren, L., Nama, N., Li, S., Li, P., Yao, X., ... Nawaz, A. A. (2015). An acoustofluidic sputum liquefier. *Lab on a Chip*, *15*(15), 3125–3131. doi:10.1039/C5LC00539F PMID:26082346

Hu, L., Qiu, M., Song, J., Hossain, M. S., & Ghoneim, A. (2015). Software defined healthcare networks. *IEEE Wireless Communications*, *22*(6), 67–75. doi:10.1109/MWC.2015.7368826

Hussain, A., Wenbi, R., da Silva, A. L., Nadher, M., & Mudhish, M. (2015). Health and emergency-care platform for the elderly and disabled people in the Smart City. *Journal of Systems and Software*, *110*, 253–263. doi:10.1016/j.jss.2015.08.041

Idowu, B., Adagunodo, R., & Adedoyin, R. (2006). Information technology infusion model for health sector in developing country: Nigeria as a case. *Technology and Health Care*, *14*(2), 69–77. PMID:16720950

Imadali, S., Karanasiou, A., Petrescu, A., Sifniadis, I., Vèque, V., & Angelidis, P. (2012, October). eHealth service support in IPv6 vehicular networks. In *2012 IEEE 8th International Conference on Wireless and Mobile Computing, Networking and Communications (WiMob)* (pp. 579-585). Piscataway, NJ: IEEE.

Integrated Cloud Applications & Platform Services. (2017). Retrieved from https://www.oracle.com/assets/hc-cloud-technologies-br-3432373.pdf

International Telecommunication Union. (2005). *The Internet of Things*. Retrieved from http://www.itu.int/osg/spu/publications/internetofthings/InternetofThings_summary.pdf

IoTWF. (2017). Received From https://www.iotwf.com/

Irdeto organization. (2017). Irdeto Global Consumer Piracy Survey.

Irfan Husain, M. D. (2014, Feb. 14). *New Healthpatch biosensor captures a wide range of information with just an adhesive, disposable patch*. Retrieved from https://www.imedicalapps.com/2014/02/vital-connect-wearable-biosensor-healthpatch/

Islam, S. R., Kwak, D., Kabir, M. H., Hossain, M., & Kwak, K. S. (2015). The internet of things for health care: A comprehensive survey. *IEEE Access: Practical Innovations, Open Solutions*, *3*, 678–708. doi:10.1109/ACCESS.2015.2437951

Jagadish, H. V., Ooi, B. C., Tan, K.-L., Yu, C., & Zhang, R. (2005). Idistance: An adaptive bþ-treebased indexing method for nearest neighbor search [TODS]. *ACM Transactions on Database Systems*, *30*(2), 364–397. doi:10.1145/1071610.1071612

Jakkula, V., & Cook, D. (2010, July). Outlier detection in a smart environment structured power datasets. In *Sixth International Conference on Intelligent Environments* (pp. 29-33). Piscataway, NJ: IEEE. 10.1109/IE.2010.13

Jalaliniya, S. & Pederson, T. (2012, October). A wearable kids' health monitoring system on smartphone. In *Proceedings of the 7th Nordic Conference on Human-Computer Interaction: Making Sense Through Design* (pp. 791-792). New York, NY: ACM. 10.1145/2399016.2399150

Jara, A. J., Zamora, M. A., & Skarmeta, A. F. (2012, June). Knowledge acquisition and management architecture for mobile and personal health environments based on the internet of things. In *2012 IEEE 11th International Conference on Trust, Security and Privacy in Computing and Communications (TrustCom)*, (pp. 1811-1818). Piscataway, NJ: IEEE. 10.1109/TrustCom.2012.194

Jara, A. J., Genoud, D., & Bocchi, Y. (2014, May). Big data in smart cities: from poison to human dynamics. In *28th International Conference on Advanced Information Networking and Applications Workshops* (pp. 785-790). Piscataway, NJ: IEEE. 10.1109/WAINA.2014.165

Jara, A. J., Zamora-Izquierdo, M. A., & Skarmeta, A. F. (2013). Interconnection framework for mHealth and remote monitoring based on the internet of things. *IEEE Journal on Selected Areas in Communications*, *31*(9), 47–65. doi:10.1109/JSAC.2013.SUP.0513005

Jason Brownlee. (2016, August). *What is Deep Learning?* Retrieved from https://machinelearningmastery.com/what-is-deep-learning/

Jia, X., Chen, H., & Qi, F. (2012, October). Technical models and key technologies of e-health monitoring. In *2012 IEEE 14th International Conference on e-Health Networking, Applications and Services (Healthcom)* (pp. 23-26). Piscataway, NJ: IEEE.

Jiawei, H., & Kamber, M. (2017). *Data Mining: Concepts and Techniques*. Morgan Kaufmann.

Jin Kang, J., Sdibi, S., Larkin, H., & Luan, T. (2015). Predictive data mining for Converged Internet of things: A Mobile Health perspective. *International Telecommunication Networks and Application Conference (ITNAC)*, Sydney, Australia, pp. 5-10. 10.1109/ATNAC.2015.7366781

Jipeng, Z., Liyang, P., Yuhui, D., & Jianzhu, L. (2012). An on-demand routing protocol for improving channel use efficiency in multichannel ad hoc networks. *Journal of Network and Computer Applications*, *35*(5), 1606–1614. doi:10.1016/j.jnca.2012.03.003

Jolliffe, I. (2011). Principal component analysis (pp. 1094–1096). Berlin, Germany: Springer.

Joon-Soo, J.-Y. (2016). A Design Characteristics of Smart Healthcare System as the IoT Application. *Indian Journal of Science and Technology*, *9*(37), 1–8.

Joyia, G. J., Liaqat, R. M., Farooq, A., & Rehman, S. (2017). Internet of medical things (IoMT): Applications, benefits and future challenges in healthcare domain. *Journal of Communication*. doi:10.12720/jcm.12.4.240-247

Jumutc, V., Langone, R., & Suykens, J. A. (2015, October). Regularized and sparse stochastic k-means for distributed large-scale clustering. In *2015 IEEE International Conference on Big Data (Big Data)* (pp. 2535-2540). Piscataway, NJ: IEEE. 10.1109/BigData.2015.7364050

Jung, B. H., Akbar, R. U., & Sung, D. K. (2012, September).Throughput, energy consumption, and energy efficiency of IEEE 802.15. 6 body area network (BAN) MAC protocol. In *2012 IEEE 23rd International Symposium on Personal, Indoor and Mobile Radio Communications-(PIMRC)* (pp. 584-589). Piscataway, NJ: IEEE.

Juxtology. (2018). Received From https://juxtology.com/iot-transformation/

Kafi, M. A., Challal, Y., Djenouri, D., Doudou, M., Bouabdallah, A., & Badache, N. (2013). A study of wireless sensor networks for urban traffic monitoring: Applications and architectures. *Procedia Computer Science*, *19*, 617–626. doi:10.1016/j.procs.2013.06.082

Kaiser Permanente, Sepsis. (2015). Risk Prediction Model Decreases Use of Antibiotics in Newborns. Author.

Kale, S., & Khandelwal, C. S. (2013, March). Design and implementation of real time embedded tele-health monitoring system. In *2013 International Conference on Circuits, Power and Computing Technologies (ICCPCT)* (pp. 771-774). Piscataway, NJ: IEEE. 10.1109/ICCPCT.2013.6528842

Kamal, M. S., Dey, N., & Ashour, A. S. (2017). Large scale medical data mining for accurate diagnosis: A blueprint. In S. U. Khan, A. Y. Zomaya, & A. Abbas (Eds.), *Handbook of Large-Scale Distributed Computing in Smart Healthcare* (pp. 157–176). Cham: Springer. doi:10.1007/978-3-319-58280-1_7

Karlof, C., Sastry, N., & Wagner, D. (2004, November). TinySec: a link layer security architecture for wireless sensor networks. In *Proceedings of the 2nd international conference on Embedded networked sensor systems* (pp. 162-175). New York, NY: ACM.

Karthick, G. S., & Pankajavalli, P. B. (2019). Healthcare IoT Architectures, Technologies, Applications, and Issues: A Deep Insight. In N. Bouchemal (Ed.), *Intelligent Systems for Healthcare Management and Delivery* (pp. 235–265). Hershey, PA: IGI Global. doi:10.4018/978-1-5225-7071-4.ch011

Karthikeyan, S., Patan, R., & Balamurugan, B. (2019). Enhancement of Security in the Internet of Things (IoT) by Using X. 509 Authentication Mechanism. In *Recent Trends in Communication, Computing, and Electronics* (pp. 217–225). Singapore: Springer. doi:10.1007/978-981-13-2685-1_22

Khalifa, A. (2014). ZIGBEE BASED WEARABLE REMOTE HEALTHCARE MONITORING SYSTEM FOR EL-DERLY PATIENTS. *International Journal of Wireless & Mobile Networks*, *6*(3), 53–67. doi:10.5121/ijwmn.2014.6304

Khoi, N. M., Saguna, S., Mitra, K., & Åhlund, C. (2015, October). IReHMo: An efficient IoT-based remote health monitoring system for smart regions. In *2015 17th International Conference on E-health Networking, Application & Services (HealthCom)*, (pp. 563-568). Piscataway, NJ: IEEE.

Kirtana, R. N., & Lokeswari, Y. V. (2017). An IoT Based Remote HRV Monitoring System for Hypertensive Patients. *IEEE International Conference on Computer, Communication, and Signal Processing*. 10.1109/ICCCSP.2017.7944086

Klonoff, D. C. (2013). Twelve modern digital technologies that are transforming decision making for diabetes and all areas of health care. *Journal of Diabetes Science and Technology*, *7*(2), 291–295. doi:10.1177/193229681300700201 PMID:23566983

Kodali, R. K., Swamy, G., & Lakshmi, B. (2015). An implementation of IoT for healthcare. *IEEE Conference Paper*. 10.1109/RAICS.2015.7488451

Ko, J., Lu, C., Srivastava, M. B., Stankovic, J. A., Terzis, A., & Welsh, M. (2010). Wireless sensor networks for healthcare. *Proceedings of the IEEE*, *98*(11), 1947–1960. doi:10.1109/JPROC.2010.2065210

Kolodner, E. K., Tal, S., Kyriazis, D., Naor, D., Allalouf, M., Bonelli, L., . . . Harnik, D. (2011, November). A cloud environment for data-intensive storage services. In *2011 IEEE third international conference on cloud computing technology and science* (pp. 357-366). Piscataway, NJ: IEEE. 10.1109/CloudCom.2011.55

Kostkova, P. (2015). Grand challenges in digital health. *Frontiers in Public Health, 3*, 134. doi:10.3389/fpubh.2015.00134 PMID:26000272

Kothmayr, T., Schmitt, C., Hu, W., Br¨unig, M., & Carle, G. (2013). Dtls based security and two-way authentication for the internet of things. *Ad Hoc Networks, 11*(8), 2710–2723. doi:10.1016/j.adhoc.2013.05.003

Krawczyk, H., Canetti, R., & Bellare, M. (1997). KHAC: Keyedhashing for message authentication.

Kriegel, H. P., Kröger, P., Sander, J., & Zimek, A. (2011). Density-based clustering. *Wiley Interdisciplinary Reviews. Data Mining and Knowledge Discovery, 1*(3), 231–240. doi:10.1002/widm.30

Krishna, K. D., Akkala, V., Bharath, R., Rajalakshmi, P., & Mohammed, A. M. (2016). *Computer Aided Abnormality Detection for Kidney on FPGA Based IoT Enabled Portable Ultrasound Imaging System.* AGBM, Published by Elsevier Masson SAS. doi:10.1016/j.irbm.2016.05.001

Kulkar, A., & Sathe, S. (2014). Healthcare applications of the Internet of things: A review. *International Journal of Computer Science and Information Technologies, 5*(5), 6229–6232.

Kumar, J. S., & Patel, D. R. (2014). A survey on internet of things: Security and privacy issues. *International Journal of Computers and Applications, 90*(11).

Kumar, K. B. S., & Bairavi, K. (2016). IoT based health monitoring system for autistic patients. *Proc. Symposium on Big Data and Cloud Computing Challenges, Smart Innovation, Systems and Technologies.* 10.1007/978-3-319-30348-2_32

Kunnath, A. T., Nadarajan, D., Mohan, M., & Ramesh, M. V. (2013, August). Wicard: A context aware wearable wireless sensor for cardiac monitoring. In *2013 International Conference on Advances in Computing, Communications and Informatics (ICACCI)* (pp. 1097-1102). Piscataway, NJ: IEEE. 10.1109/ICACCI.2013.6637330

Lamprinos, I. E., Prentza, A., Sakka, E., & Koutsouris, D. (2006, January). Energy-efficient MAC protocol for patient personal area networks. In *2005 IEEE Engineering in Medicine and Biology 27th Annual Conference* (pp. 3799-3802). Piscataway, NJ: IEEE.

Landstra, T., Zawodniok, M., & Jagannathan, S. (2007, October). Energy-efficient hybrid key management protocol for wireless sensor networks. In *32nd IEEE Conference on Local Computer Networks (LCN 2007)* (pp. 1009-1016). Piscataway, NJ: IEEE.

LeCun, Y., Bottou, L., Bengio, Y., & Haffner, P. (1998). Gradient-based learning applied to document recognition. *Proceedings of the IEEE, 86*(11), 2278–2324. doi:10.1109/5.726791

Lee, H., Park, K., Lee, B., Choi, J., & Elmasri, R. (2008, July). Issues in data fusion for healthcare monitoring. In *Proceedings of the 1st international conference on PErvasive Technologies Related to Assistive Environments* (p. 3). New York, NY: ACM. 10.1145/1389586.1389590

Lee, H. C., & Yoon, H.-J. (2017). Medical big data: Promise and challenges. *Kidney Research and Clinical Practice, 36*(1), 3–11. doi:10.23876/j.krcp.2017.36.1.3 PMID:28392994

Lee, J., Kapitanova, K., & Son, S. H. (2010). The price of security in wireless sensor networks. *Computer Networks, 54*(17), 2967–2978. doi:10.1016/j.comnet.2010.05.011

Lee, Y. D., & Chung, W. Y. (2009). Wireless sensor network based wearable smart shirt for ubiquitous health and activity monitoring. *Sensors and Actuators B: Chemical, 140*(2), 390–395. doi:10.1016/j.snb.2009.04.040

LeHong, H. & Velosa, A. (2014). Hype cycle for the Internet of Things. Gartner Group, 21.

Leicher, A., Kuntze, N., & Schmidt, A. U. (2009, May). Implementation of a trusted ticket system. In *IFIP International Information Security Conference* (pp. 152-163). Springer.

Leister, W., Abie, H., Groven, A. K., Fretland, T., & Balasingham, I. (2008, April). Threat assessment of wireless patient monitoring systems. In *2008 3rd International Conference on Information and Communication Technologies: From Theory to Applications* (pp. 1-6). Piscataway, NJ: IEEE. 10.1109/ICTTA.2008.4530274

Li, Y., Thai, M., & Wu, W. (2008). Wireless Sensor Networks and Applications. Berlin, Germany: Springer. doi:10.1007/978-0-387-49592-7

Likas, A., Vlassis, N., & Verbeek, J. J. (2003). The global k-means clustering algorithm. *Pattern Recognition, 36*(2), 451–461. doi:10.1016/S0031-3203(02)00060-2

Li, M., Lou, W., & Ren, K. (2010). *Data security and privacy in wireless body area networks. Wireless Communications.* Piscataway, NJ: IEEE.

Linda. (2016). *10 Smart Medical Devices That Are Changing HealthCare.* Retrieved from http://www.appcessories.co.uk/connected-smart-medical-devices-that-are-changing-healthcare/

Lindeman, T. (2018). *How hospitals are using predictive analytics.* Academic Press.

Li, S., Da Xu, L., & Zhao, S. (2015). The internet of things: A survey. *Information Systems Frontiers, 17*(2), 243–259. doi:10.100710796-014-9492-7

Liu, T., Kamthe, A., Jiang, L., & Cerpa, A. (2009). Performance Evaluation of Link Quality Estimation Metrics for Static Multihop Wireless Sensor Networks.

Liu, T., Kamthe, A., Jiang, L., & Cerpa, A. (2009, June). Performance evaluation of link quality estimation metrics for static multihop wireless sensor networks. In *2009 6th Annual IEEE Communications Society Conference on Sensor, Mesh and Ad Hoc Communications and Networks* (pp. 1-9). Piscataway, NJ: IEEE. 10.1109/SAHCN.2009.5168959

LM35 Temperature Sensor. (n.d.). Retrieved from http://www.dnatechindia.com/LM35-Temperature-Sensor-Basics.html

Loh, W. Y. (2011). Classification and regression trees. *Wiley Interdisciplinary Reviews. Data Mining and Knowledge Discovery, 1*(1), 14–23. doi:10.1002/widm.8

Lorincz, K., Malan, D. J., Fulford-Jones, T. R., Nawoj, A., Clavel, A., Shnayder, V., ... Moulton, S. (2004). Sensor networks for emergency response: Challenges and opportunities. *IEEE Pervasive Computing, 3*(4), 16–23. doi:10.1109/MPRV.2004.18

Lounis, A., Hadjidj, A., Bouabdallah, A., & Challal, Y. (2012, July). Secure and scalable cloud-based architecture for e-health wireless sensor networks. In *2012 21st International Conference on Computer Communications and Networks (ICCCN)* (pp. 1-7). Piscataway, NJ: IEEE. 10.1109/ICCCN.2012.6289252

Maastricht Instruments. (n.d.). *ECG Necklace.* Retrieved from http://www.maastrichtinstruments.nl/portfolio/ecg-necklace-body-area-network/

Machanavajjhala, A., Gehrke, J., Kifer, D., & Venkitasubramaniam, M. (2006, April). l-diversity: Privacy beyond k-anonymity. In *22nd International Conference on Data Engineering (ICDE'06)* (pp. 24-24). IEEE. 10.1109/ICDE.2006.1

Maciuca, A., Popescu, D., Strutu, M., & Stamatescu, G. (2013, September). Wireless sensor network based on multi-level femtocells for home monitoring. In *2013 IEEE 7th International Conference on Intelligent Data Acquisition and Advanced Computing Systems (IDAACS)* (Vol. 1, pp. 499-503). Piscataway, NJ: IEEE. 10.1109/IDAACS.2013.6662735

Mainetti, L., Patrono, L., Secco, A., & Sergi, I. (2016, July). An IoT-aware AAL system for elderly people. In *International Multidisciplinary Conference on Computer and Energy Science (SpliTech)*, (pp. 1-6). Piscataway, NJ: IEEE. 10.1109/SpliTech.2016.7555929

Majumder, A. J. A., Zerin, I., Uddin, M., Ahamed, S. I., & Smith, R. O. (2013, October). SmartPrediction: A real-time smartphone-based fall risk prediction and prevention system. In *Proceedings of the 2013 Research in Adaptive and Convergent Systems* (pp. 434-439). New York, NY: ACM. 10.1145/2513228.2513267

Malasinghe, L. P., Ramzan, N. & Dahal, K. J. (2017). Ambient Intell Human Comput. doi:10.100712652-017-0598-x

Malima, A., Siavoshi, S., Musacchio, T., Upponi, J., Yilmaz, C., Somu, S., ... Busnaina, A. (2012). Highly sensitive microscale in vivo sensor enabled by electrophoretic assembly of nanoparticles for multiple biomarker detection. *Lab on a Chip*, *12*(22), 4748–4754. doi:10.1039/c2lc40580f PMID:22983480

Manoj, A. S., Hussain, M. A., & Teja, P. S. (2019). Patient Health Monitoring Using IoT. Mobile Health Applications for Quality Healthcare Delivery, 30.

Mano, L. Y., Faiçal, B. S., Nakamura, L. H., Gomes, P. H., Libralon, G. L., Meneguete, R. I., ... Ueyama, J. (2016). Exploiting IoT technologies for enhancing Health Smart Homes through patient identification and emotion recognition. *Computer Communications*, *89*, 178–190. doi:10.1016/j.comcom.2016.03.010

Maradugu, A. (2015). Android based health care monitoring system. *2015 International Conference on Innovations in Information, Embedded and Communication Systems (ICIIECS)* (pp. 1-5). Coimbatore, India: IEEE.

Marco Varone. (2017, April). *Machine learning, Technology*. Retrieved from https://www.expertsystem.com/machine-learning-definition/

Matar, G., Lina, J., Kaddoum, G., & Riley, A. (2016). Internet of things in sleep monitoring: An application for posture recognition using supervised learning. *Proc. International Conference on IEEE Healthcom*. 10.1109/HealthCom.2016.7749469

Mattern, F., & Floerkemeier, C. (2010). From the Internet of Computers to the Internet of Things. In *From active data management to event-based systems and more* (pp. 242–259). Berlin: Springer. doi:10.1007/978-3-642-17226-7_15

Ma, X., Wu, Y.-J., Wang, Y., Chen, F., & Liu, J. (2013). Mining smart card data for transit riders 'travel patterns. *Transportation Research Part C, Emerging Technologies*, *36*, 1–12. doi:10.1016/j.trc.2013.07.010

MbientLab. (2017). *MetaWear Android API*. Retrieved from https://mbientlab.com/androiddocs/latest/

MbientLab. (n.d.). *MetaHealth*. Retrieved from https://mbientlab.com/product/metahealth-bundle/

MbientLab. (n.d.). *MetamotionC*. Retrieved from https://mbientlab.com/product/metamotionc/

McCallum, A. & Nigam, K. (1998, July). A comparison of event models for naive bayes text classification. In AAAI-98 workshop on learning for text categorization, 752(1), (pp. 41-48).

MCHobby. (n.d.). *Câble pro ECG-EKG/EMG pour électrode gel*. Retrieved from https://shop.mchobby.be/shields/695-cable-pro-ecg-ekgemg-pour-electrode-gel-3232100006959-olimex.html

MCHobby. (n.d.). *ECG-EKG/EMG shield pour Arduino*. Retrieved from https://shop.mchobby.be/shields/693-ekg-emg-shield-pour-arduino-3232100006935-olimex.html

MCHobby. (n.d.). *Electrode ECG à gel*. Retrieved from http://shop.mchobby.be/shields/696-electrode-ecg-a-gel-3232100006966.html

Medaglia, C. M., & Serbanati, A. (2010). An overview of privacy and security issues in the internet of things. The internet of things.

Mehrotra, P. (2016). Biosensors and their applications–A review. *Journal of Oral Biology and Craniofacial Research*, *6*(2), 153–159.

Mehta, M., & Ghosh, K. (2016, April). Effect of Looping On the Lifetime Of A Multi-Sink Wireless Sensor Network Deployed For Healthcare Monitoring System. [IJERCSE]. *International Journal of Engineering Research in Computer Science and Engineering*, *3*(4).

Minaie, A., Sanati-Mehrizy, A., Sanati-Mehrizy, P., & Sanati-Mehrizy, R. (2013). Application of wireless sensor networks in health care system. age, *23*(1).

Miorandi, D., Sicari, S., De Pellegrini, F., & Chlamtac, I. (2012). Internet of things: Vision, applications and research challenges. *Ad Hoc Networks*, *10*(7), 1497–1516. doi:10.1016/j.adhoc.2012.02.016

MIT Technology Review. (2015, June 22). *The Struggle for Accurate Measurements on Your Wrist*. Retrieved from https://www.technologyreview.com/s/538416/the-struggle-for-accurate-measurements-on-your-wrist/

Miyazaki, S. (1997). Long-term unrestrained measurement of stride length and walking velocity utilizing a piezoelectric gyroscope. *IEEE Transactions on Biomedical Engineering*, *44*(8), 753–759. doi:10.1109/10.605434 PMID:9254988

Mohammadzadeh, N., & Safdari, R. (2014). Patient monitoring in mobile health: Opportunities and challenges. *Medicinski Arhiv*, *68*(1), 57. doi:10.5455/medarh.2014.68.57-60 PMID:24783916

Mohammed, J., Lung, C. H., Ocneanu, A., Thakral, A., Jones, C., & Adler, A. (2014, September). Internet of Things: Remote patient monitoring using web services and cloud computing. In *2014 IEEE International Conference on Internet of Things (iThings), and Green Computing and Communications (GreenCom), IEEE and Cyber, Physical and Social Computing (CPSCom), IEEE* (pp. 256-263). Piscataway, NJ: IEEE.

Monekosso, D. N., & Remagnino, P. (2013). Data reconciliation in a smart home sensor network. *Expert Systems with Applications*, *40*(8), 3248–3255. doi:10.1016/j.eswa.2012.12.037

Montenegro, G., Kushalnagar, N., Hui, J., & Culler, D. (2007). Transmission of IPv6 packets over IEEE 802.15. 4 networks (No. RFC 4944).

Montgomery, D. C., Peck, E. A., & Vining, G. G. (2012). *Introduction to linear regression analysis* (Vol. 821). Hoboken, NJ: John Wiley & Sons.

Morris, D., Coyle, S., Wu, Y., Lau, K. T., Wallace, G., & Diamond, D. (2009). Bio-sensing textile based patch with an integrated optical detection system for sweat monitoring. *Sensors and Actuators B: Chemical*, *139*(1), 231–236. doi:10.1016/j.snb.2009.02.032

Motwani, Mirchandani, Rohra, Tarachandani, & Yeole. (2016). Smart nursing home patient monitoring system. Imperial Journal of Interdisciplinary Research, *2*(6).

MtM+ Technology Corporation (n.d.). *IoT Development Kit*. Retrieved from https://www.mtmtech.com.tw/kit.html

Murphy, K. P. (2012). *Machine learning: a probabilistic perspective*. Cambridge, MA: MIT Press.

MySignals. (n.d.). *eHealth and Medical IoT Development Platform*. Retrieved from http://www.my-signals.com/

Na, H., & Choi, Y. (2013, October). Conceptual design of personal wellness record for mobile health monitoring. In *2013 IEEE 2nd Global Conference on Consumer Electronics (GCCE)* (pp. 410-411). Piscataway, NJ: IEEE. 10.1109/GCCE.2013.6664873

Nate Drake. (2019, June). Best cloud storage of 2019 online: free, paid and business options. *Cloud Services*. Retrieved from https://www.techradar.com/

National Alliance for Health Information Technology. NAHIT releases HIT definitions. Electronic health records. Available at https://www.healthcare-informatics.com/news-item/nahit-releases-hit-definitions

Nausheen, F., & Begum, S. H. (2018, January). Healthcare IoT: Benefits, vulnerabilities and solutions. In *2018 2nd International Conference on Inventive Systems and Control (ICISC)* (pp. 517-522). IEEE.

Neter, J., Kutner, M. H., Nachtsheim, C. J., & Wasserman, W. (1996). *Applied linear statistical models* (Vol. 4). Chicago, IL: Irwin.

Neves, P., Stachyra, M., & Rodrigues, J. (2008). Application of wireless sensor networks to healthcare promotion.

Ni, P., Zhang, C., & Ji, Y. (2014, August). A hybrid method for short-term sensor data forecasting in Internet of things. In *11th International Conference on Fuzzy Systems and Knowledge Discovery (FSKD)* (pp. 369-373). Piscataway, NJ: IEEE. 10.1109/FSKD.2014.6980862

Ni, Z. (2015). Bridging e-Health and the Internet of things: The SPHERE Project. *IEEE Intelligent Systems, 30*(4), 39–46. doi:10.1109/MIS.2015.57

Noury, N., Herve, T., Rialle, V., Virone, G., Mercier, E., Morey, G., . . . Porcheron, T. (2000, October). Monitoring behavior in the home using a smart fall sensor. *Proceedings of IEEE-EMBS Special Topic Conference on Microtechnologies in Medicine and Biology,* Lyon, France. (pp. 607–610). 10.1109/MMB.2000.893857

Office for Civil Rights (OCR). (2013, July 26). Summary of the HIPAA Privacy Rule. *Health Information Privacy*. Retrieved from https://www.hhs.gov/

Omega Engineering. (n.d.). *Precision Thermistor Sensors for Surface Temperature Measurements*. Retrieved from http://www.omega.com/pptst/ON-409_ON-909.html

Orlando, P. (2014). An efficient and low cost Windows Mobile BSN monitoring system based on TinyOS. *Telecommunication Systems, 55*(1), 115–124. doi:10.100711235-013-9756-4

Orsini, M., Pacchioni, M., Malagoli, A., & Guaraldi, G. (2017, September). My smart age with HIV: an innovative mobile and IoMT framework for patient's empowerment. In *2017 IEEE 3rd International Forum on Research and Technologies for Society and Industry (RTSI)* (pp. 1-6). IEEE. 10.1109/RTSI.2017.8065914

Özdemir, A. T., & Barshan, B. (2014). Detecting Falls with Wearable Sensors Using Machine Learning Techniques. *Sensors (Basel), 14*(6), 10691–10708. doi:10.3390140610691 PMID:24945676

Páez, D. G., Aparicio, F., de Buenaga, M., & Ascanio, J. R. (2014, December). Big data and IoT for chronic patients monitoring. In *International Conference on Ubiquitous Computing and Ambient Intelligence* (pp. 416-423). Cham, Switzerland: Springer. 10.1007/978-3-319-13102-3_68

Pang, Z. (2013). Ecosystem analysis in the design of open platform-based in-home healthcare terminals towards the internet-of-things. In *15th international conference on advanced communication technology (ICACT)*. IEEE.

Pang, Z., Zheng, L., Tian, J., Kao-Walter, S., Dubrova, E., & Chen, Q. (2015). Design of a terminal solution for integration of in-home health care devices and services towards the Internet-of-Things. *Enterprise Information Systems*, *9*(1), 86–116. doi:10.1080/17517575.2013.776118

Papakostas, D., Eshghi, S., Katsaros, D., & Tassiulas, L. (2018). Energy-aware backbone formation in military multilayer ad hoc networks. *Ad Hoc Networks*, *81*, 17–44. doi:10.1016/j.adhoc.2018.06.017

Paschou, M., Sakkopoulos, E., Sourla, E., & Tsakalidis, A. (2013). Health Internet of Things: Metrics and methods for efficient data transfer. *Simulation Modelling Practice and Theory*, *34*, 186–199. doi:10.1016/j.simpat.2012.08.002

Pasluosta, C., Gassner, H., Winkler, J., Klucken, J., & Eskofier, B. M. (2015). An emerging era in the management of Parkinson's disease: Wearable Technologies and the Internet of things. *IEEE Journal of Biomedical and Health Informatics*, *19*(6), 1873–1881. doi:10.1109/JBHI.2015.2461555 PMID:26241979

Patel, M., & Wang, J. (2010). *Applications, challenges, and prospective in emerging body area networking technologies. Wireless communications.* Piscataway, NJ: IEEE.

Patel, S., Park, H., Bonato, P., Chan, L., & Rodgers, M. (2012). A review of wearable sensors and systems with application in rehabilitation. *Journal of Neuroengineering and Rehabilitation*, *9*(1), 21. doi:10.1186/1743-0003-9-21 PMID:22520559

Pauthkey: A pervasive authentication protocol and key establishment scheme for wireless sensor networks in distributed IoT applications. (2014). International Journal of Distributed Sensor Networks.

Pearson, K. (1901). LIII. On lines and planes of closest fit to systems of points in space. *The London, Edinburgh and Dublin Philosophical Magazine and Journal of Science*, *2*(11), 559–572. doi:10.1080/14786440109462720

Perera, C., Zaslavsky, A., Christen, P., & Georgakopoulos, D. (2014). Context aware computing for the internet of things: A survey. *IEEE Communications Surveys and Tutorials*, *16*(1), 414–454. doi:10.1109/SURV.2013.042313.00197

Perkins, M. D., & Kessel, M. (2015). What Ebola tells us about outbreak diagnostic readiness. *Nature Biotechnology*, *33*(5), 464–469. doi:10.1038/nbt.3215 PMID:25965752

Perrig, A., Stankovic, J., & Wagner, D. (2004). Security in wireless sensor networks. Prezi. Retrieved from https://prezi.com/ok_gznayh-ex/bandwidth-efficiency/

Pfaller, M. A., Wolk, D. M., & Lowery, T. J. (2016). T2MR and T2Candida: Novel technology for the rapid diagnosis of candidemia and invasive candidiasis. *Future Microbiology*, *11*(1), 103–117. doi:10.2217/fmb.15.111 PMID:26371384

Philipose, M., Consolvo, S., Choudhury, T., Fishkin, K., Perkowitz, M., Fox, I. S. D., & Patterson, D. (2004). Fast, detailed inference of diverse daily human activities. *Demonstrations at UbiComp*, *7*.

Pinto, S., Cabral, J., & Gomes, T. (2017). *We-Care: An IoT-based Health Care System for Elderly People.* IEEE.

Piwek, L., Ellis, D. A., Andrews, S., & Joinson, A. (2016). The rise of consumer health wearables: Promises and barriers. *PLoS Medicine*, *13*(2). doi:10.1371/journal.pmed.1001953 PMID:26836780

Polar Electro. (n.d.). *H10 heart rate sensor.* Retrieved from https://www.polar.com/us-en/products/accessories/h10_heart_rate_sensor#features

Pololu (n.d.). *AltIMU-10 v5 Gyro, Accelerometer, Compass, and Altimeter (LSM6DS33, LIS3MDL, and LPS25H Carrier).* Retrieved from https://www.pololu.com/product/2739

Porambage, P., Schmitt, C., Kumar, P., Gurtov, A., & Ylianttila, M. (2014). Two-phase authentication protocol for wireless sensor networks in distributed iot applications. *Wireless Communications and Networking Conference (WCNC).* 10.1109/WCNC.2014.6952860

Pranam Ben. (2018). Retrieved from www.predictivemodelingnews.com

Prasad, A. M., Iverson, L. R., & Liaw, A. (2006). Newer classification and regression tree techniques: Bagging and random forests for ecological prediction. *Ecosystems (New York, N.Y.), 9*(2), 181–199. doi:10.100710021-005-0054-1

Price, K., Bird, S. R., Lythgo, N., Raj, I. S., Wong, J. Y., & Lynch, C. (2017). Validation of the Fitbit One, Garmin Vivofit and Jawbone UP activity tracker in estimation of energy expenditure during treadmill walking and running. *Journal of Medical Engineering & Technology, 41*(3), 208–215. doi:10.1080/03091902.2016.1253795 PMID:27919170

Proceedings of the International Conference on Intelligent Sustainable Systems (ICISS 2017) IEEE Xplore Compliant - Part Number:CFP17M19-ART, ISBN:978-1-5386-1959-9.

Psychoula, I., Merdivan, E., Singh, D., Chen, L., Chen, F., Hanke, S., … Geist, M. (2018, March). A deep learning approach for privacy preservation in assisted living. In *2018 IEEE International Conference on Pervasive Computing and Communications Workshops (PerCom Workshops)* (pp. 710-715). Piscataway, NJ: IEEE. 10.1109/PERCOMW.2018.8480247

Pub, N. F. (2001). *Advanced encryption standard (aes)*. Federal Information Processing Standards Publication.

Qin, Y., Sheng, Q. Z., Falkner, N. J., Dustdar, S., Wang, H., & Vasilakos, A. V. (2016). When things matter: A survey on data-centric internet of things. *Journal of Network and Computer Applications, 64*, 137–153. doi:10.1016/j.jnca.2015.12.016

Raghavendra, C. S., Sivalingam, K. M., & Znati, T. (Eds.). (2006). Wireless sensor networks. Berlin, Germany: Springer.

Raghupathi, W., & Raghupathi, V. (2014). Big data analytics in healthcare: Promise and potential. *Health Information Science and Systems, Springer, 2*(3), 2–10. PMID:25825667

Raja, S. (2018). Chronic Health Patient Monitoring System Using IOT. International Journal on Recent and Innovation Trends in computing and communication, 6(3), 114-119.

Ramkumar, J. & Vadivel, R. (n.d.). Improved frog leap inspired protocol (IFLIP) – for routing in cognitive radio ad hoc networks (CRAHN). World Journal of Engineering, 15, 306-311.

Rao, G. S. V., Sundararaman, K., & Parthasarathi, J. (2010, October). Dhatri-A Pervasive Cloud initiative for primary healthcare services. In *2010 14th International Conference on Intelligence in Next Generation Networks* (pp. 1-6). Piscataway, NJ: IEEE. 10.1109/ICIN.2010.5640918

Raspberry Pi Foundation. (n.d.). *Raspberry Pi — Teach, Learn, and Make with Raspberry Pi*. Retrieved from https://www.raspberrypi.org/

Rätsch, G., Mika, S., Schölkopf, B., & Müller, K. R. (2002). Constructing boosting algorithms from SVMs: An application to one-class classification. *IEEE Transactions on Pattern Analysis and Machine Intelligence, 24*(9), 1184–1199. doi:10.1109/TPAMI.2002.1033211

Ravi, D., Wong, C., Lo, B., & Yang, G. Z. (2016). A deep learning approach to on-node sensor data analytics for mobile or wearable devices. *IEEE Journal of Biomedical and Health Informatics, 21*(1), 56–64. doi:10.1109/JBHI.2016.2633287 PMID:28026792

Razzaq, M. A., Gill, S. H., Qureshi, M. A., & Ullah, S. (2017). Security issues in the Internet of Things (IoT): A comprehensive study. *International Journal of Advanced Computer Science and Applications, 8*(6), 383–388.

RedBear. (n.d.). *BLE Shield - Retired*. Retrieved from https://redbear.cc/product/retired/ble-shield.html

Redmond, S. J., Lovell, N. H., Yang, G. Z., Horsch, A., Lukowicz, P., Murrugarra, L., & Marschollek, M. (2014). What does big data mean for wearable sensor systems? *Yearbook of Medical Informatics, 23*(01), 135–142. doi:10.15265/IY-2014-0019 PMID:25123733

Rescorla, E. & Modadugu, N. (2012). Datagram transport layer security version 1.2.

Reuters. (2017). Received from https://www.reuters.com/brandfeatures/venture-capital/article?id=16545

RF Design. (2016, Sept. 1). *Nordic-powered Bluetooth low energy development kit offers complete turnkey solution for rapid Internet of Things product development.* Retrieved from http://rf-design.co.za/nordic-powered-bluetooth-low-energy-development-kit-offers-complete-turnkey-solution-rapid-internet-things-product-development/

Rhea, S., Wells, C., Eaton, P., Geels, D., Zhao, B., Weatherspoon, H., & Kubiatowicz, J. (2001). Maintenance-free global data storage. *IEEE Internet Computing, 5*(5), 40–49. doi:10.1109/4236.957894

Riggins, F. J. & Wamba, S. F. (2015, January). Research Directions on the Adoption, Usage, and Impact of the Internet of things through the Use of Big Data Analytics. (2015). Presented at *2015 48th Hawaii International Conference on System Sciences,* Kauai, HI, p. 40. doi:10.1109/HICSS.2015.186

Rodrigues, J. P. C., de la Torre, I., Fernández, G., & López-Coronado, M. (2013). Analysis of the Security and Privacy Requirements of Cloud-Based Electronic Health Records Systems. *Journal of Medical Internet Research, 15*(8), e186. doi:10.2196/jmir.2494 PMID:23965254

Roetenberg, D. (2006). Inertial and magnetic sensing of human motion. University of Twente, 18.

Rolim, C. O., Koch, F. L., Westphall, C. B., Werner, J., Fracalossi, A., & Salvador, G. S. (2010, February). A cloud computing solution for patient's data collection in health care institutions. In *2010 Second International Conference on eHealth, Telemedicine, and Social Medicine* (pp. 95-99). Piscataway, NJ: IEEE. 10.1109/eTELEMED.2010.19

Roman, R., Najera, P., & Lopez, J. (2011). Securing the internet of things. Computer. SEC4: Elliptic Curve Qu-Vanstone Implicit Certificate Scheme (ECQV), version 0.97. Retrieved from www.secg.org

Sadiku, M. N., Musa, S. M., & Momoh, O. D. (2014). Wireless sensor networks: Opportunities and challenges. *Journal of Engineering Research and Applications, 4*(1), 41–43.

Saleem, S., Ullah, S., & Kwak, K. S. (2011). A study of IEEE 802.15.4 security framework for wireless body area networks. *Sensors (Basel), 11*(2), 1383–1395. doi:10.3390110201383 PMID:22319358

Sanfilippo, F. & Pettersen, K. Y. (2015, November). A sensor fusion wearable health-monitoring system with haptic feedback. In *2015 11th International Conference on Innovations in Information Technology (IIT)* (pp. 262-266). Piscataway, NJ: IEEE. 10.1109/INNOVATIONS.2015.7381551

Santos, A., Macedo, J., Costa, A., & Nicolau, M. J. (2014). Internet of things and smart objects for M-health monitoring and control. *Procedia Technology, 16,* 1351–1360. doi:10.1016/j.protcy.2014.10.152

Sarfraz, F. K. (2017). Health care monitoring system in Internet of things (IoT) by using RFID. *2017 6th International Conference on Industrial Technology and Management (ICITM)* (pp. 198-204). Cambridge, UK: IEEE.

Schneier, B. (2005). Schneier on security: Sha-1 broken. Retrieved from http://www.schneier.com/blog/archives/2005/02/sha1 broken.html

Schölkopf, B., Platt, J. C., Shawe-Taylor, J., Smola, A. J., & Williamson, R. C. (2001). Estimating the support of a high-dimensional distribution. *Neural Computation, 13*(7), 1443–1471. doi:10.1162/089976601750264965 PMID:11440593

Scholkopf, B., & Smola, A. J. (2001). *Learning with kernels: support vector machines, regularization, optimization, and beyond.* Cambridge, MA: MIT Press.

Schröder, U. C., Bokeloh, F., O'Sullivan, M., Glaser, U., Wolf, K., Pfister, W., ... Neugebauer, U. (2015). Rapid, culture-independent, optical diagnostics of centrifugally captured bacteria from urine samples. *Biomicrofluidics, 9*(4). doi:10.1063/1.4928070 PMID:26339318

Schweitzer, N., Stulman, A., Hirst, T., Margalit, R. D., & Shabtai, A. (2019). Network bottlenecks in OLSR based ad-hoc networks. *Ad Hoc Networks, 88*, 36–54.

Seber, G. A., & Lee, A. J. (2012). *Linear regression analysis* (Vol. 329). Hoboken, NJ: John Wiley & Sons.

Sekhar, Y. R. Android based health care monitoring system. Department Of ECE, Vignan's University, Vadlamudi, India.

Sengiz, C., Congur, G., & Erdem, A. (2015). Development of ionic liquid modified disposable graphite electrodes for label-free electrochemical detection of DNA hybridization related to Microcystis spp. *Sensors (Basel), 15*(9), 22737–22749. doi:10.3390150922737 PMID:26371004

Sha, K., Du, J., & Shi, W. (2006). WEAR: A balanced, fault-tolerant, energy-aware routing protocol in WSNs. *International Journal of Sensor Networks, 1*(3-4), 156–168. doi:10.1504/IJSNET.2006.012031

Sha, K., & Shi, W. (2005). Modeling the lifetime of wireless sensor networks. *Sensor Letters, 3*(2), 126–135. doi:10.11661.2005.017

Shanin, F., Das, H. A., Krishnan, G. A., Neha, L. S., Thaha, N., Aneesh, R. P., ... Jayakrishan, S. (2018, July). Portable and Centralised E-Health Record System for Patient Monitoring Using Internet of Things (IoT). In *2018 International CET Conference on Control, Communication, and Computing (IC4)* (pp. 165-170). Piscataway, NJ: IEEE. 10.1109/CETIC4.2018.8530891

Shaojie, W., & Chuanhe, H. (2019). Asynchronous distributed optimization via dual decomposition for delay-constrained flying ad hoc networks. *Computer Communications, 137*, 70–80. doi:10.1016/j.comcom.2019.02.006

Sharma, A., Choudhury, T., & Kumar, P. (2018, June). Health monitoring & management using IoT devices in a Cloud Based Framework. In *2018 International Conference on Advances in Computing and Communication Engineering (ICACCE)* (pp. 219-224). Piscataway, NJ: IEEE. 10.1109/ICACCE.2018.8441752

Shih-Hao, C., .-D.-J.-T. (2016). Enabling Smart Personalized Healthcare: A Hybrid Mobile-Cloud Approach for ECG Telemonitoring. IT Professionals, 18(3), 14-22.

Shilton, A., Rajasegarar, S., Leckie, C., & Palaniswami, M. (2015). A dynamic planar one-class support vector machine for internet of things environment. In *International Conference on Recent Advances in Internet of things (RIoT)*. Piscataway, NJ: IEEE. pp. 1–6. 10.1109/RIOT.2015.7104904

Shimmersensing. (n.d.). *Wearable body sensors | Wearable technology*. Retrieved from http://shimmersensing.com/products/

Shirehjini, A., Yassine, A., & Shirmohammadi, S. (2012). Equipment Location in Hospitals Using RFID-Based Positioning System. *IEEE Transactions on Information Technology in Biomedicine, 16*(6), 1058–1069. doi:10.1109/TITB.2012.2204896 PMID:24218700

Shojaei, T. R., Salleh, M. A. M., Tabatabaei, M., Ekrami, A., Motallebi, R., Rahmani-Cherati, T., ... Jorfi, R. (2014). Development of sandwich-form biosensor to detect Mycobacterium tuberculosis complex in clinical sputum specimens. *The Brazilian Journal of Infectious Diseases, 18*(6), 600–608. doi:10.1016/j.bjid.2014.05.015 PMID:25181404

Shukla, M., Kosta, Y., & Chauhan, P. (2015). Analysis and evaluation of outlier detection algorithms in data streams. In *International Conference on Computer, Communication and Control (IC4) (pp. 1–8)*. Piscataway, NJ: IEEE.

Sicari, S., Rizzardi, A., Grieco, L., & Coen-Porisini, A. (2015). Security, privacy and trust in internet of things: The road ahead. *Computer Networks*, *76*, 146–164. doi:10.1016/j.comnet.2014.11.008

Simon, G., Maróti, M., Lédeczi, Á., Balogh, G., Kusy, B., Nádas, A., . . . Frampton, K. (2004, November). Sensor network-based countersniper system. In *Proceedings of the 2nd international conference on Embedded networked sensor systems* (pp. 1-12). New York, NY: ACM.

Sinha, A., & Chandrakasan, A. (2001). Dynamic power management in wireless sensor networks. *IEEE Design & Test of Computers*, *18*(2), 62–74. doi:10.1109/54.914626

Smola, A. J., & Schölkopf, B. (2004). A tutorial on support vector regression. *Statistics and Computing*, *14*(3), 199–222. doi:10.1023/B:STCO.0000035301.49549.88

Sohrabi, K., Gao, J., Ailawadhi, V., & Pottie, G. J. (2000). Protocols for self-organization of a wireless sensor network. IEEE personal communications, 7(5), 16-27.

Solangi, Z. A., Solangi, Y. A., Chandio, S., Abd-Aziz, M. S., Hamzah, M. S., & Shah, A. (2018, May). The future of data privacy and security concerns in Internet of things. *2018 IEEE International Conference on Innovative Research and Development (ICIRD)*. 10.1109/ICIRD.2018.8376320

Souza, A. M., & Amazonas, J. R. (2015). An outlier detect algorithm using big data processing and internet of things architecture. *Procedia Computer Science*, *52*, 1010–1015. doi:10.1016/j.procs.2015.05.095

SparkFun Electronics. (n.d.). *LilyPad Accelerometer – ADXL335 - DEV-09267*. Retrieved from https://www.sparkfun.com/products/9267

SparkFun Electronics. (n.d.). *LilyPad Temperature Sensor - DEV-08777*. Retrieved from https://www.sparkfun.com/products/8777

SparkFun Electronics. (n.d.). *Pulse Sensor - SEN-11574*. Retrieved from https://www.sparkfun.com/products/11574

SparkFun Electronics. (n.d.). *SparkFun Digital Temperature Sensor Breakout – TMP102*. Retrieved from https://www.sparkfun.com/products/11931

Spinelle, L., Gerboles, M., Villani, M. G., Aleixandre, M., & Bonavitacola, F. (2015). Field calibration of a cluster of low-cost available sensors for air quality monitoring. Part A: Ozone and nitrogen dioxide. *Sensors and Actuators B: Chemical*, *215*, 249–257. doi:10.1016/j.snb.2015.03.031

Stroulia, E., Chodos, D., Boers, N. M., Huang, J., Gburzynski, P., & Nikolaidis, I. (2009, May). Software engineering for health education and care delivery systems: The Smart Condo project. In *2009 ICSE Workshop on Software Engineering in Health Care* (pp. 20-28). Piscataway, NJ: IEEE. 10.1109/SEHC.2009.5069602

Sundaravadivel, P., Kesavan, K., Kesavan, L., Mohanty, S. P., & Kougianos, E. (2018). Smart-Log: A deep-learning based automated nutrition monitoring system in the IoT. *IEEE Transactions on Consumer Electronics*, *64*(3), 390–398. doi:10.1109/TCE.2018.2867802

Sung, W. T., & Chiang, Y. C. (2012). Improved particle swarm optimization algorithm for android medical care IOT using modified parameters. *Journal of Medical Systems*, *36*(6), 3755–3763. doi:10.100710916-012-9848-9 PMID:22492176

Sun, J., Fang, Y., & Zhu, X. (2010). Privacy and emergency response in e-healthcare leveraging wireless body sensor networks. *IEEE Wireless Communications*, *17*(1), 66–73. doi:10.1109/MWC.2010.5416352

Sun, W., Cai, Z., Li, Y., Liu, F., Fang, S., & Wang, G. (2018). Security and privacy in the Medical Internet of things: A review. *Hindawi Security and Communication Networks*, 1–9. doi:10.1155/2018/5978636

Surajit, B., & Tamaghna, A. (2017). Cross layer optimization for outage minimizing routing in cognitive radio ad hoc networks with primary users outage protection. *Journal of Network and Computer Applications*, *98*, 114–124. doi:10.1016/j.jnca.2017.09.004

Surfix. (2018). Retrieved from https://www.surfix.nl/applications/biosensors

Sweeney, L. (2002). k-anonymity: A model for protecting privacy. *International Journal of Uncertainty, Fuzziness and Knowledge-based Systems*, *10*(05), 557–570. doi:10.1142/S0218488502001648

Szczechowiak, P., Oliveira, L. B., Scott, M., Collier, M., & Dahab, R. (2008). Nanoecc: Testing the limits of elliptic curve cryptography in sensor networks. Wireless sensor networks.

Taitsman, J. K., Grimm, C. M., & Agrawal, S. (2013). Protecting patient privacy and data security. *The New England Journal of Medicine*, *368*(11), 977–979. doi:10.1056/NEJMp1215258 PMID:23444980

Takeda, R., Tadano, S., Todoh, M., Morikawa, M., Nakayasu, M., & Yoshinari, S. (2009). Gait analysis using gravitational acceleration measured by wearable sensors. *Journal of Biomechanics*, *42*(3), 223–233. doi:10.1016/j.jbiomech.2008.10.027 PMID:19121522

Tan, J., Wen, H. J., & Awad, N. (2005). Health care and services delivery systems as complex adaptive systems. *Communications of the ACM*, *48*(5), 36–44. doi:10.1145/1060710.1060737

Tartarisco, G., Baldus, G., Corda, D., Raso, R., Arnao, A., Ferro, M., ... Pioggia, G. (2012). Personal Health System architecture for stress monitoring and support to clinical decisions. *Computer Communications*, *35*(11), 1296–1305. doi:10.1016/j.comcom.2011.11.015

TechTarget. Confidentiality, integrity, and availability (CIA triad). Available at https://whatis.techtarget.com/definition/Confidentiality-integrity-and-availability-CIA

Toshniwal, D. (2013). Clustering techniques for streaming data-a survey. In IEEE 3rd International Advance Computing Conference (IACC). Piscataway, NJ: IEEE. pp. 951–956.

Toshniwal, D. (2013, February). Clustering techniques for streaming data-a survey. In *3rd IEEE International Advance Computing Conference (IACC)* (pp. 951-956). Piscataway, NJ: IEEE.

Tran, T. S., Hoa, L., & Nauman, A. (2016). MSAR: A metric self-adaptive routing model for Mobile Ad Hoc Networks. *Journal of Network and Computer Applications*, *68*, 114–125. doi:10.1016/j.jnca.2016.04.010

Triantafyllidis, A. K., Koutkias, V. G., Chouvarda, I., & Maglaveras, N. (2013). A pervasive health system integrating patient monitoring, status logging, and social sharing. *IEEE Journal of Biomedical and Health Informatics*, *17*(1), 30–37. doi:10.1109/TITB.2012.2227269 PMID:23193318

Tsai, C. W., Lai, C. F., Chiang, M. C., & Yang, L. T. (2013). Data mining for the internet of things: A survey. *IEEE Communications Surveys and Tutorials*, *16*(1), 77–97. doi:10.1109/SURV.2013.103013.00206

Turkanovi'c, M., Brumen, B., & H'olbl, M. (2014). A novel user authentication and key agreement scheme for heterogeneous ad hoc wireless sensor networks, based on the internet of things notion. *Ad Hoc Networks*, *20*, 96–112. doi:10.1016/j.adhoc.2014.03.009

Ullah, M. & Ahmad, W. (2009). Evaluation of routing protocols in wireless sensor networks.

Uttarkar, R., & Kulkarni, R. (2014). Internet of Things: Architecture and Security. *International Journal of Computers and Applications*, *3*(4).

Veltink, P. H. & Boom, H. B. K. (1995, November). 3D movement analysis using accelerometry-Theoretical concepts. In Topical workshop of the concerted action RAFT (pp. 45-50).

Venkatasubramanian, K. K., & Gupta, S. K. (2010). Physiological value-based efficient usable security solutions for body sensor networks. [TOSN]. *ACM Transactions on Sensor Networks*, 6(4), 31. doi:10.1145/1777406.1777410

Vippalapalli, V., & Ananthula, S. (2016). Internet of things (IoT) based smart health care System. *International conference on Signal Processing, Communication, Power and Embedded System (SCOPES)*, 1229 – 1233. 10.1109/SCOPES.2016.7955637

Virone, G., Wood, A., Selavo, L., Cao, Q., Fang, L., Doan, T., . . . Stankovic, J. (2006, April). An advanced wireless sensor network for health monitoring. In Transdisciplinary conference on distributed diagnosis and home healthcare (D2H2) (pp. 2-4).

Vojas, J. (2016). Demystifying the internet of things. *Computer*, 49(6), 80–83. doi:10.1109/MC.2016.162

Wang, C., Liu, C., & Wang, T. (2013). A remote health care system combining a fall down alarm and biomedical signal monitor system in an android smart-phone. Int. J. Adv. Comput. Sci. Appl, 4.

Wang, R., Blackburn, G., Desai, M., Phelan, D., Gillinov, L., Houghtaling, P., & Gillinov, M. (2017). Accuracy of wrist-worn heart rate monitors. *JAMA Cardiology*, 2(1), 104–106. doi:10.1001/jamacardio.2016.3340 PMID:27732703

Wang, X., Gui, Q., Liu, B., Jin, Z., & Chen, Y. (2014). Enabling smart personalized healthcare: A hybrid mobile-cloud approach for ECG telemonitoring. *IEEE Journal of Biomedical and Health Informatics*, 18(3), 739–745.

Watchguard. Retrieved from http://customers.watchguard.com/articles/Article/How-is-jitter-calculated

Waziri, V. O., Alhassan, J. K., Ismaila, I., & Egigogo, R. A. (2016). Securing file on cloud computing system using encryption software: a comparative analysis. *International Conference on Information and Communication Technology and Its Applications (ICTA 2016)*. 97-104.

Werner-Allen, G., Lorincz, K., Ruiz, M., Marcillo, O., Johnson, J., Lees, J., & Welsh, M. (2006). Deploying a wireless sensor network on an active volcano. *IEEE Internet Computing*, 10(2), 18–25. doi:10.1109/MIC.2006.26

What is GSR (galvanic skin response) and how does it work? (n.d.). Retrieved from https://imotions.com/blog/gsr/

World Famous Electronics. (n.d.). *Heartbeats in your projects*. Retrieved from http://pulsesensor.com/

World Health Organization. (2015). *Ageing and health*. Available at http://www.who.int/mediacentre/factsheets/fs404/en/

Wu, D., Bleier, B. S., Li, L., Zhan, X., Zhang, L., Lv, Q., ... Wei, Y. (2018). Clinical phenotypes of nasal polyps and comorbid asthma based on cluster analysis of disease history. *The Journal of Allergy and Clinical Immunology. In Practice*, 6(4), 1297–1305. doi:10.1016/j.jaip.2017.09.020 PMID:29100865

Xtelligent. (n.d.). *Healthcare Media Health IT Analytics*. Retrieved from http://www.xtelligentmedia.com/network/HealthITAnalytics

Xuan, L., Zhuo, L., Peng, Y., & Yongqiang, D. (2017). Information-centric mobile ad hoc networks and content routing: A survey. *Ad Hoc Networks*, 58, 255–268. doi:10.1016/j.adhoc.2016.04.005

Xu, S., Zhang, Y., Jia, L., Mathewson, K. E., Jang, K. I., Kim, J., ... Bhole, S. (2014). Soft microfluidic assemblies of sensors, circuits, and radios for the skin. *Science*, 344(6179), 70–74. doi:10.1126cience.1250169 PMID:24700852

Xu, X., Shu, L., Guizani, M., Liu, M., & Lu, J. (2015). A survey on energy harvesting and integrated data sharing in wireless body area networks. *International Journal of Distributed Sensor Networks*, 11(10).

Yang, Y. & Wang, J. (2008, April). Design guidelines for routing metrics in multihop wireless networks. In *IEEE IN-FOCOM 2008-The 27th Conference on Computer Communications* (pp. 1615-1623). Piscataway, NJ: IEEE. 10.1109/INFOCOM.2008.222

Yang, G., Xie, L., Mäntysalo, M., Zhou, X., Pang, Z., Da Xu, L., ... Zheng, L. R. (2014). A health-iot platform based on the integration of intelligent packaging, unobtrusive bio-sensor, and intelligent medicine box. *IEEE Transactions on Industrial Informatics, 10*(4), 2180–2191. doi:10.1109/TII.2014.2307795

Yen, C. W., de Puig, H., Tam, J. O., Gómez-Márquez, J., Bosch, I., Hamad-Schifferli, K., & Gehrke, L. (2015). Multi-colored silver nanoparticles for multiplexed disease diagnostics: Distinguishing dengue, yellow fever, and Ebola viruses. *Lab on a Chip, 15*(7), 1638–1641. doi:10.1039/C5LC00055F PMID:25672590

Yick, J., Mukherjee, B., & Ghosal, D. (2005, October). Analysis of a prediction-based mobility adaptive tracking algorithm. In *2nd International Conference on Broadband Networks*, 2005. (pp. 753-760). Piscataway, NJ: IEEE. 10.1109/ICBN.2005.1589681

Yick, J., Mukherjee, B., & Ghosal, D. (2008). Wireless sensor network survey. *Computer Networks, 52*(12), 2292–2330. doi:10.1016/j.comnet.2008.04.002

Yu, J., Fu, B., Cao, A., He, Z., & Wu, D. (2018, December). EdgeCNN: A Hybrid Architecture for Agile Learning of Healthcare Data from IoT Devices. In *2018 IEEE 24th International Conference on Parallel and Distributed Systems (ICPADS)* (pp. 852-859). Piscataway, NJ: IEEE. 10.1109/PADSW.2018.8644604

Yuehong, Y. I. N., Zeng, Y., Chen, X., & Fan, Y. (2016). The internet of things in healthcare: An overview. *Journal of Industrial Information Integration, 1*, 3–13. doi:10.1016/j.jii.2016.03.004

Zanella, A., Bui, N., Castellani, A., Vangelista, L., & Zorzi, M. (2014). Internet of things for smart cities. IEEE Internet of things journal, 1(1), 22-32.

Zhang, H. (2004). The optimality of naive Bayes. AA, 1(2), 3.

Zhang, X. M., & Zhang, N. (2011). An open, secure and flexible platform based on internet of things and cloud computing for ambient aiding living and telemedicine. In 2011 international conference on computer and management (CAMAN). IEEE.

Zhang, Y. & Sun, S. (2013, April). Real-time data driven monitoring and optimization method for IoT-based sensible production process. In 2013 10th IEEE international conference on networking, sensing and control (ICNSC) (pp. 486-490). Piscataway, NJ: IEEE.

Zhang, W., Passow, P., Jovanov, E., Stoll, R., & Thurow, K. (2013, August). A secure and scalable telemonitoring system using ultra-low-energy wireless sensor interface for long-term monitoring in life science applications. In *2013 IEEE International Conference on Automation Science and Engineering (CASE)* (pp. 617-622). Piscataway, NJ: IEEE. 10.1109/CoASE.2013.6653979

Zhao, W., Wang, C., & Nakahira, Y. (2011). *Medical application on internet of things*. Academic Press.

Zhou, H. (2012). *The internet of things in the cloud: a middleware perspective*. CRC Press. doi:10.1201/b13090

ZigBee Alliance, San Ramon, "ZigBee Specification v1.0,"CA, USA2005.

About the Contributors

P. B. Pankajavalli has received merit certificate for topping the list of candidates in Database Management Systems during her Post Graduation at Vellalar College for Women, Bharathiar University. She was an Assistant Professor, Department of Computer Science from 2003 to 2013 in Kongu Arts and Science College, Erode. She served as Assistant professor (SG) in PSG College of Technology, Coimbatore till 2015. Now she is as an Assistant Professor in the Department of Computer Science, Bharathiar University, Coimbatore. She is actively doing projects from DST and has filed an Indian patent. She is very active in research and has published more than 100 papers in International Journals, International Conference and has edited research volumes. She has supervised 8 MPhils and 40 postgraduates. She is also a member of Board of Studies in PSG College of Technology, Affiliated colleges of Periyar University and Bharathiar University. She has actively peer-reviewed many journals. Her research interest includes Ad-hoc, Sensor Networks, and the Internet of Things.

G. S. Karthick is working as a Junior Research Fellow under DST-ICPS project and a full-time Ph.D. Research Scholar in the Department of Computer Science, Bharathiar University, Coimbatore, India. His current research interests focus on the recent developments in IoT-Based Healthcare. Previously, he worked as an Assistant Professor in the Department of Computer Science, Sri Ramakrishna College of Arts and Science, Coimbatore, India. He has topped the Post-Graduation with Gold Medal in 2017 from Bharathiar University, Coimbatore, India. He has topped Under-Graduation with the exemplary performance from SNR Sons College, Coimbatore, India and also aced three subjects to receive gold medals in 2015. He has published research papers in International Journals and presented papers in International and National Conferences. He has published many book chapters and filed an Indian Patent. His area of specializations and research interests are Wireless Sensor Networks, Internet of Things and Analysis of Algorithms.

* * *

Sankar A. received his Ph.D in Computer Science from Bharathiar University, Coimbatore, India in 2003. He is currently working as Professor in the Department of Computer Applications, PSG College of Technology, Coimbatore, India. He has more than 25 years of teaching experience and ten years of research experience. His research interest includes agile software engineering, networks, e-learning and data mining.

Jayanthi Jagannathan is working as an associate professor in the department of Computer Science and Engineering, Sona College of Technology (SCT), Salem, Tamilnadu, India. She is having three years of Industrial experience as a software engineer and 17 years of teaching experience in SCT. Her area of interest includes web technologies, software engineering, Software Testing, Artificial Intelligence, Internet of Things, Data mining and Big Data Analytics. She has published more than fifty papers in the national and international journals and conferences. She is one of the co-investigator of the DST funded project on CDSS for Breast Cancer for rural women community. She has received many appreciation awards for the teaching and learning and Research and Development activities.

Vidhya Kandasamy received her M.E. degree with First Class - Distinction from Government College of Technology,Coimbatore and B.E degree with First Class from Muthayammal Engineering College, Rasipuram. Currently she is pursuing her Ph.D under Anna University, Chennai. She is having 10.8 years of experience in teaching and 1.4 years of experience in industry. Her research area includes Cloud Computing, Data Analytics-Machine learning, Internet of Things and its integration with Cloud and also Artificial Intelligence. She has published 8 research papers in International Journals and 4 papers in International Conferences and 6 papers in various national level conferences. She is certified by EMC Academic Professional Associate in Cloud Infrastructure Services. She is the member of ISTE and IEEE.

S. Vijayarani Mohan is a Assistant Professor, Department of Computer Science, Bharathiar University, Coimbatore, India. She has 11 years of teaching/research and technical experience. Her research interests include data mining, privacy data mining, image mining, text mining, web mining, data streams, and information retrieval. She has published more than 100 research articles in national/international journals and conferences.

A. Muniyappan has completed M.Sc in Computer Science. He is currently pursuing his PhD in Computer Science in the School of Computer Science and Engineering, Bharathiar University, Coimbatore, Tamil Nadu, India.

Geetha N. graduated from Bharathiar University in 1999 with a B.Sc in Physics. She completed her post graduate degree MCA from Bharathiar University. She has 15 years of teaching experience. She is currently working as Assistant Professor (Selection Grade) in Department of Computer Applications, PSG College of Technology. She published 2 papers in international journals, 4 papers in international conference and a review member for various conferences. Her research interest includes, Internet of Things, routing in ad hoc networks, wireless sensor network.

N. Priya is a Ph.D. Research Scholar in the Department of Computer Science, School of Computer Science and Engineering, Bharathiar University, Coimbatore, Tamilnadu. She has received M.Sc Information Technology from Madras University, Chennai and M.Phil Computer Science from Sri Chandrasekharendra Saraswathi Viswa Mahavidyalaya University. Her main research work focuses on Wireless Sensor Networks and Fault Tolerance Mechanisms in Distributed Environments.

Rajkumar Rajaseskaran has completed his Ph.D. from Vellore Institute of Technology University, Vellore in Computer Science and Engineering. Her research area includes Data Analytics, Data Mining, Big Data and Machine learning. He has been teaching from last 17 years with emphasis on Data Analytics, Data Mining, Sentimental Analysis, Machine Learning, Social and Information Network Analysis, and Learning Analytics. He has filed a Patent on Holographic keyboard for smart Devices. Presently, he is working at Vellore Institute of Technology Vellore. He is Main Editor of the Book entitled "Contemporary Applications on Mobile Computing in Healthcare Settings" published by IGI Global. He is the Deputy Editor Asia for Public Health in Africa (Springer). Editorial Board Member for International Journal of IOT and Cyber Assurance, Associate Editor for International Journal of Social Computing and Cyber Physical Systems (Inderscience). He is working on various projects assigned from American Association of Advancement of Sciences (AAAS). He was the Head of Department for Data Analytics, Coordinator for Apple University Development Program.

Sivaramakrishnan Rajendar received his B.E. Computer Science Engineering and M.E. Computer Science Engineering from Anna University Chennai. Currently he is pursuing his Ph.D in the area of cyber physical systems. He has 8 years of experience in teaching. His areas of interest also include Cloud Computing, Deep Learning, Theory of Computation and Compiler Design. He presented and published several papers in National and International Conferences and Journals. He is a life time member of ISTE and IEANG.

J. Ramkumar working as an Assistant Professor in Post Graduate and Research Department of Computer Science at VLB Janakiammal College of Arts and Science, Coimbatore, Tamilnadu, India. He has completed M.C.A., and M.Phil in Computer Science. He is currently pursuing his Ph.D degree (in part time) in Bharathiar University, and working closely with Dr. R. Vadivel. His area of interest includes ad hoc networks, routing, decision support system and Internet of Things. He acted as board member in more than 200 international conferences and journals. He has 9 memberships in internationally reputed professional bodies. He has published more than 20 research articles in international conferences and journals, which includes Scopus and other indexed publication.

M. Sridhar has completed M.Sc in Computer Science. He is currently pursuing his PhD in Computer Science in the School of Computer Science and Engineering, Bharathiar University, Coimbatore, Tamil Nadu, India. His fields of interest are Wireless Sensor Network and Internet of Things.

Rajasekaran Thangaraj received B.E and M.E Degree in Computer Science Engineering from Anna University, India in 2008 and 2011 respectively. He is currently pursuing Ph.D in Information and Communication Engineering department. He held Lecturer Position at Sasurie College of Engineering during 2011-2012. At present he is working as Assistant Professor at KPR Institute of Engineering and Technology, India. His research area of interest include Machine learning, Deep learning, Computer Vision and Internet of Things. He is currently working on developing computer vision and deep learning algorithms for object recognition, animal recognition, plant classification and disease identification. He has published 10 research papers in International Journals,4 papers in International Conference and 16 papers in National Conferences. He is a Life Member of the Indian Society for Technical Education (ISTE).

V. Jeevika Tharini received the B.C.A degree from Mother Teresa Women's University, Tamilnadu, India, in 2016, and the M.Sc. Computer Science from Bharathiar University, Coimbatore, Tamilnadu, India, in 2018. She is a full-time M.Phil. Research Scholar with the Department of Computer Science from Bharathiar University, Coimbatore, Tamilnadu, India. Her current research interests include utility mining, privacy preserving, and optimization techniques. She has published papers in international journals and conferences.

R. Vadivel completed his B.E. in Periyar University, Salem and M.E. in Annamali University, Chidambaram. He obtained his PhD degree from Manonmaniam Sundaranar University, Thirunelvely, Tamilnadu. At present he is working as an Assistant Professor in the Department of Information Technology, Bharathiar University, Coimbatore. He has published more than 50 research papers in National, International Journals and Conferences. He is guiding M.Phil and Ph.D. research scholars. His research interest lies in the area of Computer Networks & Security, Mobile Computing, Mobile Ad-Hoc Networks, Wireless Sensor Networks, Data mining and Digital Signal Processing. He is a life member of CSI, ISTE, ACS, ISCA, AMIE, IACSIT and IAENG.

Index

T

W

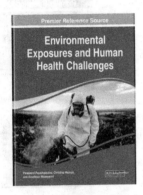
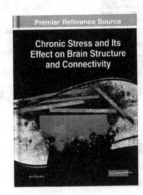
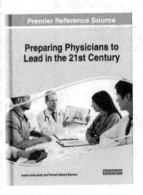
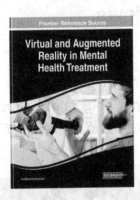
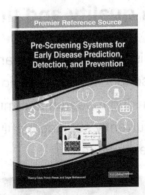
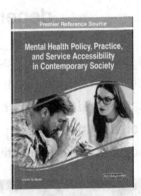
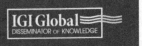

Ensure Quality Research is Introduced to the Academic Community

Become an IGI Global Reviewer for Authored Book Projects

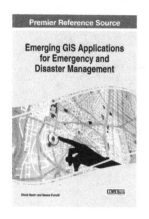

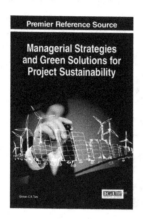

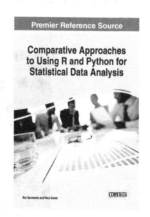

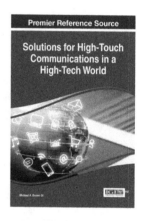

The overall success of an authored book project is dependent on quality and timely reviews.

In this competitive age of scholarly publishing, constructive and timely feedback significantly expedites the turnaround time of manuscripts from submission to acceptance, allowing the publication and discovery of forward-thinking research at a much more expeditious rate. Several IGI Global authored book projects are currently seeking highly-qualified experts in the field to fill vacancies on their respective editorial review boards:

Applications and Inquiries may be sent to:
development@igi-global.com

Applicants must have a doctorate (or an equivalent degree) as well as publishing and reviewing experience. Reviewers are asked to complete the open-ended evaluation questions with as much detail as possible in a timely, collegial, and constructive manner. All reviewers' tenures run for one-year terms on the editorial review boards and are expected to complete at least three reviews per term. Upon successful completion of this term, reviewers can be considered for an additional term.

If you have a colleague that may be interested in this opportunity, we encourage you to share this information with them.

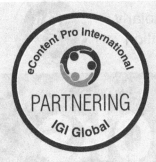

IGI Global Proudly Partners With eContent Pro International

Receive a 25% Discount on all Editorial Services

Editorial Services

IGI Global expects all final manuscripts submitted for publication to be in their final form. This means they must be reviewed, revised, and professionally copy edited prior to their final submission. Not only does this support with accelerating the publication process, but it also ensures that the highest quality scholarly work can be disseminated.

English Language Copy Editing

Let eContent Pro International's expert copy editors perform edits on your manuscript to resolve spelling, punctuaion, grammar, syntax, flow, formatting issues and more.

Scientific and Scholarly Editing

Allow colleagues in your research area to examine the content of your manuscript and provide you with valuable feedback and suggestions before submission.

Figure, Table, Chart & Equation Conversions

Do you have poor quality figures? Do you need visual elements in your manuscript created or converted? A design expert can help!

Translation

Need your documjent translated into English? eContent Pro International's expert translators are fluent in English and more than 40 different languages.

Email: **customerservice@econtentpro.com**   **www.igi-global.com/editorial-service-partners**

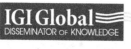

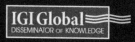

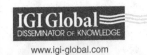
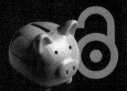
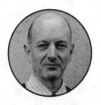

Printed in the United States
By Bookmasters